DATE DUE			
Apr 7 79			
Apr 19 79			
Apr 26 79			
May 2 79			
Mar 11 80			
Oct 12 '80			

Nutrition, Longevity, and Aging

ACADEMIC PRESS RAPID MANUSCRIPT REPRODUCTION

Proceedings of a Symposium
on Nutrition, Longevity, and Aging
Held in Miami, Florida
February 26–27, 1976

Nutrition, Longevity, and Aging

Edited by
Morris Rockstein
Marvin L. Sussman

Department of Physiology and Biophysics
University of Miami School of Medicine
Miami, Florida

ACADEMIC PRESS INC., New York San Francisco London 1976
A Subsidiary of Harcourt Brace Jovanovich, Publishers

ACADEMIC PRESS, INC.
111 Fifth Avenue, New York, New York 10003

United Kingdom Edition published by
ACADEMIC PRESS, INC. (LONDON) LTD.
24/28 Oval Road, London NW1

Library of Congress Cataloging in Publication Data
Main entry under title:

Nutrition, longevity, and aging.

Proceedings of a symposium held at the University of Miami School of Medicine, Miami, Fla., Feb. 26-27, 1976; sponsored by the Training Program in Cellular Aging of the Departments of Physiology/Biophysics and Microbiology.
Bibliography: p.

1. Aging–Nutritional aspects–Congresses. 2. Longevity–Nutritional aspects–Congresses. 3. Aged–Nutrition–Congresses. 4. Nutrition–Congresses. I. Rockstein, Morris. II. Sussman, Marvin L. [DNLM: 1. Aging–Congresses. 2. Nutrition–Congresses. 3. Longevity–Congresses. WT104 N977 1976]
QP86.N87 612'.39 76-26639
ISBN 0-12-591656-6

PRINTED IN THE UNITED STATES OF AMERICA

CONTENTS

CONTRIBUTORS

W. O. Caster, Department of Nutrition, University of Georgia, School of Home Economics, Athens, Georgia 30602

George C. Gerritsen, The Upjohn Company, Kalamazoo, Michigan 49001

William R. Hazzard, University of Washington, School of Medicine, and, Northwest Lipid Research Clinic, Harborview Medical Center, Seattle, Washington 98104

Leonard F. Jakubczak, Veterans Administration Hospital, St. Louis, Missouri 63125

Olaf Mickelsen, Department of Food Science and Human Nutrition, Michigan State University, East Lansing, Michigan 48824

Adrian M. Ostfeld, Department of Epidemiology and Public Health, Yale University School of Medicine, New Haven, Connecticut 06510

Morris Rockstein, Department of Physiology and Biophysics, University of Miami School of Medicine, Miami, Florida 33152

Robert E. Shank, Department of Preventive Medicine, Washington University School of Medicine, St. Louis, Missouri 63110

Albert J. Stunkard, Department of Psychiatry and Behavioral Sciences, Stanford University School of Medicine, Stanford, California 94305

Marvin L. Sussman, Department of Physiology and Biophysics, University of Miami School of Medicine, Miami, Florida 33152

Donald M. Watkin, Nutrition Program, Administration on Aging, Office of Human Development, Department of Health, Education and Welfare, and, Department of Medicine and Surgery, Veterans Administration, Washington, D. C. 20201

Vernon R. Young, Department of Nutrition and Food Science and Clinical Research Center, Massachusetts Institute of Technology, Cambridge, Massachusetts 02139

PREFACE

This volume is the sixth publication in a series of published proceedings of annual symposia dedicated to various aspects of biological gerontology, sponsored by the Training Program in Cellular Aging of the Departments of Physiology/Biophysics and Microbiology. Papers included here were presented by the participants in a symposium on "Nutrition, Longevity, and Aging," held on February 26 and 27, 1976 at the University of Miami School of Medicine, Miami, Florida.

Interest in the relationship of diet to life span is not new. In 1842, John Bell wrote in his book *On Regimen and Longevity,* "The food of those most remarkable for their longevity. . . is all important . A man's health will suffer, by using promiscuously, various articles of food, any one or two of which, alone, would sustain him in all plentitude of bodily vigour, for a lifetime." This simple observation made in the middle of the last century has been followed by great scientific progress in the field of nutrition as exemplified by the now classic studies of Clive McCay, and more recently, of Morris Ross (discussed by several participants in this symposium).

Clinicians and research scientists working in the field of nutrition and closely related specialities were invited to relate their expertise on specific problems in the study of gerontology as well as to general aspects of the aging process. Some of the papers employ animal models, a basic tool in gerontological research, to investigate the relationship of nutrition to aging. Others discuss the effects of diet on increasing longevity as well as reducing the incidence or severity of diseases common in the aging human population (e.g., diabetes mellitus, stroke, atherosclerosis, obesity). It is hoped that the various papers reporting well-controlled studies will help to separate fact from fantasy in a field where new fads receive major publicity in the news media and rapid public acceptance, often before any scientific merit for them can be established.

Aside from presenting detailed facts and findings concerning this important subject matter area, the Editors hope that the contents of this volume will serve to stimulate clinical researchers as well as basic scientists to undertake investigations involving the nutritional basis of many of the basic problems encountered in the study of aging.

Morris Rockstein

Marvin L. Sussman

ACKNOWLEDGMENTS

The Editors owe special thanks to Mrs. Estella Cooney for her continued dedication to producing the final published version of these proceedings, in both editing and typing the camera copy for this publication.

The Training Program acknowledges the generosity of the Mead Johnson Research Center-Medical Division; E. R. Squibb and Sons, Inc.—The Squibb Institute for Medical Research; Johnson and Johnson; and the Hoffmann-LaRoche, Inc. Research Division, whose contributions helped to make this a successful symposium and the publication of these proceedings possible.

The symposium from which this publication resulted was supported, for the most part, by funds from the National Institute on Aging (Training Program in Cellular Aging) Grant # AG 00013, and also in part by the Department of Physiology and Biophysics, University of Miami School of Medicine (Professor Werner R. Loewenstein, Chairman).

Special thanks are due to Dr. Jeffrey Chesky of the Department of Physiology and Biophysics, who co-chaired the two-day meeting in Dr. Rockstein's absence.

Morris Rockstein

Marvin L. Sussman

INTRODUCTION: FOOD FOR THOUGHT

Morris Rockstein, Ph.D.
and
Marvin L. Sussman, Ph.D.

Department of Physiology and Biophysics
University of Miami School of Medicine
Miami, Florida 33152

If one were to describe the tone of the third quarter of this century, it would have to be the prevalence of fadism of many varieties. This is evidenced by the return of the fashions of the "Gatsby" era, "environmentalism", a back-to-the-land movement, and, particularly, fads in foods.

In actual fact, this meeting was not organized to attack such dietary fads as the organic food diet, the macrobiotic diet, and the drinking man's diet, or to compare various kinds of diets. Instead, its major objective was to bring together individuals of different expertise to discuss the basic problems relating nutrition and diet to the aging process and to the problems of the aged. However, whether we are thinking of the role of nutrition in general or its particular influence in determining the course and direction of the aging process, a critical analysis must also necessarily be made of some of the claims for the life-extending properties of different nutrients or of restrictive diets involving caloric or protein intake.

By way of introduction, let us look at the titles of a number of recent newspaper and magazine articles which demonstrate the great interest the news media has for featuring controversial topics in nutrition: "Vitamin C: The Dosage Debate Goes On", "Vitamin Balance The Real Key?" (from a local newspaper), "Food For a Thought" (from Geriatrics), "Importance of Vitamins for the Elderly" (from the Merck report of January, 1956), "Good Nutrition for the Good Life" (from Modern Maturity, December-January, 1975-1976), "Sugar: Dangerous to the Heart?" (from Medical World News, February 12, 1971), "Framingham P. S. - Fat in Food May Not Count" (from Medical World News, September, 1970), "Dietary-Fat Debate - Thin on Answers" (from Medical World News, September, 1970), "Vitamins: Their Uses From A to Z" (from Moneysworth, October, 1975), "Eating to Live Longer" (from Woman's Day,

1973), "Nutrition's Best 'Pill' for Warding Off Age", "Diet and Aging" (from Modern Maturity, April-May, 1973), to name but a few. In fact, hardly a week goes by that a major magazine or newspaper does not feature at least one article on some current aspect of nutrition and diet.

Aside from proposals of nutritional intervention for the retardation, postponement or even prevention of the physical manifestations of the aging process and, secondarily, the extension of the individuals' life span through proper nutrition, it is obvious that, first and foremost, we must have a complete knowledge of the nutritional needs of humans, especially those individuals entering late middle age and early old age. Unfortunately, most of our knowledge of the nutritional requirements of man has been derived from the work on experimental lower animals, particularly the white rat. Any laboratory animal on an *ad libitum* diet under confined conditions may, at best, be compared with an overfed and underexercised human. In spite of such limitations, studies involving laboratory animals have provided valuable information as regards human nutrition and comparative gerontology. For example, classical experiments with rats have suggested that delayed physical manifestations of aging combined with life prolongation can be produced (at least in rats) by the careful restriction of proteins or calories in their diet. However, in isolated human populations during the Second World War, we do know that undernourishment resulting from and combined with poor living conditions produced individuals resembling prematurely aged adults.

On the other hand, the fact that certain diseases, particularly cardiovascular ailments, atherosclerosis, osteoporosis and others have a greater incidence in older persons, raises specific questions concerning the role of nutrition in "natural aging" and in relation to the greater prevalence and increased severity of certain diseases in individuals 60 years of age and older. Such questions include whether or not calcium or vitamin E supplementation can, indeed, prevent or even cure true osteoporosis; and also the question of the role of various dietary components (particularly lipids) in determining the differential, age-related progression of atherosclerosis in some individuals, but not in others. These questions also include the consideration of the importance of obesity in determining longevity, aside from the genetic factors which may indeed be responsible for a combination of familial tendencies toward obesity associated with shortened life span, and, therefore, whether or not mechanisms underlying life-shortening in the overweight persons are clearly definable.

Malnutrition - A Problem With Epidemic Proportions

Environmental factors play a major role in the determination of an animal's life span and, equally or even more important, the quality of life it experiences. Perhaps the most important environmental factor is diet, since the satisfaction of hunger is a basic biological drive common to all animals. In a man's life, food intake may be one of the most significant variables. Improper nutrition is probably one of the major factors causing, either directly or indirectly, poor health in Western society. Dietary problems in old age may arise from changes in metabolic requirements due to the onset of senescence and factors related to it or, even more likely, may be the continuation of the individual's life-long dietary habits. In spite of the significant role played by nutrition, few physicians pay proper attention to diet for the prevention and treatment of nutritionally-related diseases.

Many people have the misconception that malnutrition is brought about solely as the effect of undernourishment. On the contrary, overnourishment (which may be a greater cause of morbidity than undernourishment) must also be included in a proper definition of malnutrition. A wide spectrum of problems arises as a consequence of inadequacies in dietary intake, from those associated with undernourishment at one end (ranging from mild avitaminoses to acute starvation) to complications related to overnourishment and obesity on the other. It is highly probable that chronic malnutrition has always been an important factor in sharply limiting survival in ancient populations, just as it does in underdeveloped societies in Asia and Africa today. So-called overnourishment, an undesirable by-product of modern Western civilizations' dependence on labor-saving technology, can also lead to a serious reduction in longevity. A superabundance of calorically unbalanced food intake leads to obesity which has been correlated statistically with high mortality rates in the middle-aged and aged population.

On a worldwide scale, undernourishment accounts for reduced longevity and an increase in the incidence of nutritionally-related diseases. In the elderly American population, semistarvation (i.e., the inadequate intake of essential nutrients) due to a lack of money to purchase food is not an uncommon occurrence. In this area, old people living on South Miami Beach have been known to rummage through garbage cans for food to supplement their diet. Even with the availability of an adequate supply of food (often with the help of local welfare agencies or federally-supported programs such as food stamps) and no physiological problems involving the absorption and utilization of nutrients in the gastrointestinal tract of the body, the causes of malnutrition may be classified in three principal categories:

(1) Rejection of food due to a number of reasons (such as a lack of interest to buy and prepare food or poor dentition). Such rejection of food may lead to a variety of symptoms in the elderly such as mental dullness, apathy, withdrawal, muscular weakness, changes in the skin and mucous membranes, anemia, lowered serum albumin and lowered vitamin levels, to name only a few.

Rejection of food may be the reaction of the elderly individual to any one of a number of changes in his life-style. These may include a loss of status (i.e., retirement, marriage of children, loss of a mate). The older person confronted by such a situation may have feelings that he is no longer needed or wanted. Such dejection and depression may be manifested by little or no attention being paid to personal needs, one of which is diet.

(2) Unbalanced intake with adequate calories may arise from the selective rejection of meats and other important dietary constituents, even though the nutritional intake is otherwise calorically balanced. The aged individual, often living alone, may find it difficult to prepare adequate meals for himself. Accordingly, the elderly tend to make use of food products which are prepackaged and easily consumable with little or no further preparation. These foods include cakes, breads, crackers, potato chips, etc. Moreover, the American business community makes such foods readily available at relatively modest cost. Thus, the elderly rely on such food products as a quick, easy and inexpensive way to satisfy their hunger. Even with vitamin and mineral supplementation of such a diet, a high-quality source of protein may be lacking.

(3) Excessive caloric intake may result from an overconsumption of foods high in caloric content simultaneous with the rejection of foods rich in protein (particularly meat). Obesity, equated with prosperity in some cultures, may be defined as a relative excess of body fat content. This excess may be caused by too much readily available food combined with little will power and sedentary activity, or to a diet high in carbohydrates and fats. Obesity may also be linked with an underlying emotional disturbance, in extreme cases requiring psychiatric attention.

The overweight individual may be more prone to

conditions such as dyspnea, bronchitis, diabetes mellitus, gallstones, gout, hypertension, generalized atherosclerosis (with elevated risk of angina pectoris and cardiac failure), increased tendency toward accidents from a loss of balance and greater resulting trauma when such accidents do occur. Statistics, chiefly derived from commercially insurable risks, indicate that obesity reduces life expectancy; e.g., a 25-pound increase in weight above the standard reduces the expectation of life of a 45-year-old man by about 25 percent. It has been estimated that if all cancers could be eliminated, the average life span of an individual might be increased by about two years, while the elimination of obesity and its related diseases would result in a four-year increase. Indeed, this increase in longevity might be even greater, since many conditions known to decrease longevity are less severe when uncomplicated by obesity.

The Probable Solution

What can be done to eliminate the problems of malnutrition in America? It should be of prime concern that every elderly individual receives a balanced diet. Even more important, the diet of pregnant women would be carefully monitored and then proper nutrition begun at birth, so that by the time middle and old age were reached, the individual might have a reduced incidence of risk factors leading to diseases related to nutrition.

In this connection, The White House Conference on Aging held in 1971 made six recommendations for the improvement of the nutritional status of elderly Americans, as follows:

1. Initiate funding programs and research, which would be supported in part by the Federal Government, for the rehabilitation of those elderly people who are malnourished and for the prevention of malnutrition among those people approaching old age. Allocation of sufficient funds was recommended to begin a major research effort involving the influence of nutrition on the aging process and the diseases of the elderly.

2. Standards for food and nutrition services should be established and strictly enforced by the Federal Government with specific regulations for the nutrition and food services given by home-care agencies and institutions receiving Federal funds. These standards should include the quality and nutritive value of foods, food handling methods, and methods for the preparation and serving of food and special dietary needs

of such individuals. Nutritional counseling should be available and readily accessible.

3. Consumer education in nutrition was recommended for all consumers, especially the aged, as was the education by qualified nutritionists of those who serve the consumer (teachers in elementary and secondary schools, doctors, dentists, nurses, etc.).

4. Food services in elderly housing projects was proposed, as was the encouragement and support to provide services and facilities for the purchase of food, preparation of meals, and home delivery of prepared meals (e.g., the Meals-On-Wheels program) for eligible persons living outside of housing developments or in isolated areas.

5. Elimination of hunger and malnutrition through a guaranteed, minimum, adequate income, etc., was likewise recommended.

6. Food safety and wholesomeness should be assured through the establishment and enforcement by the Federal Government of standards necessary to insure and to improve the nutritive value of the national food supply. Labelling of the nutrient and other ingredient contents of food products was suggested as a means of achieving greater consumer awareness and understanding, especially in the direction of protecting the elderly.

The Outlook

Individual variations in nutritional requirements for the elderly arise as a result of a lifetime of different disease insults and differences in body structure and metabolism. Therefore, in reality, there can be no single solution to the nutritional problems associated with old age. However, through the combined efforts of scientists such as those participating in this symposium, the basic information about the dietary requirements of people in all age segments of the population may be determined. Eventually, through their combined efforts, and through the efforts of clinicians and basic scientists on an international scale, the ways will be found to manipulate the diet, so as to increase the human life span through a reduction in the incidence and severity of nutritionally-related diseases. This possibility is not unrealistic, since it is estimated that approximately one-half to one-third of the health problems experienced by the older individual are believed to be directly or indirectly related to nutrition, particularly in the early years. Elimination of malnutrition early in life would have a profound affect on increasing the average longevity, particularly, as well as improving the quality of life throughout each person's lifetime.

In closing this brief introductory comment on what we consider to be one of the most timely as well as significant meetings in the field of aging, we should like to emphasize that some of our speakers will be detailing, in the chapters which follow, the still poorly understood nutritional needs of the human species in general and of older persons in particular. In the latter case, the role of nutrition *per se* becomes secondarily obscured by such important affects in older persons as economic limitations of diet (especially in the case of retired individuals) and the solitary living arrangements of single, old persons, eating irregularly and without the appropriate social atmosphere conducive to good appetite and proper food habits. Similarly, loss of appetite with diminishing capacities of taste and smell typical of the aged and, finally, the possible secondary influences of such elements as ill-fitting dentures affecting food intake, constipation and, of course, chronic debilitating illnesses, may singly or in combination be responsible for poor eating habits and, therefore, malnutrition in such individuals. In the last connection, the chronic intake of drugs prescribed for long-term, serious illnesses and chronic, minor conditions in older persons may likewise serve to reduce the normal appetite for food and thus contribute, secondarily, to poor nutrition and even malnutrition, in the case of this large segment of well over 10% of our population, our 65 years and older Americans.

NUTRITIONAL CHARACTERISTICS OF THE ELDERLY-AN OVERVIEW

Robert E. Shank, M.D.

Danforth Professor and Head
Department of Preventive Medicine
Washington University School of Medicine
St. Louis, Missouri

The significance of nutrition for long life or slowing of the aging process is of great public and medical interest. Most everyone holds an opinion, but the evaluation of factual knowledge of this relationship is a large and complex undertaking. This, however, is the responsibility assigned the participants in this symposium. It is likely that in many areas to be addressed we shall find that the sum of knowledge is relatively small while the need for new information and research is large (Shank, 1975). Nevertheless, to recognize the limits of our knowledge and to identify promising avenues for investigation in this important health area is obviously a worthy objective. Although we meet in Florida, we are not likely to find a fountain of youth at this time. Perhaps we can point a way or ways by which other investigators will bring a larger measure of health and longer life for future generations of older persons.

The objective of this paper is to provide a descriptive overview or introduction of the health and nutritional characteristics of the aged. This will be done in relatively broad terms. Hopefully, a framework will be provided on which the speakers to follow can build and add the details of structure.

A first characteristic to be noted is that the number and proportion of older persons in the population of the United States are expanding at a rapid rate. Most of us are well aware of this fact, since the rate of increase is of such proportions that the financial base of the Social Security system is threatened, or so we are cautioned through the news media. There are in excess of 22 million persons 65 years of age or older in our population (Metropolitan Life Ins. Co., 1975a,b) (Table I). They represent 10% of the total population. In Florida the percentage is larger, of the order of 15%. Men are a minority, comprising but 40% of this older group of persons and only 27% of the population older than age 75 years.

It is to be expected that the disparity between the sexes will widen in the future because of the more favorable survival record of women throughout life.

TABLE I

Population at Ages 65 and Over, By Sex and Age United States, 1960-1980

Sex and Age	Population in 1,000's April 1 1960	April 1 1970	July 1 1974	July 1 1980	Percent Increase 1960-1970	1970-1980
Male						
65+	7,503	8,366	8,966	9,914	11.5	18.5
65-69	2,931	3,124	3,473	3,827	6.6	22.5
70-74	2,185	2,316	2,411	2,818	6.0	21.7
75+	2,387	2,926	3,082	3,269	22.6	11.7
Female						
65+	9,057	11,605	12,849	14,609	28.1	25.9
65-69	3,327	3,872	4,362	4,836	16.4	24.9
70-74	2,554	3,130	3,291	3,931	22.6	25.6
75+	3,176	4,603	5,196	5,842	44.9	26.9

Source of basic data: Various reports of the Bureau of the Census.

A notable point concerning the recent rate of growth of aged populations is the fact that during the 1960's the oldest age group, 75 years and older, increased at 1-1/2 to 2 times the rate of the group as a whole. During the current decade, the increase is comparable for all age and sex groups, except that the group of oldest men is expected to increase at only half the rate of the past decade, and half that of other age groups of older men in the present decade.

If we look backward in time, we find that the population of the United States has doubled in the last half century and that the median age has increased from 25.3 to 28.3 years (Table II). During this time interval, females have moved to predominance in number and have made larger gains than males in life expectancy measured at birth. Currently, the female has an expected life span of 74.0 years, while the male expectancy is 66.6 years.

As to other descriptive characteristics of our oldest age group (Table III), 9 percent of the men and 8.2 percent of women are non-white. Like proportions of men and women are described as single or divorced. In contrast, the proportion of men who are married is twice that of women and the proportion of widowed women is three times that of the men. A rather stark reality in these facts is that only slightly more than a third of the women have a surviving husband while more than two-thirds of the men have a wife who is still living.

The 1970 census data also indicate that about 96% of older men and 94% of women live in households, with the remainder in institutions and group quarters. An important development of the last two decades has been the growing independence of older persons, and the numbers who choose to live in communities comprised of and planned for older people. The census data provide no clue as to the proportion now living in such communities. This fact has other meaning since it implies a preference of younger generations to separate themselves from their parents and the responsibilities for their care.

TABLE II

Life Expectancy and Sex Ratios at Various Ages of United States Population in 1920 and 1970

	1920	1970
Total Population	105,710,000	203,166,000
Median Age (yrs)	25.3	28.3
Male/Female Ratio	104.1	94.8
Life Expectancy at Birth (yrs)		
Male -	58.1	66.6
Female -	61.6	74.0
Population-45 years of age & over		
Percent of Total Population	21.0	19.3
Male/Female Ratio	115.4	91.6
Life Expectancy (yrs)		
Male -	29.9	31.8
Female -	30.9	37.8
Population-65 years of age & over		
Percent of Total Population	4.8	10.0
Male/Female Ratio	101.5	72.2
Life Expectancy (yrs)		
Male -	12.2	12.8
Female -	12.7	16.4

TABLE III

Selected Social Characteristics of Population of Age 65 Years and Over (United States - 1970)

	Percent	
	Male	Female
Color		
White	91.0	91.8
Non-white	9.0	8.2
Marital Status		
Single	7.5	8.1
Married	72.4	36.5
Widowed	17.1	52.2
Divorced	3.0	3.2
Living Arrangements		
In households	95.7	93.7
In group quarters	4.3	6.3
Labor Force Participation		
In labor force	24.8	10.0
Employed	23.7	9.5
Unemployed	1.1	0.5
Not in labor force	75.2	90.0

Data derived from 1970 Census of Population.

Available income and economic status changes greatly as persons enter the latter half of the seventh decade of life. Nearly a quarter of the men and one-tenth of the women in the age group above 65 years continue employment. The extent of the reduction in expendable income is demonstrated in Table IV. The median income of families headed by a white person 55 to 64 years of age is $14,137, a figure which is reduced to $7,518 according to 1974 data if the family head is 65 years of age or older. Comparable median incomes for families headed by a black person are substantially lower and are $8,218 and $4,909, respectively. For both races there is a marked increase in the proportion of families with incomes less than $5,000 per year when the head of the family reaches or exceeds 65 years of age. One-quarter of such white families and one-half of black families currently are in this lowest income class. A group of older persons at largest disadvantage in terms of income are those individuals who are living outside of family relationships. Median annual income for such white persons in 1974 was $3,073 and for black individuals, $2,152. Other information indicates that the economic status of the average older person living in the United States has improved

TABLE IV

Total Money Income in 1974 for Older Persons Living in Families or Separately*

	Median Family Income	Percent Distribution of Family Income: Up to $5,000	$5,000-$10,000	$10,000-$15,000	Above $15,000	Median Individual Income of Persons Living Outside of Families
White Persons						
55-64 years	$14,137	9.3	19.8	25.4	45.5	$5,277
65+ years	7,518	26.4	38.9	18.2	16.7	3,073
Black Persons						
55-64 years	$ 8,218	28.7	29.9	24.4	16.9	$2,896
65+ years	4,909	51.4	33.4	8.0	7.4	2,152

*Data taken from Current Population Reports, Series P-60, No. 101, Jan. 1976, U. S. Bureau of the Census.

markedly in recent decades. Actually, ninety-five billion dollars, or 11.2% of the 850 billion dollar aggregate household income in 1974, was accounted for by families headed by a person 65 years or more of age. Despite this fact, a large proportion of older persons are severely limited in income and may, therefore, be unable to afford the living arrangements, food choices and medical care which would be most supportive of sustained good health and function.

In summary then, demographic and census information offers the following general description of this important segment of our population, the oldest age group. It has been growing more rapidly than most other age segments, has a substantial preponderance of women, includes a relatively large proportion of individuals removed from family relationships (in one sense this represents movement to greater independence, but in another to social isolation), and is characterized by relatively low income. Each of these facts has significance for the health and nutritional experience of our elder citizens.

The occurrence of disease and illness in the aged is importantly determined by earlier health events, conditions of working and living, and exposures of a variety of kinds. What then is the experience of aged persons relative to illness and the need for medical care? One measure is the annual frequency of health incidents, a statistic available through the National Center for Health Statistics (Table V). Examining representative measures, we find that the aged experience acute illnesses or conditions at a much lower rate than does the population at large - 109 against 220 events per year (Metropolitan Life Ins. Co., 1974). However, hospitalization for acute or short term care occurs at twice the rate in groups of older persons as it does for all ages combined. The frequency of hospitalization is slightly greater for older men than women. Accidental injuries account for approximately twenty percent of acute events in the aged, and more than half of these occur in the home. In seeking medical care, persons 65 years of age and older average about seven visits per year to their physicians. The comparable rate for physician usage by the entire population is five visits per year.

Another important measure of illness experience is the average number of days of confinement to bed for acute and chronic illnesses per 100 persons per year. In the oldest segment of the population this rate is 1411 days per 100 persons per year which compares with a rate of about 650 for the entire population. However, acute conditions account for only one-third of bed confinements in the aged, and with a higher proportion for women (39%) than for men (25%).

TABLE V

Health Incidents and Average Number of Days of Bed Confinement in the Total Population and in the Aged

	Number of All Ages	Health Incidents Events/100 Persons/Year 65 Years of Age and Over		
		Total	Male	Female
All Acute Conditions	220	109	98	117
Accidental Injuries, Total	31	21	22	21
Home Injuries	12	12	13	11
Discharges from Short Term Hospitals	14	26	28	25
Annual Physicians Visits	498	690	633	730
Average Number of Days of Bed Confinement/100 Persons/Year				
Acute & Chronic Conditions	646	1,411	1,330	1,468
All Acute Conditions	405	474	341	570
Accidental Injuries, Total	80	195	172	212
Home Injuries	25	97	38	140

Also revealing of the medical care needs of the elderly are the statistics which record the frequency of chronic conditions (Table VI). Approximately six percent of persons under 45 years of age have limitation in activity and 0.6 percent are unable to carry on major activities. Contrasting rates for the age group 45-64 years are 21 percent with activity limitation and 4.5 percent with inability to function in major duties. However, for the aged, 43 percent have limitations and 16 percent are unable to carry major activities. These deficits are much greater in men than in women, with a rate of major limitations four times that of females.

If the types of diseases responsible for activity limitation in the elderly are listed in terms of their relative importance, we find that approximately 20 percent of women and of men have heart disease as a cause (Table VII). Various forms of arthritis and rheumatism account for activity limitation in 27 percent of women and 14 percent of men. Visual impairments are the cause in about 7 percent of both sexes. Hypertension is given as the responsible disorder in 8.5 percent of women and 4 percent of men. Mental and nervous conditions account for activity limitation or confinement of three percent of the elderly. This category includes senile psychosis, one of the scourges and fears of the aged and their families.

TABLE VI

Frequency of Chronic Conditions
United States, 1969-1970, 1972

Health Status	Percent Distribution					
	All Ages	Under 45	45-64	65 and Over		
				Total	Male	Female
	All Persons					
Total	100.0	100.0	100.0	100.0	100.0	100.0
With no activity limitation	87.3	94.1	78.9	56.8	53.0	59.5
With activity limitation	12.7	5.9	21.1	43.2	47.0	40.5
With limitation in major activity	9.6	3.5	16.6	37.9	43.3	34.1
Unable to carry on major activity	3.0	0.6	4.5	16.3	28.3	7.7

TABLE VII

Frequency of Chronic Conditions
United States, 1969-1970

Type of Chronic Condition	Persons Limited in Activity					
	All Ages	Under 45	45-64	Elderly		
				Total	Male	Female
Total	100.0	100.0	100.0	100.0	100.0	100.0
Heart conditions	15.5	6.3	19.0	20.5	21.8	19.3
Arthritis and rheumatism	14.1	4.4	15.7	21.2	14.4	27.1
Visual impairments	4.8	3.6	3.8	7.0	7.0	7.0
Hypertension without heart involvement	4.6	1.8	5.2	6.4	4.0	8.5
Mental and nervous conditions	4.4	5.3	5.0	3.0	2.6	3.4

At this point I shall reiterate some of the characteristics of the aged as they relate to illness and compromises in health and independent activity. The purpose will be to indicate possible nutritional significances. About one-fourth of the aged are admitted to hospitals each year and the elderly average seven visits to their physicians annually. In these events there are opportunities for evaluation of the general health status and for obtaining information about dietary practices and the adequacy of nutrient intakes. The disabilities and restricted activity resulting from accidents and the chronic diseases prevalent in the elderly may impair food choice and intake. Moreover, certain of these events influence the need for nutrients or for diet planning. For instance, nitrogen and calcium losses may be substantial with but a few days of immobilization or confinement to bed. Or in another instance, the use of sodium-restricted diets in the treatment and care of patients with heart disease can bring about appetite failure or greatly decreased intake of usual and desirable foods. Cardiac failure, when it occurs, is accompanied by loss of appetite as well as by an increase in basal metabolic rate(BMR). As a result, weight loss may be rapid and extreme. Drugs utilized in treating the chronic illnesses of later life may also influence nutrient requirements in a variety of ways. For instance, digitalization may produce nausea and vomiting; the use of diuretics may induce urinary loss of potassium and hypokalemia; steroid hormones may cause water and salt retention.

While attempting to afford a description of the illness experiences of the aged in statistical terms, it should also be pointed out that important changes have occurred in mortality rates for common causes of death in the last decade (Metropolitan Life Ins. Co., 1975a,b). Of particular note is the persistent decline in death rates for ischemic heart disease or coronary atherosclerosis - the chief cause of death in later life (Table VIII). Standardized death rates for males of all ages have fallen by 6.6% in the decade ending in 1973. Older men have shared in this more favorable outlook, as demonstrated by the 10.3 percent decrease in death rates for men aged 65-69 years. Similarly, mortality rates for cerebrovascular disease have fallen 13.1% overall, with comparable decreases even in men past age 70 years. For comparison, the changes in death rates for diabetes are also given in Table VIII.

The mortality experience of women in the U.S. has been even more favorable with lessening overall death rates for ischemic heart disease, cerebrovascular disease and diabetes. In each instance the lower death rates continue into the oldest age groups of women. Certainly there is no ready explanation for these changes nor agreement on the factors responsible. Two possible considerations, however, for declining mortality rates for ischemic heart disease and cerebrovascular disease are the earlier recognition and more effective treatment of hypertension and the changes in American diet favoring reduced intake of animal fat and cholesterol, as well as the increased consumption of vegetable oils. Still other factors of nutritional significance that may have had a role in lowering mortality for diabetes and hypertension in women have been recent fads as well as health information which encourage weight control in earlier life and the avoidance or correction of obesity. However, the validity of these explanations can be questioned. Certainly they lack statistical proof. Nevertheless, if we are to look for nutritional factors important for longevity and health in old age, these are diseases of great importance.

TABLE VIII

Percent Changes in Standardized Mortality Rates
1962 - 1973

Age Group	Ischemic Heart Disease	Cerebrovascular Disease	Diabetes
	Men		
All	- 6.6	-13.1	+ 1
45-49	- 8.6	-12.7	- 1
65-69	-10.3	-16.5	+ 2
70-74	- 4.3	-10.7	+ 4
75+	+ 2.3	- 6.7	+17
	Women		
All	-12.3	-18.1	-10
45-49	- 0.2	- 5.6	+11
65-69	-18.8	-25.6	-22
70-74	-14.9	-22.2	-17
75+	- 3.1	- 9.5	+ 9

The metabolic and physiological changes which parallel the passage of years and are concomitants of aging have nutritional significance. We would like to refer to certain of these. Studies of basal metabolic rates undertaken early in this century demonstrated that rates were related most importantly to body size as measured by square meters of body surface. Rates are higher for males than for females at all ages. In both sexes the rates are highest in infancy and early childhood, decreasing during late adolescence to plateau in early adulthood. There then is gradual reduction of about 15 percent between the ages of 20 and 70 years. The decreasing BMR combined with the reduced expenditure of physical energy in work and/or recreation which is usual in older adults calls for decreased intake of calories as food.

During adulthood important changes occur in body composition, including a progressive increase in body fat and a decrease in lean body mass (Table IX). Data from body counter measurements of the isotope ^{40}K demonstrate these changes (Forbes and Reina, 1970). In men these investigators recorded average lean body mass (LBM) of 59 kg at age 25 years, with decrease to 47 kg by age 65-70 years. During this age span the average quantity of body fat increased from 14 to 26 Kg. Accordingly, the proportion of body weight as fat increased from 19% at age 25 to 35% at age 65 years. Comparable data for women indicated an increase in body fat from 33% to 49% of body weight in the same age interval. This was associated with an average increase in total body fat of 15 kg and a decrease in lean body mass of 5 kg. These data were obtained by weighing many persons for each age group and are, therefore, cross-sectional in type. Relatively few longitudinal observations have been made of the same adults over periods of decades. Of the few that are recorded, comparable changes in lean body mass and body fat have been recorded.

TABLE IX

Mean Values - Body Weight, Lean Body Mass and Body Fat of Adults of Various Ages *

Age	No.	Weight (kg)	LBM (kg)	Fat (kg)	Fat (%)
		Men			
25	585	73	59	14	19
45	881	76	56	20	26
55	835	74	52	22	30
65-70	234	73	47	26	35
		Women			
25	267	59	40	19	33
45	391	67	39	28	42
55	373	70	39	31	44
65-70	144	69	35	34	49

*Forbes and Reina, 1970.
LBM = Lean Body Mass

Figure 1 depicts in graphic fashion the observed and expected changes in body composition in males between age 25 and 70 years. In addition to the changes in lean body mass or cell mass and in body fat, it demonstrates the loss in bone mineral. The process of demineralization is a general phenomenon and is more marked in older women than in men, and may produce osteoporosis and bone pain.

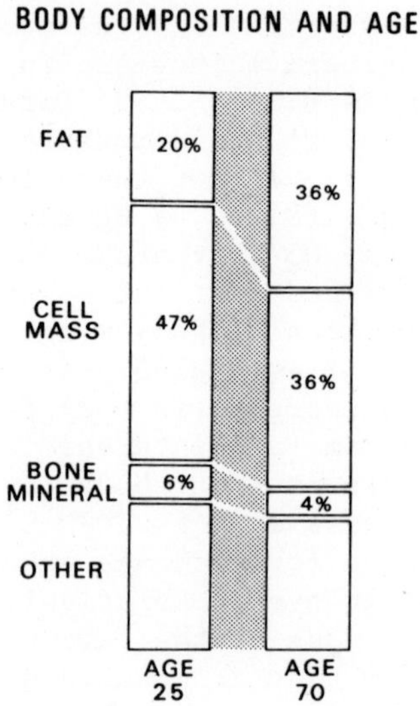

Fig. 1 Body composition and age of men. Body fat increases, while cell mass and bone mineral decrease as age progresses after maturity. (From Gregerman and Bierman, 1974.)

Studies by Shock and his associates (1963) have demonstrated an age-associated decrease in body water, paralleled by reduced oxygen consumption. The reductions in basal metabolic rate, lean body mass, and body water suggest that there is loss in the total number of body cells with increasing age. Evidence in experimental animals supports this contention, while in man an age-related decrease has been demonstrated in the numbers of non-glial cells in the cerebral cortex as well as the number of nephrons within the kidney, the latter being associated with reduction in glomerular and tubular functions, at least in some reports.

The changes in organ system functions which relate to aging could also be explained by reduction in cell metabolism. Many investigators have sought evidence of this by studies of enzyme function in animals. A few pertinent observations might be considered here. Although reduced activity of a number of enzymes (alkaline and acid phosphatase, D-amino acid oxidase, succinoxidase and pseudocholinesterase) has been reported in metabolically important tissues of old rats (i.e., heart, kidney and liver), most of these are unchanged when related to the DNA content (Barrows and Roeder, 1962). On the other hand, cathepsin and tryptophan peroxidase activity in relation to DNA content of tissue is increased. Moreover, the RNA content of cells of aged mice is increased with evidence of more rapid rates of turnover of protein.

Much attention has been given to the relative roles of DNA and RNA in the aging process. Several interesting hypotheses have been advanced. One hypothesis is that somatic mutations occurring in DNA produce RNA which cannot effectively synthesize protein and enzymes. According to this concept, cell death occurs when the activity of key enzymes decrease below a critical level.

The changes in protein metabolism referred to pertain to proteins with relatively short half-lives. The proteins contained in structural components of tissues are of much longer half-life. Two such proteins are collagen and elastin. These proteinaceous materials have been studied in both young and old animals and humans. Maturation of collagen was found in measurable quantities. Old collagen when contrasted to young has greater contractility when heated to 65°C and takes a longer time to relax. In rats, underfeeding or intermittent feeding and fasting inhibits the maturation of tendon or tail collagen (Verzar, 1963).

Verzar (1963) believes the modification in collagen produced by or associated with aging is due to the increase in number of crosslinks between molecules formed by hydrogen and ester bonds. Other investigators (Milch and Murray, 1962) have provided evidence that aldehydes are the intermediary metabolites which stabilize the lattice structure of collagen. Glyceraldehyde is the most potent stabilizer. It has been suggested that if procedures could be formulated to reduce tissue concentration of this important intermediary of carbohydrate metabolism, an approach might be provided for slowing down the molecular aging of collagen. Since collagen is included in all connective tissue and makes up 40% of total body protein, it is a body constituent worthy of consideration and additional evaluation for studies of aging.

Clinical experience supports the view that changes occur in the function of various other organ systems as the result of years of living. In general, the responses to physiological stresses are enhanced and reserves are limited. This is demonstrated by the age-related adaptations in the cardiopulmonary system. Resting systolic and diastolic blood pressure tends to increase, as does the pulse rate in response to exercise. Cardiac output is reduced and heart size increases. Vital capacity and maximum breathing capacity diminishes, while thorax size or çircumference decreases.

Of particular importance to the health and nutritional status of older persons are the modifications which occur with time along the enteric canal, since this is the avenue of access for digestion, absorption and elimination of food and its products. One of the frequent and unfortunate concomitants of old age is reduced perception of smell and taste. Therefore, appetite and desire for food is reduced and food preferences change, usually in the direction of simpler and relatively unseasoned items.

Most of us are well aware of the toll that the years take in teeth. Edentulousness is a common characteristic and the choice and enjoyment of foods may be greatly narrowed by the lack of dentures or by those which are ill fitting. Since gingival atrophy continues after removal of teeth, dentures which were totally appropriate at first fitting may become loose and troublesome. Atrophy of the gastric and intestinal mucosa as well as achlorhydria in older persons decreases rates of absorption of essential nutrients and reduces the quantities of intestinal mucous secreted. Intestinal motility becomes less active and constipation is likely to be a frequent complaint. The prevalence of intestinal diverticulae is age related and accounts for episodes of diverticulitis.

A recent study focused on the digestive disorders occurring in and reported by older persons during the National Health Survey of 1968 (Wilson, 1974). Of importance are the following facts (Table X):

1) Peptic ulcer is about as prevalent in persons older than 65 years as in middle-aged adults, 45-64 years.

2) Abdominal herniae occur in twice as many older persons as in their middle-aged counterparts.

3) The most frequent complaint in both age groups is constipation but the prevalence is nearly three times as great in the oldest group of persons.

4) Most other gastrointestinal disorders and complaints occur at higher rates in oldest subjects.

Of all the organ systems, the gastrointestinal tract is the most likely to be symptomatic among the aged. It is, therefore, the site and cause of concern for many older persons in their evaluation of their health status. It also becomes the reason for modification of long established food habits and for diets which may or may not be nutritionally adequate. Choice of foods may be determined more importantly by comfort or discomfort following a meal.

TABLE X

Prevalence of Selected Chronic Digestive Conditions in U.S. Population - 1968 *

Condition	Number per 1,000 population	
	Aged 45-64	Aged 65+
Peptic ulcer	33.4	29.0
Hernia	28.3	58.8
Functional and symptomatic upper G.I. disorder	23.5	37.7
Gallbladder condition	21.4	32.8
Chronic enteritis	17.9	34.0
Gastritis and duodenitis	16.2	24.0
Frequent constipation	35.0	96.3
Intestinal conditions	8.1	12.5
Liver conditions	2.4	6.2
Stomach trouble NOS	5.2	5.3

*Data from DHEW Publication No. (HRA) 74-1510, 1968.

Among the previously proposed bases for aging was the suggestion that advancing age produces a deficiency in availability or activity of hormones. About the only hormone for which in reality this holds true is the estrogen lack which follows the menopause. Other changes of endocrine function are, however, age related and may produce a variety of effects on hormone production, secretion and action. Gregerman and Bierman (1974) point out that standards of normality in clinical tests of endocrine function require consideration of age-associated effects occurring throughout populations. They assert that failure to appreciate this phenomenon in connection with age-related changes in glucose tolerance has led to probable overestimation of the incidence of diabetes in the adult population and to the frequent initiation of unnecessary therapeutic procedures. In an explicit and detailed review of the subject of aging and hormones, they state:

> "Aging affects many aspects of endocrine regulation but does not affect all the endocrine glands or all the different hormones secreted by the same gland to the

> same extent. Diminished secretion is sometimes a primary phenomenon, but age-related decreases of the rate of metabolic disposal of some hormones also leads to decreased hormone secretion rates as secondary or homeostatic mechanisms. Age not only can affect the concentration of a specific plasma protein involved in hormone transport but also can influence the concentration of the free or metabolically active portion of that hormone in the blood. Target-tissue sensitivity to hormonal effects is sometimes age related and in certain instances appears to involve hormone receptor mechanisms."

The variety and complexity of the hormonal changes identified and associated with aging are listed in figure 2. Later papers will deal with certain of these in more detail. Therefore, I would like to point to but a few examples. Growth hormone, although unmodified in terms of its concentration in blood, is produced with stimulation in smaller quantities and has less end-organ effect in older persons. Gonadotrophins are increased in blood in postmenopausal women but are not known to be otherwise functionally modified by age. Thyroxin exhibits enhanced end-organ sensitivity and is more rapidly disposed of in the older person. The primary modification in insulin activity is that of decreased secretion with dietary or other stimulus. The overall effects of these alterations in hormone function imply a variety of changes in requirements and utilization of nutrients associated with aging.

	HORMONE CONCENTRATION IN BLOOD	RESPONSE TO PHYSIOLOGIC OR PHARMACOLOGIC STIMULATION	METABOLISM (DISPOSAL RATE)	END-ORGAN SENSITIVITY
GROWTH HORMONE	↔	↓		↓
GONADOTROPINS	↑*			
THYROTROPIN (TSH)	↔	↓		↔
THYROXINE (T4)	↔	↔	↓	↑
TRIIODOTHYRONINE (T3)	↓			
PARATHYROID HORMONE	↓			↑
CORTISOL	↔	↔	↓	
ADRENAL ANDROGENS	↓	↓		
ALDOSTERONE	↓		↓	
INSULIN	↔	↓	↔	↔
GLUCAGON	↔	↔		
TESTOSTERONE	↓		↓	
ESTROGENS	↓		↓	

Fig. 2 Changes in plasma hormones during aging in man. ↑= increase; ↓= decrease; ↔ = no change; * = postmenopausal; blank spaces indicate that no data are available. (From Gregerman and Bierman, 1974.)

The guide or standard for planning nutrient intakes and diet for healthful living of all age groups in the United States is provided by the National Research Council in its Recommended Dietary Allowances (1974). Allowances for selected nutrients in the diets of older persons are listed in Table XI. It is of interest that the only explanation given for these allowances pertains to the caloric allowances. It is stated that energy intakes for persons above 50 years of age should be reduced to levels 90 percent of the allowance for mature adults. Certainly this would seem to be appropriate in view of decreased basal or resting metabolic rates. However, as with all such allowances, there must be adaptation not only for age but also for body size, physical activity and the specific additional needs of the person. The allowances for individuals past 50 years of age do not call for reduction in the intake of other nutrients, i.e. protein, vitamins and minerals, comparable to the 10 percent decrease in energy consumption. In essence, this implies or calls for nutrient enrichment of the diet of the older person, providing somewhat larger quantities of these other nutrients per 1,000 kcal. If this is to be accomplished, the aged must have nutritional knowledge and motivation for most appropriate choice of foods.

TABLE XI

Recommended Dietary Allowances*
(NRC - 1974)

For Persons Older Than 50 Years		
	Women	Men
Calories (kcal)	1,800	2,400
Protein (gm)	46	56
Vitamin A (I.U.)	4,000	5,000
Vitamin E (I.U.)	12	15
Ascorbic Acid (mg)	45	45
Niacin (mg)	12	16
Riboflavin (mg)	1.1	1.5
Thiamin (mg)	1.0	1.2
Calcium (mg)	800	800
Iron (mg)	10	10

*Recommended Dietary Allowances, 8th Revised Ed., National Academy of Science, Washington, D. C., 1974.

The information available concerning food consumption and the nutrient quality of diets consumed by older persons is limited. However, a source is available in the Household Food Consumption Survey of the U. S. Department of Agriculture (1972). The data in Table XII are taken from the reports of the survey of 1965 and 1966 and demonstrate the decreasing mean nutrient intake with advancing age in men. Energy intakes decreased from a mean value of 2.465 kcal in the decade from 55 to 64 years of age, to 2.051 kcal for men aged 65 to 74 years, and to 1.866 kcal at age 75+ years. The mean intake of other nutrients also decreased with age. However, only for calcium intake at age 75+ years is the mean value well below the recommended allowance. The data, recorded as mean intake, fails to disclose the important proportion of the older population whose consumption of one or more nutrients falls to levels well below the recommended allowances.

TABLE XII

Mean Nutrient Intake Per Day*
(Males)

	Age in Years			
	35-54	55-64	65-74	75+
Calories (kcal)	2,643	2,465	2,051	1,866
Protein (gm)	107	99	82	72
Fat (gm)	133	124	100	90
Carbohydrate (gm)	244	228	204	191
Calcium (gm)	0.77	0.70	0.67	0.60
Iron (mg)	16.9	16.2	13.4	11.3
Vitamin A (I.U.)	6,560	9,740	5,640	4,720
Thiamine (mg)	1.4	1.4	1.2	1.1
Ascorbic acid (mg)	75	78	67	54

*U.S. Dept. of Agriculture - Household Food Consumption Survey, 1965 - 1966.

An accessory finding of some importance deriving from the 1965-66 survey was the observation that about 35 percent of men and women 75 years of age and older used vitamin or mineral supplements. This is a proportion of users greater than for any other age group, except infants and youngest children. Use of such supplements by men and women aged 65 to 74 years was at a level of 26 percent. This would seem to indicate that oldest people do have a concern about their diets and the possible benefits in health to come from added intake of vitamins and minerals.

A nutritional survey undertaken in 1968 to 1970 in ten states by the Center for Disease Control (1972) involved populations which were in the lowest quartile of income at the time of the 1960 census. The oldest age segment of the populations sampled included persons above 60 years of age. Nutritional deficits of greatest prevalence included iron in both sexes, vitamin A in Spanish-American men and women, riboflavin in black and Spanish-Americans of both sexes, and vitamin C in males of all racial origins. Physical examinations and anthropometric measurements demonstrated that obesity occurred commonly in white and black older women in the lowest income brackets.

Utilizing similar or the same techniques of measurement, a first health and nutrition examination survey was undertaken on a scientifically-designed sample representative of U.S. civilian populations aged 1 to 74 years in 1971-72 (Abraham et al., 1974, 1975). The observations of persons older than 60 years indicated that the most frequent deficits were those of dietary iron, vitamin A, vitamin C and calcium. Low hemoglobin and hematocrit values occurred frequently in black older persons as contrasted to white. This was not associated, however, with the same high prevalence of low serum iron and transferrin saturation values as evidence of iron deficiency in the aged black persons. Clinical signs or laboratory evidence of other nutrient deficiency was of very low frequency in this survey, but obesity was recorded as occurring commonly in older women, with higher rates in black than in white women. In contrast, more older white men were obese than older black men.

This paper has attempted to present in broad perspective the health needs of older persons and the nutritional considerations which derive from or relate to them. Undoubtedly, the aged have particular nutritional characteristics. With the extension of our research efforts, there is a likely possibility that nutritional factors and diet itself will be shown to play significant roles in the process of aging or turn out to be determinants of longevity.

REFERENCES

Abraham, S., Lowenstein, F. W. and Johnson, C. L. (1974). "Preliminary Findings of the First Health and Nutrition Examination Survey, United States, 1971-1972: Dietary Intake and Biochemical Findings". DHEW Publ. No. (HRA) 74-1219-1, Rockville, Maryland.

Abraham, S., Lowenstein, F. W. and O'Connell, D. E. (1975). "Preliminary Findings of the First Health and Nutrition Examination Survey, United States, 1971-1972: Anthropometric and Clinical Findings". DHEW Publ. No. (HRA) 75-1229, Rockville, Maryland.

Barrows, C. H., Jr. and Roeder, L. M. (1962). In "Biological Aspects of Aging" (N. W. Shock, ed.), pp. 290-295, Columbia University Press, New York.

Center for Disease Control (1972). "Ten State Nutrition Survey, 1968-70". DHEW Publ. No. (HSM) 72-8130.

Forbes, G. B. and Reina, J. C. (1970). Metabolism 19, 653.

Gregerman, R. I. and Bierman, E. I. (1974). In "Textbook of Endocrinology" (R. H. Williams, ed.), pp. 1059-1070, W. B. Saunders Co., Philadelphia.

Metropolitan Life Ins. Co. (1974). Stat. Bull. 55 (July), 9.

Metropolitan Life Ins. Co. (1975a). Stat. Bull. 56 (April), 8.

Metropolitan Life Ins. Co. (1975b). Stat. Bull. 56 (June) 3; (August) 3; (November) 3.

Milch, R. A. and Murray, R. A. (1962). Proc. Soc. Exp. Biol. Med. 111, 551.

National Research Council (1974). "Recommended Dietary Allowances - Eighth Revised Edition". National Academy of Sciences, Washington, D. C.

Shank, R. E. (1975). In "Epidemiology of Aging" (A. M. Ostfeld and D. C. Gibson, eds.), pp. 199-213, DHEW Publ. No. (NIH) 75-711, Bethesda, Maryland.

Shock, N. W., Watkin, D. M., Yiengst, M. J., Norris, A. H., Gaffney, G. W., Gregerman, R. I., and Falzone, J. A., Jr. (1963). J. Gerontol. 18, 1.

U. S. Dept. Agriculture (1972). Household Food Consumption Survey, 1965-66, Report No. 11.

Verzar, F. (1963). Sci. Am. 208, 104.

Wilson, R. W. (1974). "Prevalence of Selected Chronic Digestive Conditions - United States, July - December, 1968". Vital Health Stat., Ser. 10, No. 83.

THE ROLE OF NUTRITION IN HUMAN AGING

W. O. Caster, Ph.D.

Professor of Nutrition
School of Home Economics
University of Georgia
Athens, Georgia 30602

Nutrition plays an important role in controlling the rate of human aging -- at least many nutritionists would affirm this as an article of faith. Occasionally we even see convincing demonstrations that this principle operates in the lives of those about us.

My mother, Rena, was known as an excellent cook. We visited her one winter, some three to four months after father died, and were horrified to see how she had changed -- had deteriorated. It shortly became clear that she was not eating at all properly. She had had a cold and did not feel like walking to the grocery store, some three blocks away. The less she ate, the weaker she felt. She had slowed down physically and was less alert mentally. She looked and acted much older.

As you might guess, we promptly changed her living arrangements to a situation that assured three meals per day, under dietetic controls. Within the next few weeks, Rena returned to a much more vigorous and alert state of being. The changes were quite dramatic. Was it nutrition alone that made the change? I could certainly convince myself that nutrition was among the more important of the controlling variables. It is nevertheless true that before one can speak with certainty about nutritional effects, and indicate precisely which nutrients are critical, it becomes necessary to limit the discussion to experimental data obtained under more rigorously defined conditions.

A difficult issue relates to the need to define the aging process in precise and quantitative terms. At first glance, one is overwhelmed by the multidimensionality of this problem. Watkin (1964) has stated that, "Strictly speaking, a study in man of any parameter as a function of age _per se_ is impossible. Aging in man at least is not merely the passing of years, but also the accumulation of insults." He goes on to list some of the common "insults" of living and then points out that, "no two individuals have ever traversed 65 years of living to acquire them in exactly the same quantity and quality."

Any work with the human is beset with problems and sources of variability, and the study of aging certainly has more than its share of these. Nevertheless, there are those physiological and biochemical trends that are related to "the passage of years" and are reasonably common to all persons.

It will be the purpose of this discussion to focus attention on some of these consistent, age-related trends, and to examine the evidence suggesting that these trends are influenced by the nutritional status of the subject. In doing this, it is recognized that aging is a highly multivariate entity, and that one must look simultaneously at a variety of age-related trends in order to grasp the overall picture. The deterioration that we refer to as "aging" can be measured by observing physical, mental and psychomotor performance changes and it can be measured by considering the biochemical and clinical changes associated with the progress of degenerative diseases characteristic of the aged. Notable among these diseases are diabetes, cardiovascular disease and cancer.

DIABETES

With increasing age there is an impaired ability to utilize glucose, and there is an ever-increasing probability of diabetes mellitus developing. It seems generally true that, following a test dose, the rate at which the excess glucose disappears from the blood stream is a function of the age of the subject. The disappearance is most rapid in the young, somewhat slower (perhaps 75 percent as fast) in the middle aged, and slowest (about 50 percent as fast) in the aged. This observation has been reported under a variety of experimental conditions (Unger, 1957; Silverstone *et al.*, 1957; Hayner *et al.*, 1965), and is measurable in terms of the elevated shape of the glucose tolerance curve.

National public health data (U. S. Dept. HEW, 1970), in figure 1, show that the death rate from diabetes increases progressively with age. This is true in both the black and white populations of this country, although the incidence of diabetes in the black population is considerably greater than is observed among the white. These racial differences are, in turn, strongly correlated with economic and dietary differences.

It is the economic and the dietary differences, rather than purely racial factors, which appear to be critical in relation to diabetes. One evidence of this is seen in the fact that a major part of this increase seen in the black has occurred since 1955 (U. S. Dept. HEW, 1970). Similar differences have been noted in other populations. Brunner _et al_. (1964) found an incidence of diabetes of 0.05 percent in Yemenite Jews who had recently arrived in Israel, compared with 0.55 percent in the Yemenite Jews who had been living in Israel for longer than ten years. Here is an even more clear cut case in which diet and the way of life, rather than racial factors, altered the incidence of diabetes by a factor of about 10-fold.

In general then, one measure of aging is the decrease ability to utilize glucose (as shown by an elevated glucose tolerance curve) and an increased tendency toward diabetes. Population statistics suggest that diet can be critically important in this matter.

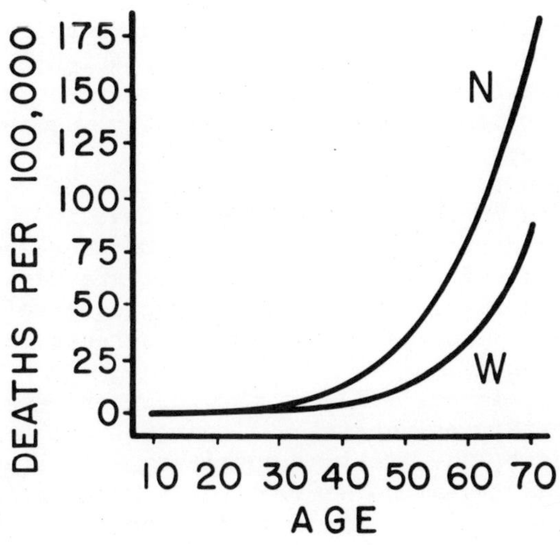

Fig. 1 Death rate per 100,000 for diabetes in white (W) and non-white (N) populations in the United States, as observed for different age groups ranging from 10 to 70 years.

Recent data from our own laboratory (Caster and Bleecker, 1975) point to certain specific nutrients as being important in relation to this effect. Caproic acid (present in butterfat and coconut oil) and certain of its amino derivatives (norleucine, leucine, methionine, glutamate and norvaline), under chronic feeding conditions, can produce a marked hyperglycemia and an elevated glucose tolerance curve in work with experimental animals. Caproic acid and/or some of its amino derivatives were fed as 0.1 - 1.0 percent of the diet. The initial effect, seen in the first day or two was to reduce the plasma glucose level. When this feeding was continued for 30 - 40 days, the plasma glucose level returned to normal and then slowly increased to a near-diabetic range (170 - 190 mg of glucose per dl), and the glucose tolerance curve was simultaneously displaced upward.

One of our observations suggests that the plasma insulin level was also elevated at this time. This would suggest that this dietary modification tends to produce an insulin-resistant type of diabetes.

We searched for commercially-available foods that might provide elevated levels of caproic acid derivatives. One diet that was fed consisted of corn grits (high in leucine) and chicken skin (a good source of lysinonorleucine). Within a month, the rats developed a marked hyperglycemia (plasma glucose levels of 190 mg/dl).

In relation to later discussion, it may be worth noting that the protein in this diet resembles that in the grits-greens-fat back diet characteristic of the poor and black of the southeastern United States since pellagra days (Ridlon, 1916; Bailey and Mize, 1961). It is precisely this population group (see Fig. 1) that shows a marked increase in the incidence of diabetes.

Here, then, is one index of the aging process that is clearly susceptible to nutritional control. In experimental animals, at least, the critical nutrients are related to caproic acid and its amino derivatives. Other relationships undoubtedly are yet to be discovered. For those interested in this search, I might suggest one additional direction. It is known that one way of producing Sekoke disease, a diabetes-like disease seen in carp, is to feed products containing rancid oil (Yokote, 1970). In further work relating to diabetes, it might be wise to keep records on the consumption of potato chips and other sources of heated or oxidized fats, as well as to look for interactions relating to vitamin E and other antioxidants.

OBESITY

Obesity is a condition that is associated with, and tends to complicate, diabetes and other degenerative diseases of later life. Starting with the teenage period there is a progressive tendency for an increase in subcutaneous fat as measured by skin-fold thickness (Brozek et al., 1953; Mayer, 1968). Here again we have age-related trends that are susceptible to dietary control. The extent to which excess body fat accumulates is quite generally considered to be related to diet and energy expenditure. In the case of the chicken, some simple dietary rules have been developed for the control of body fat (Fraps, 1942; Donaldson et al., 1956). These relate to the relative proportions of the various nutrients, protein in particular, in the diet. In the case of mammalian systems, the situation is not this simple.

In the human, small changes in food intake do not produce the clear-cut changes in body weight and body fat that the theorists would expect to see, even if these changes persist over a long period of time. Rose and Williams (1961) describe two groups of young men with a substantial (nearly two-fold) difference in food intake, but apparently equal energy output, that showed no difference in body weight, basal metabolic rate or other pertinent characteristics. Miller and Mumford (1967) clearly demonstrated that the production of obesity by increasing food consumption experimentally is not as easy a process as one might imagine.

There are some indications that a change in nutrient composition of the diet may have more effect. Mickelsen et al. (1955) were able to produce obesity in one strain of rats by feeding a high-fat diet. Sims et al. (1973) have shown that, with a judicious choice of diet, human body weight can be increased by controlled over-feeding. On a high carbohydrate or high protein diet something of the order of a two-fold increase in calories was required to produce a 10 kg increase in body weight, and a continued elevated intake (about 50 percent above normal) was required to maintain this excess weight. A return to a normal caloric intake resulted in a prompt loss of this excess weight.

By contrast, when a high-fat diet was fed, the body weight could be increased and maintained at elevated levels with only a moderate increase in caloric consumption.

From all of these observations, it appears that the percentage of fat in the diet is critical in the production and control of obesity.

In our own work (Caster et al., 1975) it was found that four of the common saturated fatty acids, (caproate, caprate, myristate, and stearate), when fed under defined conditions, had some tendency to increase the food intake and feed efficiency of a rat diet. Even more importantly, the inclusion of linoleate (the most common polyunsaturated fatty acid) in dietary fat was even more effective in producing an increase in carcass fat. The amount of oleate (mono-unsaturated fatty acid) in dietary fat had significant systematic effects in controlling the amount of DNA (or the number of adipose tissue cells) in abdominal fat pads (Caster and Resurreccion, 1972).

From these data it appears that diet composition can indeed have a marked influence on the tendency to develop a "middle-age spread". Most critical among the nutrients is the amount and chemical composition of the fat component.

CARDIOVASCULAR DISEASE

Diseases of the heart and vascular system constitute the age-related changes that have probably excited more interest and concern than any of the other health factors. With increasing age there is a progressive increase in high blood pressure, elevated plasma cholesterol level, and a tendency toward coronary heart disease and stroke. The relationship between the incidence of each of these conditions and advancing age resembles the curves shown in figure 1. There is a more rapid increase in later years, and the poor and black in southeastern United States show an unusually high incidence of some of these conditions (Tyroler, 1970).

Smoking, exercise and emotional stress are known to influence the incidence and severity of cardiovascular disease, but diet is also important. There have been strong suggestions (Council on Foods and Nutrition, 1972) to the effect that it would be prudent for the entire middle-aged population in this country to change the nature of the lipid in its diet. Much of the saturated animal fat should be replaced with polyunsaturated vegetable oils.

There are numerous reviews of the literature supporting this suggestion, but there is still no unanimous agreement concerning the interpretation of the basic data in this field (see Reiser, 1973 *vs*. Keys *et al*., 1974, for example). A detailed review of this conflict is beyond the scope of this discussion. Suffice it to say that substantial evidence suggests that human diets high in butterfat, coconut oil and whole egg tend to elevate the blood cholesterol level, and that populations with high cholesterol levels are characterized by a high incidence of coronary heart disease.

Data from our own laboratory (Caster *et al*., 1975) tend to suggest that caproic acid esters are more important than had previously been appreciated, and that cholesterol, when fed at reasonably low levels, may be of little importance in controlling blood cholesterol levels.

The relationship between dietary fat and hypertension or stroke is much less clear. In our own work with experimental animals (Resurreccion and Caster, 1972) it was found that a small but statistically significant decrease in systolic pressure occurred when the amount of fat in the diet was increased from 10 percent to 25 percent of the diet weight, and this pressure attained a minimum value when the dietary fat contained 19 percent stearate. These data seem to minimize the emphasis on dietary fat as it relates to blood pressure.

The most reliable way that we have found to increase the blood pressure in rats is by feeding a cereal grain diet (Caster _et al._, 1974). A number of the common breakfast cereals, either hot or ready-to-eat, raised the systolic pressure of the rat to 170 - 200 mm Hg within 30 - 40 days. This is a nutritional effect that needs considerably more study.

Probably the highest incidence of hypertension and death due to cerebrovascular disease is to be found in the southeastern stroke belt (Tyroler, 1970). This is particularly true of the poor and black population living in the coastal plains of North and South Carolina and Georgia. This population, for good economic reasons, is not known for eating unusually large amounts of butter and prime beef. Their diet may however contain an unusually large proportion of corn grits.

Some studies of this "stroke belt" have focused attention on the mineral content of the drinking water. The general finding is that soft-water areas have higher death rates from cardiovascular disease than do hard-water areas (Schroeder, 1960). The possible importance of mineral nutrition is made more credible by the well known finding that any increase in dietary sodium tends to increase blood pressure in an almost linear fashion (Meneely and Dahl, 1961).

In a study of the waters of Evans County, Georgia, we found (Chah _et al._, 1976) that cardiovascular disease patients drank from water supplies containing significantly higher concentrations of phosphate, cobalt and iron, and significantly less cadmium than did matched controls. Likewise, stroke patients on the average drank water containing significantly more sodium than did their matched controls. These data would tend to confirm reports of others to the effect that the trace mineral content of drinking water may be correlated in a statistically significant way with the health records of the patients drinking that water.

Our work did not stop at this point, however. Mixed diets were collected from this same area, and analyzed for trace minerals. It was found that, in the case of all of the elements studied, the diet provided perhaps 100-fold (ranging from 10- to 5000-fold) more of each element per day than did the drinking water (Chah et al., 1976). This makes it appear highly unlikely that any of the correlations relating drinking water composition to health problems are physiologically meaningful.

If trace minerals are indeed crucial to cardiovascular disease, this is a matter than can be explored more fruitfully in relation to studies of diet composition rather than in relation to drinking water -- which provides only a fraction of a percent of the trace minerals consumed per day.

If nothing else, these data suggest a note of caution in relation to the interpretation of epidemiological correlation studies. Perhaps this should be the central theme of any review of the relationship between diet and heart disease. While there are a number of interesting looking correlations, considerably more work needs to be done before causality is established.

CANCER

An even more difficult health area to discuss is that relating diet to cancer. There is a growing literature suggesting that gastrointestinal cancer, at least, may be related to the diet consumed by the patient.

Kmet and Mahbourbi (1972) have pointed to the very unusual geographical distribution of esophageal cancer in Iran, without suggesting any specific dietary cause. Haenszel (1967) has listed 19 different specific foods that, on an epidemiological basis, might be related to gastric cancer.

Other dietary factors have been discussed in relation to cancer of the intestinal tract (Wynder et al., 1969; Gregor et al., 1971; Walker, 1971) and cancer of the bladder (Yoshida et al., 1971).

Currently there is considerable interest centered on neoplastic disease of the colon, and its possible relationship to either the amount of crude fiber in the diet (Burkitt, 1973) or to the amount of fat and meat (Haenszel et al., 1973; Wynder and Reddy, 1974) in the diet.

Nitrosamines, associated with bacon, preserved meat products, and certain other products (Shapley, 1976), are potent carcinogens and are capable of inducing cancer in many different parts of the body (Jijinsky, 1970; Wolff and Wasserman, 1972). There is also evidence relating polyunsaturated fatty acids, particularly after heating, to several aspects of the cancer story (Sugai et al., 1962; Michael et al., 1966; Andia and Street, 1975). If one were to include the topic of pesticides, and include several other non-nutrient materials that may be present in trace amounts in foods, the recital could be extended to include a major part of the cancer literature. There is also a vitamin-nutrition aspect to this story, that will probably be discussed later.

In reviewing the diet-cancer literature, one is strongly reminded of the definition of the aging process as the accumulation of insults. It becomes a question of how many carcinogenic insults one can absorb before cancer appears. A number of these are clearly associated with items in the diet.

PHYSICAL FITNESS

Undoubtedly the factor most universally associated with aging, in the public mind, is the generalized deterioration in physical performance that is observed in the elderly. In the course of a few years there is a noticeable decline in vigor, in physical strength and coordination, and in general work abilities (Buskirk, 1966; Norris and Shock, 1974). Figure 2 shows the typical pattern of change seen in some of the experimental data related to performance.

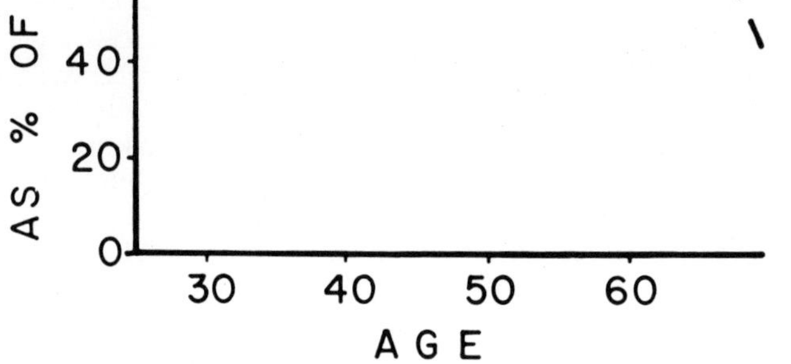

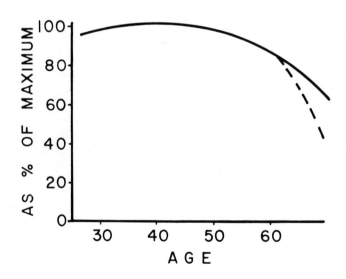

Fig. 2 Changes in muscle strength as a measure of physical performance with age.

By using exhaustion tests with treadmill equipment, one can measure a person's maximum work output in terms of the maximum rate of oxygen consumption. The highest work rates are observed at about age 30. In confirmation of this, Lehman (1951) has pointed out that the distance runners sent to the Olympic Games by the United States have had an average age of 31.5 years and that championships in many sports were won by contestants in the age range 28 - 36 years. There is a slow but progressive decline in maximum work output from age 30 to 60. At some point, beyond age 60, the rate of decline becomes much more rapid.

With a hand dynamometer, one can measure hand grip strength. Burke et al. (1953) and Miles (1950) did this using over 1000 men and women at different ages. A maximum strength was observed at about age 30, and there was a slow, progressive decline until age 60 - 70. Beyond this, strength declined more rapidly.

Various organs and systems in the body show a similar pattern of deterioration with age. In the eye, with increasing age, there is a progressive yellowing and decreased transparency of lens tissue (Said and Weale, 1959). Along with this is a progressive decrease in the size of the pupil (Robertson and Yudkin, 1944; Birren et al., 1948; Luria, 1960). Together these effects lead to a progressive decrease in dark adaptation (Steven, 1946) and may help to explain decreased visual abilities on such tests as flicker fusion frequency (Brozek and Keys, 1945; Weale, 1963).

Similarly one could measure finger dexterity, eye-hand coordination, a variety of pyschomotor functions (Birren and Botwinick, 1955), cardiovascular function and the function of a variety of organs and systems in the body. In many cases in which this was done, a maximum performance was observed around age 30, and a linear decrement occurred to, or beyond, age 60. Depending upon the nature of the performance task and the experimental subject, the relative loss from age 30 to 60 varied somewhat (Norris et al., 1953, 1956; Norris and Shock, 1974; Brandfonbrener et al., 1955) but in many cases it represented an over-all decrease to a level that was 50 - 70 percent of maximal. In most instances the changes observed with advancing age were large enough to be easily measurable. The age at which a more rapid decline begins varies somewhat from person to person, but the general pattern seems universal enough to provide a useful basis for a systematic study of the aging process.

Unfortunately, so far as I can find, nutrition has not been used as a controlling variable in relation to any systematic study relating aging to physical function. It would seem that this is an area of investigation that needs to be pursued.

BONE DENSITY

Closely related to muscle strength is the strength of ligament, tendon (Zuckerman and Stull, 1969), bone and other supportive tissues associated with that muscle. Parallel changes in muscle strength and bone density have been demonstrated in a variety of ways (Howell, 1917; Tower, 1939). As a muscle is strengthened, bone density increases. Conversely, inactivity leads to a parallel demineralization of skeleton and loss of muscle mass (Asher, 1947).

Figure 2 describes the systematic loss of muscle strength with aging. Associated with this one would expect a parallel loss of bone density.

The solid curve in figure 3 summarizes the changes in bone density observed in some 1000 men and 3000 women at different ages (Albanese, 1975). Since this work was limited to "normal" people, it is presumed that cases showing the osteoporosis of old age were systematically excluded. A broken line is appended to represent this situation.

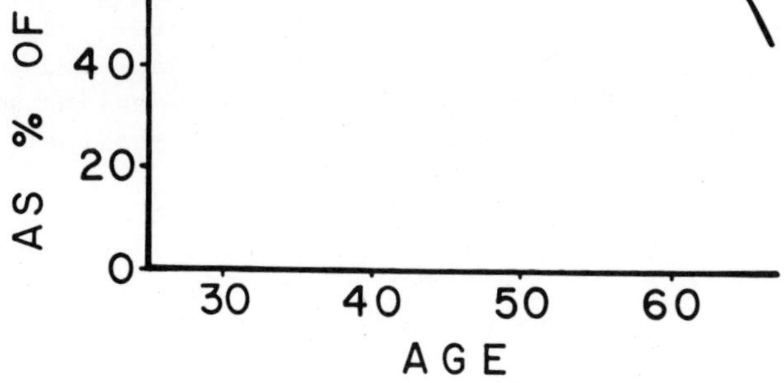

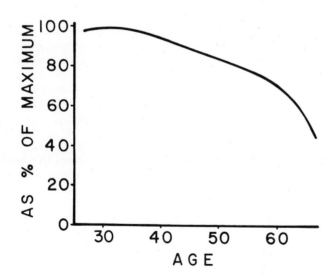

Fig. 3 Changes in bone density in men and women with age. (The broken line represents bone density for individuals with osteoporosis, excluded from this study.)

There are slight differences between the curves seen for men and women. The maximum bone density is seen in women around age 40 and for men around age 50. Both age groups were somewhat later than the 30-year age level corresponding to the time of maximal muscular strength. Hence, in the aging musculoskeletal system, the loss of strength in the active muscle mass preceeds the loss of skeletal strength by some 10 - 20 years.

Clinicians and nutritionists have been concerned about the demineralization of the skeleton that occurs with advanced age. It is suggested that an increased intake of fluoride might harden the bone mineral and thus delay the process of skeletal demineralization (Rich et al., 1964; Goggin, 1965; Cass et al., 1966; Cohen and Gardner, 1966). From a comparison of figures 2 and 3, it appears that exercise and nitrogen metabolism may be as important as mineral nutrition in maintaining normal bone density. This is further confirmed by the work of Garn et al. (1967) who studied the relationship between bone density and age in populations with quite different calcium intakes and found surprisingly similar age-response curves.

ECONOMICS AND DIET

Before closing any discussion of the role of nutrition in human aging, it would seem appropriate to make note of certain dietary changes that frequently accompany the aging process. Beyond the age of 50 or 60, there are often progressive and predictable changes in diet. Part of these may be for health reasons, and part may be for economic reasons. Dietary choices are limited by a lack of functional teeth, and by medical restrictions imposed by diabetes, hypertension, hypercholesteremia, gout, gallbladder problems, kidney stones and perhaps other conditions. The food intake and energy output normally decline with age, but this decline may be further accelerated by arthritis and dizziness that rapidly decrease the ability to walk and exercise.

Not the least of the disabilities of the aged is their lack of money. A large proportion of the elderly must subsist on a poverty diet. In Georgia, one quarter of the elderly are trying to subsist on incomes of less than $1000 per year. Hence, physical and medical changes are not the only factors to act as controls on the diet of the elderly. In many cases the crucial control is economic.

With this in mind it is well to turn again to figure 1, and to the data relating to diabetes and heart disease. The poor and black have a much higher incidence of diabetes and cardiovascular disease, on an age-adjusted basis, than do the more affluent white population. When experimental animals are fed a diet of corn grits and chicken skin (which mimics the protein component of the poverty diet of this region) the animals shortly develop hyperglycemia (Caster and Bleecker, 1975) and hypertension (Caster and Parthemos, 1976).

It, therefore, seems appropriate to ask if part of the increase in diabetes and heart disease seen characteristically in elderly populations might be associated with the change toward a poverty diet -- which, in turn, exacerbates physiological trends that are already present at this age.

CONCLUSION

In summary, there is such a thing as aging. We all see it and recognize it, but have difficulty defining it in quantitative terms. It is seen as a consistent pattern of changes that each of us undergoes, starting slowly around age 30 and progressing at a more rapid rate beyond the age of 60 or so.

Aging is a multifactorial phenomenon, characterized by a progressive degeneration in physical performance and an increasing tendency toward diabetes, heart disease and other health problems. We have considered some of the data describing the relationship between nutrition and these age-related factors. In each case in which positive results were reported, the pattern was quite consistent from one population to another -- sufficiently consistent so that it would seem possible to construct, from these data, a physiological scale of aging that would have wide utility.

Among these various studies is a substantial body of data suggesting that diet influences the rate of aging -- at least it influences many if not all of the major components of this aging scale. Certain specific foods and nutrients are importantly involved.

There is a major disagreement between workers relative to the identity of those foods and nutrients which are most critically involved in raising blood cholesterol levels and predisposing one to cardiovascular disease. Most workers point to some component of dietary lipid. Our own work emphasizes the importance of caproic acid, which is present in butterfat and coconut oil. In addition, caproate and certain amino acids related to caproate (such as the leucine of corn protein and the lysinonorleucine of connective tissue) tend to raise the blood sugar level, elevate the glucose tolerance curve and perhaps predispose animals to diabetes.

Dietary fat, particularly the polyunsaturated vegetable oil, tends to promote obesity, and high fat diets seem to be correlated with an increased incidence of bowel cancer.

For a variety of reasons, therefore, dietary fats and oils of almost any chemical description seem to provide potential problems when added to the diet of an aging person.

The progressive decrease in skeletal strength that occurs in the later years of life is the cause of some concern. Thus far the only nutrient that has proven helpful in preventing this is fluoride. It is suggested that exercise and the slowing of nitrogen loss are items that should be considered further in this regard.

Some of the most serious problems related to hypertension, stroke, and diabetes seem to be associated with a poverty diet -- which in the Southeast tends to be corn grits, greens, fat back (salt pork) and molasses. Here, the nutrient relationships have not been defined. Obviously, there is in this area a large open field for human nutrition studies.

In this discussion, aging has been defined in two phases, a slow degenerative phase extending roughly from age 30 to 60, and a more rapid phase beginning sometime around or after age 60. The transition point between these phases is undoubtedly determined in large part by the accumulations of those insults of living (metabolic and otherwise) that come with the passage of years. The evidence that we have considered suggests that nutrition also plays a role in determining the age at which rapid degeneration begins.

Opinions are expressed to the effect that changes in diet and living conditions can delay or hasten the age at which this second phase begins and perhaps can even influence the rate at which degenerative changes proceed. Hard evidence on this point, observed in actual work with older persons, is needed but, unfortunately, is lacking.

REFERENCES

Albanese, A. A. (1975). Food Nutr. News 47, 1.

Andia, A. G. and Street, J. C. (1975). J. Agric. Food Chem. 23, 173.

Asher, R. A. J. (1947). Brit. Med. J. 2, 967.

Bailey, B. W. and Mize, J. J. (1961). Ga. Agric. Exp. Stn. Circ. N.S. 23, 3.

Birren, J. E. and Botwinick, J. (1955). J. Gerontol. 10, 429.

Birren, J. E., Bick, M. W., and Fox, C. (1948). J. Gerontol. 3, 267.

Brandfonbrener, M., Landowne, M., and Shock, N. W. (1955). Circulation 12, 557.

Brozek, J. and Keys, A. (1945). J. Consult. Psychol. 9, 87.

Brozek, J., Chen, K. P., Carlson, W., and Bronczyk, F. (1953). Fed. Proc. 12, 21.

Brunner, D., Altman, S., Nelken, L., and Reider, J. (1964). Diabetes 13, 268.
Burke, W. E., Tuttle, W. W., Thompson, C. W., Janney, C. D., and Weber, R. J. (1953). J. Appl. Physiol. 5, 628.
Burkitt, D. P. (1973). Proc. Nutr. Soc. 32, 145.
Buskirk, E. R. (1966). In "Recreation Research" (by American Association for Health, Physical Education and Recreation and the National Recreation and Park Association), pp.62-79, National Education Association, Washington, D. C.
Cass, J. S., Croft, J. D., Perkins, P., Nye, W., Waterhouse,C., and Terry, R. (1966). Arch. Intern. Med. 118, 111.
Caster, W. O. and Bleecker, S. (1975). J. Nutr. 105, 308.
Caster, W. O. and Parthemos, M. D. (1976). Am. J. Clin. Nutr. (in press).
Caster, W. O. and Resurreccion, A. (1972). Ninth Inter. Congr. Nutr., Mexico City, Abstr. of Short Communications, pg. 185.
Caster, W. O., Parthemos, M. D., and Jones, J. B. (1974). Fed. Proc. 33, 716A.
Caster, W. O., Resurreccion, A. V., Cody, M., Andrews, J. W., Jr., and Bargmann, R. (1975). J. Nutr. 105, 676.
Chah, C. C., Caster, W. O., Combs, G. F., Hames, C. G., and Heyden, S. (1976). Fed. Proc. 35 (in press).
Cohen, P. and Gardner, F. H. (1966). J. Am. Med. Assoc. 195, 962.
Council on Foods and Nutrition (1972). J. Am. Med. Assoc. 222, 1647.
Donaldson, W. E., Combs, G. F., and Rosomer, G. L. (1956). Poultry Sci. 35, 1100.
Fraps, G. S. (1942). Poultry Sci. 22, 421.
Garn, S. M., Rohmann, C. G., and Wagner, B. (1967). Fed. Proc. 26, 1729.
Goggin, J. E. (1965). Public Health Rep. 80, 1005.
Gregor, O., Toman, R., and Prusova, F. (1971). Scand. J. Gastroenterol. 6, 79.
Haenszel, W. (1967). In "Neoplasms of the Stomach" (G. McNeer and G. T. Pack, eds.), pp. 3-28, J. B. Lippincott Co., Philadelphia.
Haenszel, W., Berg, J. W., Sezi, M., Kurihara, M., and Sock, P. B. (1973). J. Natl. Cancer Inst. 51, 1765.
Hayner, N., Kjelsberg, M. O., Epstein, F. H., and Francis, T., Jr. (1965). Diabetes 14, 413.
Howell, J. A. (1917). Anat. Rec. 13, 233.
Jijinsky, W. (1970). Nature 225, 21.
Keys, A., Grande, F., and Anderson, J. T. (1974). Am. J. Clin. Nutr. 27, 188.
Kmet, J. and Mahbourbi, E. (1972). Science 175, 846.
Lehman, H. C. (1951). Am. J. Psychol. 64, 161.

Luria, S. M. (1960). J. Opt. Soc. Am. 50, 86.
Mayer, J. (1968). "Overweight: Causes, Cost, and Control". Prentice-Hall, Englewood Cliffs, New Jersey.
Meneely, G. R. and Dahl, L. K. (1961). Med. Clin. North Am. 45, 271.
Michael, W. R., Alexander, J. C., and Artman, N. R. (1966). Lipids 1, 353.
Mickelsen, O., Takahashi, S., and Craig, C. (1955). J. Nutr. 57, 541.
Miles, W. R. (1950). In "Methods in Medical Research" (R. W. Gerard and W. R. Miles, eds.), vol. 3, pp. 154-156, Year Book Publishers, Chicago.
Miller, D. S. and Mumford, P. (1967). Am. J. Clin. Nutr. 20, 1212.
Norris, A. H. and Shock, N. W. (1974). In "Science and Medicine of Exercise and Sport" (W. R. Johnson and E. R. Buskirk, eds.), 2nd Ed., pp. 346-365, Harper and Row, New York.
Norris, A. H., Shock, N. W., and Wagman, I. H. (1953). J. Appl. Physiol. 5, 589.
Norris, A. H., Shock, N. W., Landowne, M., and Falzone, J. A., Jr. (1956). J. Gerontol. 11, 379.
Reiser, R. (1973). Am. J. Clin. Nutr. 26, 524.
Resurreccion, A. and Caster, W. O. (1972). Fed. Proc. 31,674.
Rich, C., Ensinck, J., and Ivanovilch, P. (1964). J. Clin. Invest. 43, 545.
Ridlin, J. R. (1916). Public Health Rep. 31, 1979.
Robertson, G. W. and Yudkin, J. (1944). J. Physiol. 103, 1.
Rose, G. A. and Williams, R. T. (1961). Brit. J. Nutr. 15, 1.
Said, F. S. and Weale, R. A. (1959). Gerontologia 3, 213.
Schroeder, H. A. (1960). J. Am. Med. Assoc. 172, 1902.
Shapley, D. (1976). Science 191, 268.
Silverstone, F. A., Brandfonbrenner, M., Shock, N. W., and Yiengst, M. J. (1957). J. Clin. Invest. 36, 504.
Sims, E. A. H., Danforth, E., Jr., Horton, E. S., Bray, G. A., Glennon, J. A., and Salans, L. B. (1973). Recent Prog. Horm. Res. 29, 457.
Steven, D. M. (1946). Nature 157, 376.
Sugai, M., Witting, L. A., Tsuchiyama, H., and Kummerow, F.A. (1962). Cancer Res. 62, 510.
Tower, S. S. (1939). Physiol. Rev. 19, 1.
Tyroler, H. A. (1970). In "The Community as an Epidemiologic Laboratory" (I. I. Kessler and M. L. Morton, eds.), pp. 100-122, Johns Hopkins Press, Baltimore.
Unger, R. H. (1957). Ann. Intern. Med. 47, 1138.
U. S. Department of Health, Education and Welfare (1970). "Diabetes Mellitus Mortality in the United States, 1950-67". PHS Publ. No. 1000, Ser. 20, No. 10.

Walker, A. R. P. (1971). So. Afr. Med. J. 1971, 15.
Watkin, D. M. (1964). In "Mammalian Protein Metabolism" (H. N. Munro and J. B. Allison, eds.), Vol. II, pp. 247-263, Academic Press, New York.
Weale, R. A. (1963). "The Aging Eye". Harper and Row, New York.
Wolff, J. A. and Wasserman. A. E. (1972). Science 177, 15.
Wynder, E. L. and Reddy, B. S. (1974). Cancer 34, 801.
Wynder, E. L., Kajitani, T., Ishikawa, S., Dodo, H., and Takano, A. (1969). Cancer 23, 1210.
Yokote, M. (1970). Nippon Suisan Gakkaishi 36, 1214.
Yoshida, O., Brown, R. R., and Bryan, G. T. (1971). Am. J. Clin. Nutr. 24, 848.
Zuckerman, J. and Stull, G. A. (1969). J. Appl. Physiol. 26, 716.

BIOCHEMICAL IMPACT OF NUTRITION ON THE AGING PROCESS

Donald M. Watkin, M.D., M.P.H., F.A.C.P.[1,2]

Director
Nutrition Program
Administration on Aging
Office of Human Development
Department of Health, Education and Welfare
Washington, D.C. 20201

I. INTRODUCTION

Twelve years ago in Glasgow, I delivered the Eighth Annual Ciba Foundation Lecture on Research on Aging entitled "The Impact of Nutrition on the Biochemistry of Aging in Man". Early in the course of the lecture, I posed two questions: (1) What is known of the relation of nutrition to aging in man?; and (2) Can we describe the impact of nutrition on the biochemistry of aging in man? My answers over a decade ago were "very little" and "no", respectively (Watkin, 1966).

In 1964, while espousing a nihilistic attitude toward the then-existing state of the nutrition-aging relationship, I assumed that the strides of the previous decade in molecular biology would soon be matched by equally giant steps in our understanding of nutrition's impact on aging as a biologic process. For example, in treating the major heading "Undernutrition and Longevity" (Watkin, 1966), I made the following comments:

> "It is perhaps significant that underfeeding as a means of prolonging life is practically the only positive example of the impact of nutrition on the course of aging, but even this example yields impure data, since quantifying parameters such as longevity are

---

[1]On detail from the Department of Medicine and Surgery, Veterans Administration.

[2]Mailing address: 21 Primrose Street, Chevy Chase, Maryland 20015

> affected by phenomena other than aging *per se*. How underfeeding influences the biochemistry of aging has yet to be explained, but it is encouraging to know that various laboratories are presently working toward an explanation in terms of modern molecular biology. This search for an explanation in chemical terms represents a new spirit in gerontology and may herald the end of the search for descriptive differences between young and old which has so dominated gerontologic investigation."

The conclusions of my Glasgow lecture began by echoing my nihilistic attitude (Watkin, 1966):

> "....let me reemphasize that our present knowledge of the nutrition-aging relationship in man is so limited as to preclude recommendations for general clinical application by any responsible nutritionist or gerontologist. Individualized nutritional advice, whether preventive or curative in intent, by physicians and their paramedical colleagues, advice which takes into account the medical, emotional and socio-economic status as well as the age of each patient, has no substitute at the present time."

These remarks continued by exhorting all working in the fields of nutrition and gerontology to "....discourage by every means at our command efforts by food-faddists, charlatans, deliberate swindlers and even ethical profit-seeking enterprises to promote nutritional products or regimens as panaceas for the problems of old age".

They stressed our responsibility to educate all - including ourselves - in the value of preventive nutrition and urged all scientists to work in our own specialties and in concert with those in other disciplines "....in pursuit of additional knowledge on the impact of nutrition on the biochemistry of aging with the expectation that such pursuits will eventually lead directly or through some unanticipated fallout to the means for the effective regulation of aging in man".

In the dozen years since my remarks in Glasgow, few of my hopes for progress in understanding the nutrition-aging relationship have been realized, and still my conclusions of 1964 stand as yet unaltered.

Personally, however, my internal set has changed. I have come to view the nutrition-aging relationship with different-hued glasses. In addition, while still an eternal optimist, I have expanded the scale of the time implosion on which I confidently depended to supply resolutions to the nutrition-aging enigmas as perceived in 1964.

In partial explanation of these changed attitudes, let me review my own experiences of the past dozen years. I have acquired a degree in public health; directed two large nutrition- and health-oriented epidemiological surveys, one in Paraguay (Watkin _et al._, 1969) and one in New York State (DHEW, 1972); served as program chief for research in nutrition and gerontology for the Veterans Administration Central Office; directed a spinal cord injury center where innumerable quadriplegics of all chronologic ages manifested the signs of "instant aging" (Watkin, 1972); studied the influence of differences in physical work load, protein and calorie intake, and age on skeletal and cardiac muscle of rats (Watkin and Munro, 1973); chaired panel and technical committee sessions on nutrition and aging for two White House Conferences (White House Conference on Food, Nutrition and Health, 1970; DHEW, 1974); and, for the past 30 months, directed the Nutrition Program for Older Americans authorized by Title VII of the Older Americans Act of 1965, as Amended (DHEW, 1976).

These experiences have convinced me that when we refer to the impact of nutrition on aging we must cease being purists seeking only "knowledge for knowledge's sake"(Watkin, 1966), as I urged in 1964, but we must really seek to relate that impact to relevant, highly visible, tangible problems in today's society of ever-increasing numbers of elderly persons.

II. NUTRITION'S IMPACT ON THE AGED OF TODAY

A. Major Nutrition-Related Problems of the Aged

Today we meet in a state which is home to 1.7 million Americans 60 years of age and over, representing over 5.5 percent of the 32 million in that age category in the United States, not to mention the tens of thousands in that age bracket who spend part of each year in Florida while maintaining residences elsewhere. These persons are already old. They are politely referred to as "the aging", but in reality the vast majority are more correctly described as "aged". They face an incredible array of major problems, _viz._, those concerned with health, education, income maintenance, consumer protection, culture, society, housing, transportation, crime and law. Each of these impinges directly on the aged's ability to use nutrition as a means of assuring their optimum physical and mental performance.

B. Health Considerations: The Top Priority

Health-related problems do not head this list by accident but rather because, by measures applied objectively by trained observers as well as subjectively by the aged themselves, health-related problems deserve the top rank order among priorities.

Aside from humanitarian considerations of the misery caused by disease and disability, health-related problems pose economic and fiscal stresses of staggering proportions. Data for 1974 published by the Social Security Administration (DHEW, 1975a) show that 40 percent of the over $100 billion dollars spent on health in the United States was spent by or in behalf of those 65 years of age and over. Add to those dollars funds spent on those 60 through 64 years of age and on others whose physiologic age justify their inclusion in the aged category and the enormity of the cost of health for the elderly even in 1974 terms is appalling. But the value of the dollar has eroded since 1974, and the needs of the elderly have multiplied. From these two factors alone, the inference may be drawn that the quantity and quality of health care for the aged have diminished since 1974, a year when quantity and quality were far from good, let alone ideal.

In addition, the elderly of today have great expectations, are increasingly vocal in the political arena, and have a voting participation record in national elections of about 80 percent, far higher than the percentage for young Americans. These 26 million elderly voters are being heard; their needs are being recognized. Federal, state and community tax dollars are being directed in ever greater quantities into programs and institutions whose intent is to serve the needs of the elderly but whose reality frequently is to serve only to expend endless resources in a losing cause.

The elderly represent a minority, less than 13 percent of the American population. Yet they consume, under present economic and political conditions and at the present application of knowledge by the health industry, an outrageously high proportion of the time and resources of that very industry, not to mention the time and resources of other organizations, individuals and family members.

"Aging" is a term which has been usurped from biological scientists and applied by social, behavioral and political scientists as a euphemism for "aged". Aging, as now perceived by the public at large, excludes consideration of those not yet aged, of those in utero and of those yet to be conceived. The problems in the health field alone of the elderly minority will continue to subsume more and more scarce resources unless the amelioration of disease and disability can become, first, effective and, second, cost-effective.

In the realm of effectiveness, nutrition has potential impact of great magnitude in relieving the health problems of those already old. By so doing, it thereby can influence favorably the attitudes and the votes of the aged toward investigations in biologic aging which may have little or no direct impact on their own well being. Moreover, if the impact of nutrition on their health can be made cost-effective, it can release untold resources for the now grossly underfunded assault on the mechanisms underlying the nutrition-aging relationship (Watkin, 1976).

Malnutrition among the aged in the United States is invariably secondary to disease and disability - physical, emotional and/or attitudinal (Watkin, 1976). Primary malnutrition - i.e., malnutrition from an absolute lack of food - does not affect this nation. Nonetheless, malnutrition is malnutrition, regardless of its causation, and can be ameliorated only by the provision of nutrition appropriate for the disease or disability at hand. The record of the health industry *per se*, and of nonhealth-oriented organizations affording supportive services, in assuring the distribution, the availability, the accessibility and the utilization of information, facilities, personnel and services, for maintaining and improving the nutritional status and thereby the health of those afflicted, is grossly inadequate (National Nutrition Policy Study Hearings, 1974).

C. Present Inadequate Management of Nutrition

The spotlight has focused during the past year on nosocomial malnutrition (Butterworth, 1974), including that quantified by a Federal investigation of nursing homes (DHEW, 1975b). While the inadequacies spotlighted are disgraceful, they represent only a wisp of steam from the seething cauldron of nutritional inadequacies among the nation's diseased and disabled aged who are not institutionalized but who reside in communities all over America.

In part, this condition is the responsibility of physicians who have had little formal training in nutrition. However, even the most skilled and motivated physician is faced with tremendous odds in efforts to assure appropriate nutrition among sick and disabled elderly living in their own places of residence.

Among the obstacles are: (1) years of inadequate patient nutrition preceding the onset of an acute phase of illness or disability, yielding a patient with depleted reserves even prior to the ravages of disease; (2) patient delay in seeking medical attention, giving the pathological condition further time to deplete body reserves (Levenson and Watkin, 1959); (3) obstinancy by patients in discarding long-held myths opposing the acceptance of modern nutritional advice; (4) failure by patients and their families to comprehend the interrelations of nutrition and disease and the need to attend to both simultaneously; (5) unavailability of personnel, equipment and supplies needed to provide patients with oral, gavage or parenteral nutrition and medication; and (6) lack of human minds and hands to assist patients in regaining optimum health.

D. What to Do; How to Do It

While it is impossible to turn back the clock for those already old, much must be done to improve the nutrition and health status of both the chronologically and physiologically old afflicted with disease and disability. The scientific knowledge underlying such improvement is known; the application of scientific knowledge is what is lacking (figure 1).

Knowledge → | Application

Fig. 1 Application of presently available scientific knowledge to improve the nutrition and health status of both the chronologically and physiologically old afflicted with diseases and disability is presently blocked.

Resolution of this conundrum is by no means impossible. One thoughtful approach designed to produce a "new American mentality", a term coined by Jean Mayer (Manoff, 1975), suggests methods for penetrating American homes by television-delivered nutrition- and health-related messages at least twice weekly. Perhaps even more important, Manoff (1975) concludes that "nutrition professionals" must go beyond the school, the laboratory and the kitchen (where traditional approaches have yielded little success) if the "new American mentality" is to be achieved.

While Manoff (1975) has appealed to the "nutrition professionals", my concern for nutrition's impact on aging throughout life leads me to make an even broader appeal. I urge all scientists investigating aging as a biological process to break out of their laboratories, classrooms, clinics and seminars, to mingle with the public, to find out what the public know, and to learn how the public translate that knowledge -- correct or incorrect -- into votes for their representatives and executives at the federal, state and community levels. Having experienced that adventure, I urge them next to begin to use modern communication technology to create new public understanding of life as a biologic process and, in so doing, to indicate how environmental factors, of which nutrition is one directly under each American's control, influence the quality of life in proportion to their good or bad affect on aging as a biologic process.

The huckster approach to such strategic objectives need offend no one from this decade on. When Watson (1968) published The Double Helix, his personal account of the personalities involved in the discovery of the structure of DNA, certain quarters of the scientific community grumbled. Recently, however, PBS broadcast in "living color" "A Rerun of the Race for DNA" (Anderson, 1976) to a national audience of millions. These millions of citizens were shown -- many for the first time -- how the adenine-thymine and the guanine-cytosine base pairs form the steps while the sugar-phosphate backbones twist about them to produce the spiral staircase of DNA in molecular model form. While the personalities as well as the faces of Watson, Crick, Wilkins, Pauling and the memories of Rosalind Franklin were major attractions, the production brought to the American public some understanding of what modern science comprises. It showed clearly how human understanding is based on knowledge and how knowledge fundamental to human health is structured on basic research. For me, at least, it was far more productive than the hundreds of media messages citing the burdens of old age and suggesting even though not so stating to all Americans that the worst is yet to come.

But scientists must do more than listen, learn, consider and perform over and in the media. They need to experience some of the frustrations of disease and disability among the aged not only during demonstrations at professional meetings, but while dealing with the aged on the front lines. One method is to volunteer a few hours a week to serving the physiologically old, preferably in their own places of residence. Watch what they select to eat, how they prepare it, with whom they dine, and how much pleasure the meal provides. Inquire about their health, their strength, their state of mind. Then see what happens when you, the scientist, begin to introduce your own knowledge, your own personality and your own physical strength into the process of improving their health and nutritional status. If your baseline data are recorded objectively and if you repeat your objective measurements a few weeks later, you will have demonstrated objectively to yourselves the impact of nutrition on the end products of the biochemistry of the diseased and disabled aged.

III. OPTIMUM NUTRITION DOES PAY OFF

A. The Aging Balance Sheet

The bottom line of the aging balance sheet is the summation of genetic endowment, environmental (including nutritional) factors, and, to be sure, a little bit of luck. An example of someone who excelled in the first and the last items is the charming 97-year-old Paraguayan lady whose face is captured in figure 2. Imagine, if you will, what she would have looked like at 97 had she benefited *in utero* from good maternal nutrition and in the early years of life from appropriate nutrition combined with modern preventive medicine. Add to such beginnings lifelong sound nutrition, regular preventive and curative medical and dental services, modern family planning, abstinence from cigar smoking and occasional trips to a *salón de belleza* and we might have before us the portrait of a beauty at least as attractive as Katherine Hepburn is today but one 30 years Miss Hepburn's senior.

B. Proof of the Payoff

All this is designed to emphasize the fact that optimum nutrition from conception to death pays off regardless of one's genetic endowment. It pays off in terms of better physical and behaviorial growth and development of children (Vega and Robles, 1962; Cravioto, 1963; Ramos-Galván *et al*., 1964; Cravioto and Robles, 1965; Cravioto *et al*., 1966); larger head and brain size, correlating with greater intellectual capacity (Nutrition Foundation, 1967; Winick, 1976); fewer diseases (National Nutrition Policy Study Hearings, 1974); less disability from accidents (Stevens *et al*., 1962); a lower incidence of neoplastic disease (Burkitt, 1973); more productive and happier lives; and, if we accept data from actuarial (Dublin and Marks, 1930) and epidemiologic (Keys, 1970) studies in man and in experimental animals (McKay, 1947; McKay *et al*., 1935, 1939, 1941, 1943; Ross, 1959, 1961, 1964, 1969, 1972; Ross and Bras, 1965, 1973, 1975; Berg and Simms, 1960, 1965; Berg *et al*., 1962; Widdowson and Kennedy, 1962), an older average age at death and a longer life span, respectively.

Some of these data were published over 40 years ago (McKay et al., 1935) and comparable data are still being published (Ross and Bras, 1975). Most of these publications were summarized in my Glasgow lecture in 1964 (Watkin, 1966) and have been updated since (Watkin, 1973).

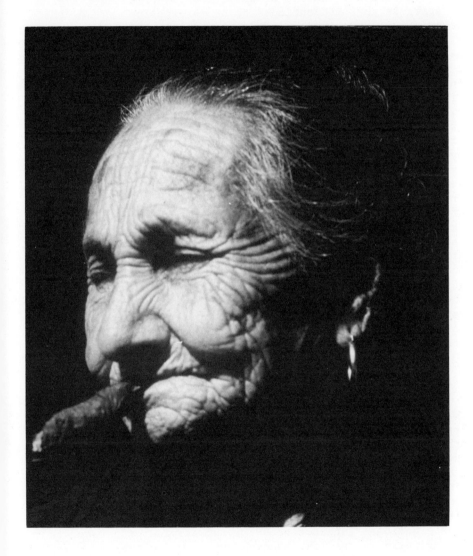

Fig. 2 A 97-year-old Paraguayan lady whose genetic endowment and good fortune have enabled her to survive to an old age in spite of absolute lack of attention to concepts of modern nutrition and preventive medicine.

IV. DESCRIPTIVE RESEARCH CONTINUES

A. Descriptions Better but Explanations Still Lacking

The striking feature of nutritionally-oriented research in aging is that it continues to be descriptive. True, the descriptions have improved in proportion to the sophistication of the experimental designs. In man, for example, longitudinal studies of nutrition-related parameters have replaced cross-sectional studies which were often subject to too many interpretations. An excellent example of this form of investigation is that conducted at the Gerontology Research Center of the National Institutes of Health in Baltimore where longitudinal studies have shown, for the first time, that regressions of height and weight on age occur not only in group-mean by-decade presentations (Stone and Norris, 1966), but also in presentations by decade cohorts from 30 to 80 years of age of mean regression slopes of height and weight on age determined from serial measurements of the same subjects over a period of eight years (Shock, 1972). Other data from the Gerontology Research Center show reductions in basal and activity calories and in total daily calorie intake with advancing age (McGandy *et al.*, 1966). These investigations confirm what many suspected was happening and establish correlations among parameters measured but still give us no explanation in biochemical terms for the observations made. In animals, as in man, the descriptions have become more sophisticated but convincing demonstrations of mechanisms are still lacking (Finch, 1972; Leto *et al.*, 1976a, b).

B. MEDLARS Search for Biochemical Mechanisms

Clinical investigations, as I have pointed out before (Watkin, 1966), are difficult, costly and, in recent years, less objective than those of earlier decades, because of the proscription of certain data gathering procedures. It seemed logical, therefore, to combine reports of studies in species other than man in the search for clues to the impact of nutrition on the biochemistry of aging.

In January, 1976, an off-line bibliographic citation list generated by MEDLARS II, the National Library of Medicine's National Interactive Retrieval Service, was requested for articles in English, Spanish, Russian and Czech, published from 1964 through 1975, dealing with the relationship of "nutrition" (including proteins, minerals, vitamins and trace elements) to "aging", "aged", "age" or "genes". The search retrieved 290 citations from a data base of approximately 2900 journals.

Table I shows a taxonomic breakdown of the 290 citations. Correlative citations are those relating specific parameters to the chronologic age or passage and to the nutrition of the species or cell line under consideration without objectively demonstrating any fundamental biochemical mechanism responsible for the reported correlations. Descriptive citations are those reviewing literature without presenting original data, expressing opinions, or dealing only with observations in those already old. Pharmacological citations are those reporting dose responses to a single nutrient or to combinations of nutrients in dose ranges in excess of known requirements for the particular species under study. They also include toxicologic studies. Tangential citations are those reporting information bearing only remotely on the interrelations of nutrition and aging. Mechanistic citations are those reporting data derived from experiments designed to reveal changes in nucleic acid synthesis, repair, metabolism and reproduction associated with specific nutritional regimens at specific chronological ages or passages of the species or cell line under consideration.

TABLE I

Taxonomy of 290 MEDLARS Citations on Nutrition and Aging, 1964-1975*

Category	n	%
Correlative	183	63.1
Descriptive	58	20.0
Pharmacologic	41	14.1
Tangential	5	1.7
Mechanistic	3	1.1
Total	290	100.0

*Taxonomic breakdown of 290 citations generated by MEDLARS II, the National Library of Medicine's National Interactive Retrieval Service, for articles in English, Spanish, Russian and Czech published from 1964 through 1975 dealing with the relationship between nutrition and aging. (n = number)

Note particularly the paucity of citations dealing with mechanisms, the preponderance of correlative and descriptive citations and the large number of pharmacologic citations.

The three mechanistic citations include one which describes changes in RNA polymerase activity and DNA metabolism in mammalian zinc deficiency (Terhune and Sandstead, 1972); the second describes chromosome aberrations in mice fed free radical reaction inhibitors (Harman _et al_., 1970); and the third measured iron levels in DNA preparations in albino rats (Goldshtein _et al_.,1966). Of these three, one deals with an outright deficiency, the second, with the effects of a dietary additive on chromosomal morphology, and the third with the correlation between age and iron levels in DNA preparations in rats. Obviously, none is particularly pertinent to the impact of nutrition on the biochemistry of the aging process.

The interpretation of these data is not difficult. It suggests clearly that, despite the high hopes of a decade ago, work designed to indicate the biochemical mechanisms through which nutrition influences the process of aging has not been published in final form. The plethora of correlative and descriptive citations and the heavy emphasis on toxicology among those falling in the pharmacologic category suggest that the investigation embarking on research in the nutrition-aging relationship have been equipped with the wrong tools.

V. GREAT POTENTIAL FOR RESEARCH ON MECHANISMS

A. Outlook More Encouraging

Fortunately, the scene is somewhat more encouraging than would appear on the basis of the MEDLARS search alone. Many laboratories are aware of the need to explore the mechanisms underlying desirable changes in morbidity and longevity associated with certain nutritional environments and the need to quantify the impact at the various phases of the life cycle. Some have begun such studies and others have plans to do so when appropriate methodology has been perfected.

B. Wide Range of Research

The range of research involved in such work is wide. It covers changes with age and their modification by nutrition in enzyme activity, in enzyme induction and adaptation, in the rate at which errors in the incorporation of amino acids into protein occur, in the duration of the specificity of DNA polymerases, in the rate of formation of faulty proteins and enzymes, in the speed with which cross-linkages develop in collagen, in the amounts of glutamine and asparagine deaminated per unit time, in the rate at which autoimmunity develops, in the control of hypothalamic and hypophyseal secretions and in the effectiveness of repair of genes damages by exogenous and endogenous factors, to mention only a few components of the range.

Laboratories who already have quantified in man, in animal species, in cell lines or in microbiologic systems changes in specific parameters with age or cell passage are ideally situated to observe changes induced by modifications in nutrition. The design used in many descriptive studies whereby dietary modifications are introduced at various phases of the life cycle is appropriate provided established parameters are measured to assure comprehension of the biochemical mechanisms involved.

C. Quantifiable Data on Nutrient Intake Desirable

Quantitative data on nutrient and fluid intake should always be obtained. While this may pose many logistic problems, the data derived permit better evaluation among experimental groups in animal studies than do data derived from studies utilizing *ad libitum* nutrient and water consumption. The same opinion, of course, is relevant to studies involving human subjects.

VI. RESEARCH IN COOPERATION WITH THE AGED OF TODAY

A. 1966 → 1976: Miami Demonstration → Nutrition Program for Older Americans (NPOA)

This presentation was begun with comments directed toward involving the scientific community in the management of many problems, particularly those in the realm of health, facing those who are already old. I would certainly be remiss if I failed to mention that research into better resolutions of these problems as well as help in the delivery of services providing temporizing solutions is badly needed. In 1966, Miami led the nation in becoming the site of a new concept in the delivery of nutrition, health and other supportive services to those already old (McKibbin, 1966). In a decade, the Miami-initiated concept has developed explosively until it now comprises the more than 7000 sites of the Nutrition Program for Older Americans (NPOA) authorized by Title VII of the Older Americans Act of 1965, as Amended. Table II presents in diagramatic form how the concept, first implemented in Miami, now operates. Note especially that dining together is the center of gravity, drawing participants to sites where they have the opportunity to take advantage of a broad spectrum of health-related and other important supportive services.

TABLE II

$\alpha \rightarrow \Omega$ CONCEPTUALIZATION OF THE NPOA*

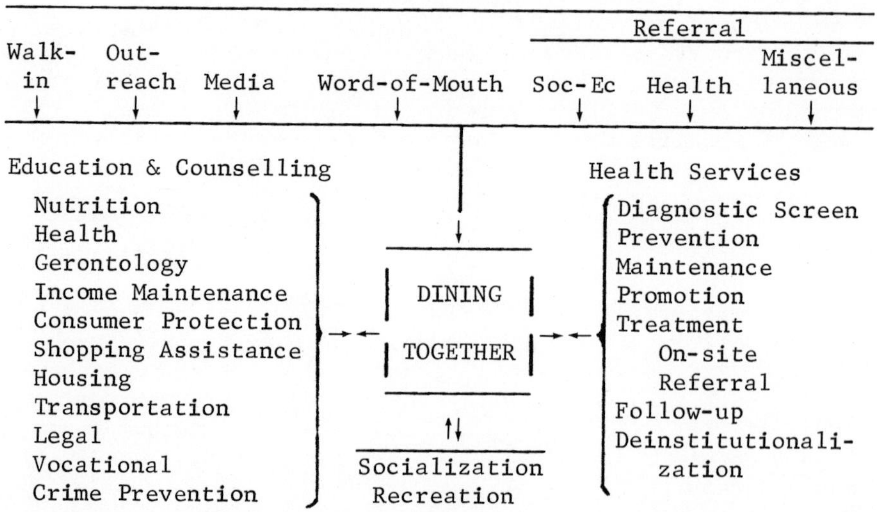

*Conceptualization of the Nutrition Program for Older Americans (NPOA) authorized by Title VII of the Older Americans Act of 1965, as Amended.

B. NPOA's Deficiency in Research and Development

All will recognize that one glaring deficiency in the NPOA concept is the lack of any specific research and development component. Explanations for this deficiency at the Federal level are numerous, and the participation of the Administration on Aging participation in research associated with the NPOA are severely restrained.

C. Productive Intra-State Research and Development

Not so, however, with intra-state research activities. State agencies on aging, state universities and state community extension services are working with the aged participants in the NPOA and finding such cooperation fertile soil for demonstrating that good nutrition, when provided in concert with other activities surrounding the center of gravity of dining together, can have a profound impact on the lives, the health, the happiness and apparently, as shown by a few studies now underway (Kohrs, 1975), on objective nutritional parameters of those already old.

D. Research and Development Needs Still Unmet

However, much more research and development is needed. The need ranges from developing more cost-effective methods of managing NPOA's meal service and supportive services and finding better methods for serving those too isolated by geography, disease or disability to join others in dining together to the collection of data indicating that good nutrition - apart from the psychosocial value of dining together - really does or does not improve the well-being, the capacity to cope with disease and disability, and the longevity of those already old.

E. Nutrition Alone No Panacea; Applying Present, Acquiring New Nutrition-Health-Aging Triad Knowledge Essential

Some may wonder why the possibility that better nutrition may not be a panacea is emphasized. The concern stems from experiences in studying host-tumor relationships in neoplastic diseases during which investigations begun over 20 years ago provided ample evidence that good nutrition for patients with active neoplastic processes, if delivered without concern for control of the neoplasms, yields more active neoplasms and more rapid demises of the patients (Tschudy *et al.*, 1959; Watkin, 1959, 1961; Watkin and Steinfeld, 1965). It is essential to reinforce with all possible emphasis the fact that nutrition is no panacea for the problems of the aged or the problems of all of us who are aging, unless it is combined with attention to what is already known about other health-related sciences and unless the nutrition-health-gerontology triad becomes the object of vigorous investigation in the field, in the clinic and in the basic science laboratory.

F. NPOA: Substrate for Research and Development

The NPOA is an institution now assured of $187,500,000 *per annum* from the Administration on Aging (AoA), an estimated $23,500,000 from the U.S. Department of Agriculture in the form of donated foods, $18,750,000 in state matching funds, from $5,000,000 to $10,000,000 from other federal and state departments and agencies and state legislative appropriations, and at least $7,800,000 from participant contributions. With this fiscal infrastructure, the NPOA serves as a substrate on which to develop investigative programs funded from other federal, state, foundation, university and private resources. The quality of the output from such investigative programs is dependent on the quality of the investigators who seek to take advantage of the substrate offered. With attention to experimental design and scrupulous attention to the details of informed consent, the NPOA substrate provides a means to the end of increasing knowledge of the impact of nutrition on the biochemistry of aging in man as well as a means of applying such knowledge on a very large scale. Productive research performed in the NPOA context would have relevance on a scale unprecedented in nutrition or aging research.

VII. PAYOFF OF NUTRITION-HEALTH-AGING TRIAD RESEARCH ASSURED

Investigations of the nutrition-health-aging relationship, regardless of the difficulties they entail, are bound to be productive. Nutrition is the most impressive environmental key to good health in man. No other environmental factor can be controlled by each American as can his or her nutrition. No other environmental factor has proven so successful in prolonging the lives of experimental animals. Even clinical investigators seeking reasons for apparent longevity, as did Alexander Leaf (1973a, b) among the elderly of Ecuador, Hunza and Transcaucasian Soviet Socialist Republics, have laid most emphasis on nutrition and its co-conspirator in plotting longevity, strenuous physical activity.

VIII. SUMMARY AND CONCLUSIONS

In spite of increases in the number of investigators devoting themselves to research in nutrition and aging, progress in the past dozen years toward better understanding of the mechanisms by which nutrition influences aging as a biochemical process has not lived up the the expectations of the middle 1960s. Descriptive and correlative investigations in a spectrum of health-related disciplines have provided data which has improved our knowledge of the natural history of aging in man, animals and cells. However, mechanisms underlying older age at death associated with nutritional modifications remain unidentified.

Nonetheless, several possible approaches to the identification of these mechanisms are at present already developed or being developed. If pursued vigorously, they promise much.

Simultaneous with and even preceding such research, attention must be paid to the positive impact which appropriate nutrition has on the health, life satisfaction and attitude toward basic investigations of those already old. For these people, the personal benefit from an altruistic view toward basic investigations may be minimal. Scientists concerned with the nutrition-health-aging triad owe it to all the people they serve and to their own professional interests to become more deeply involved in the education of, investigation of and concern for present day aged persons. The Nutrition Program for Older Americans (NPOA) now operational at more than 7000 sites throughout the United States affords one substrate for such activities on the parts of scientists concerned with the nutrition-health-aging triad.

Mechanisms responsible for the impact of nutrition on the biochemistry of aging must be spelled out if progress is to be made in convincing human beings of the virtue of judicious nutrition throughout life. Only such convincing scientific data will enable responsible investigators and practitioners to counteract effectively the tidal wave of misleading information now influencing the American public through media messages from faddists, quacks and profit-seeking corporate entities.

Meanwhile, however, much knowledge based on descriptive studies, knowledge not yet applied, can be used through improved education of the American public and greater efforts by all knowledgeable scientists to improve the health of those already old and of all Americans who are aging, through application of nutrition principles which obviously do make impact, albeit in an unknown manner, on the biochemistry of aging.

ACKNOWLEDGEMENT

The author is deeply indebted to Mrs. Diane L. Keaton of the HEW Department Library and to Mr. Silas Jackson and Dr. Anne E. Caldwell of the National Library of Medicine for their invaluable assistance in the planning, performance and interpretation of the MEDLARS search incorporated in this presentation. He is also most appreciative of the technical assistance of Mr. Edward G. Watkin whose efforts were essential in the production of this manuscript.

REFERENCES

Anderson, J. (1976). Wash. Post, Feb. 22, 1976, p. C-1.

Berg, B. N. and Simms, H. S. (1960). J. Nutr. 71, 225.

Berg, B. N. and Simms, H. S. (1965). Can. Med. Assoc. J. 93, 911.

Berg, B. N., Wolf, A., and Simms, H. S. (1962). J. Nutr. 77, 439.

Burkitt, D. P. (1973). Brit. Med. J. 1, 274.
Butterworth, C. E., Jr. (1974). Nutr. Today 9, 4.
Cravioto, J. (1963). Am. J. Pub. Health 53, 1803.
Cravioto, J. and Robles, B. (1965). Am. J. Orthopsychiat. 35, 449.
Cravioto, J., DeLicardie, E. R., and Birch, H. G. (1966). Pediatrics 38, 319.
Department HEW (1972). Publication Nos. (HSM) 72-8130, 72-8131, 72-8132, 72-8133 and 72-8134. Center for Disease Control, Atlanta.
Department HEW (1974). Publication No. (OHD) 74-20912, pp. 43-47. Superintendent of Documents, U.S.G.P.O., Washington, D. C.
Department HEW (1975a). Publication No. (SSA) 76-11910. Superintendent of Documents, U.S.G.P.O., Washington, D.C.
Department HEW (1975b). Publication No. (OS) 76-50021. Superintendent of Documents, U.S.G.P.O., Washington, D.C.
Department HEW (1976). Publication No. (OHD) 76-20170. Superintendent of Documents, U.S.G.P.O., Washington, D.C.
Dublin, L. I. and Marks, H. (1930). Human Biol. 2, 159.
Finch, C. E. (1972). Exp. Gerontol. 7, 53.
Goldshtein, B. I., Rud, S. G., and Poliakova, L. L. (1966). Vopr. Med. Khim. 12, 618.
Harman, D., Curtis, H.J., and Tilley, J. (1970). J. Gerontol. 25, 17.
Keys, A. (1970). Circulation 41-42, 1-211.
Kohrs, M. B. (1975). Preliminary Report. Missouri Office of Aging. Jefferson City, Missouri.
Leaf, A. (1973a). Nat. Geographic 143, 93.
Leaf, A. (1973b). Nutr. Today 8, 4.
Leto, S., Kokkonen, G. C., and Barrows, C. H., Jr. (1976a). J. Gerontol. 31, 144.
Leto, S., Kokkonen, G. C., and Barrows, C. H., Jr. (1976b). J. Gerontol. 31, 149.
Levenson, S. M. and Watkin, D. M. (1959). Fed. Proc. 18, 1155.
Manoff, R. K. (1975). J. Nutr. Ed. 7, 139.
McGandy, R. B., Barrows, C. H., Jr., Spanias, A., Meredith, A., Stone, J. L., and Norris, A. H. (1966). J. Gerontol. 21, 581.
McKay, C. M. (1947). Am. J. Pub. Health 37, 521.
McKay, C. M., Crowell, M. F., and Maynard, L. A. (1935). J. Nutr. 10, 63.
McKay, C. M., Maynard, L. A., Sperling, G., and Barnes, L. L. (1939). J. Nutr. 18, 1.
McKay, C. M., Maynard, L. A., Sperling, G., and Osgood, H. S. (1941). J. Nutr. 21, 45.
McKay, C. M., Sperling, G., and Barnes, L. L. (1943). Arch. Biochem. 2, 469.

McKibben, G. B. (1966). Dept. HEW/SRS R&D Grant AA-4014 (66-3). National Technical Information Service, Springfield, Virginia.
National Nutrition Policy Study-1974 (1974). Series 74/NNP-3 & 3A, NNP-4 & 4A, NNP-5 & 5A, NNP-6 & 6A and NNP-7 & 7A. Superintendent of Documents, U.S.G.P.O., Washington, D.C.
Nutrition Foundation (1967). "Proceedings of an International Conference on Malnutrition, Learning and Behavior". The Nutrition Foundation, New York.
Ramos-Galván, R., Vega, L., and Cravioto, J. (1964). Bol. Med. Hosp. Infant. Mex. 21, 157.
Ross, M. H. (1959). Fed. Proc. 18, 1190.
Ross, M. H. (1961). J. Nutr. 75, 197.
Ross, M. H. (1964). In "Diet and Bodily Constitution" (G.E.W. Wolstenholme and M. O'Conner, eds.), pp. 90-107, J. & A. Churchill, London.
Ross, M. H. (1969). J. Nutr. 97, 565.
Ross, M. H. (1972). In "Symposium on Nutrition and Aging - Part I" (D. M. Watkin, ed.), Am. J. Clin. Nutr. 25, 834.
Ross, M. H. and Bras, G. (1965). J. Nutr. 87, 245.
Ross, M. H. and Bras, G. (1973). J. Nutr. 103, 944.
Ross, M. H. and Bras, G. (1975). Science 190, 165.
Shock, N. W. (1972). In "Nutrition in Old Age" (L.A.Carlson, ed.), pp. 12-23, Almquist & Wiksell, Uppsala.
Stevens, J., Freeman, P. A., Nordin, B. E. C., and Barnett,E. (1962). J. Bone Jt. Surg. 44B, 520.
Stone, J. L. and Norris, A. H. (1966). J. Gerontol. 21, 575.
Terhune, M. W. and Sandstead, H. H. (1972). Science 177, 68.
Tschudy, D.P., Bacchus, H., Weissman, S.S., Watkin, D.M., Eubanks, M., and White, L. (1959).J. Clin. Invest.38,892.
Vega, L. and Robles, B. (1962). Salud Publ. Mex. 4, 385.
Watkin, D. M. (1959). ACTA Unio Internat. Contra Cancrum. 15, 907.
Watkin, D. M. (1961). Am. J. Clin. Nutr. 9, 446.
Watkin, D. M. (1966). In "World Review of Nutrition and Dietetics" (G. H. Bourne, ed.), Vol. 6, pp. 124-164. S. Karger, Basel/New York.
Watkin, D. M. (1972). In "Proceedings of the Joint Meeting of the U.S. Veterans Administration Spinal Cord Injury Centers and the International Medical Society of Paraplegia, Boston, 1971" (H. S. Talbot, ed.), pp. 231-232, U. S. Veterans Administration, Washington, D. C.
Watkin, D. M. (1973). In "Modern Nutrition in Health and Disease, 5th Edition" (R. S. Goodhart and M. E. Shils, eds.), pp. 681-710, Lea & Febiger, Philadelphia.
Watkin, D. M. (1976). In "World Review of Nutrition and Dietetics" (G. H. Bourne, ed.), S. Karger, Basel/New York (in press).

Watkin, D. M. and Munro, E. (1973). J. Nutr. 26, xxi (abstract).

Watkin, D. M. and Steinfeld, J. L. (1965). Am. J. Clin. Nutr. 16, 182.

Watkin, D. M., Pearson, W. N., Chichester, C. O., Weswig, P., Ferencz, C., Fischman, S., Kocher, R., Reh, E., Sheehy, R., Elsea, W., Miranda, H., Yampey, M., et al. (1969). In "Encuesta de Nutrición: República del Paraguay, Mayo-Agosto de 1965", pp. 1-482, Programa de Nutrición, Centro Nacional para el Control de Enfermedades Crónicas, Servicio de Salud Pública, Departamento de Salud, Educación y Bienestar, Bethesda.

Watson, J. D. (1968). "The Double Helix". Atheneum, New York.

White House Conference on Food, Nutrition and Health, 1969. (1970). Final Report, pp. 1-341, and Addendum, pp. 1-5, Superintendent of Documents, U.S.G.P.O., Washington, D.C.

Widdowson, E. M. and Kennedy, G. C. (1962). Proc. Roy. Soc. B 156, 96.

Winick, M. (1976). "Malnutrition and Brain Development". Oxford University Press, New York.

PROTEIN METABOLISM AND NEEDS IN ELDERLY PEOPLE

Vernon R. Young, Ph.D.*

Department of Nutrition and Food Science
and Clinical Research Center
Massachusetts Institute of Technology
Cambridge, Massachusetts 02139

INTRODUCTION

Older people comprise a significant and increasing proportion of the populations of North America and Europe. It is important, therefore, to give greater attention to the psychological and physiological requirements of the aged for food and essential nutrients, if the effective design and conduct of national public health and nutrition policies for the elderly are to be achieved. It is unfortunate, however, that the nutrient requirements and recommended daily allowances for this age group have received inadequate investigation and concern. At present, the planning and nutritional evaluation of diets for the elderly is based largely on data obtained from healthy young adults. This practice is highly unrealistic in view of the increased disease rate and changes in body metabolism and physiological function that characterize advancement of the adult years.

It may be useful to introduce the topics reviewed below by referring to results obtained in dietary surveys of older people. For this purpose, therefore, the study by Lonergan _et al_. (1975) provides a suitable example, in which weekly dietary histories and weighed-diet records were obtained for elderly men and women living in Edinburgh, Scotland. As shown in Table I, at least one-third of the 75- to 90-year-old age group consumed diets supplying energy, protein, iron and vitamin D at levels equal to, or less than, the recommended levels of intake for the United Kingdom (Department of Health and Social Security, 1969).

Although the significance of these data to nutrition and health are difficult to judge, for various reasons (_e.g_.,

*Jointly with Riccardo Uauy, M.D., Joerg C. Winterer, M.D., and Nevin S. Scrimshaw, Ph.D., M.D.

Hegsted, 1972; Beaton, 1972; Beaton and Swiss, 1974), they raise a number of issues which deserve elaboration in this review. In the first place, recommended intakes are usually intended to be above the requirements for most healthy individuals. Therefore, intakes of less than the recommended levels do not mean a deficient dietary supply for all individuals, but indicate that some individuals risk deficiency. In order to estimate the expected prevalence of "deficiency", an estimate is required of the variation in nutrient requirements among apparently similar individuals. No definitive data are available in this area, although individual variations increase with advancing age. It is unknown whether this phenomenon can be attributed directly to the molecular events responsible for aging and senescence, or whether it is secondary to disease-related effects on metabolism and nutrient utilization (e.g., Scrimshaw et al., 1968). Apart from this problem of variation, interpretation of the dietary survey data shown in Table I assumes, at present, that the protein and amino acid requirements of the elderly do not differ significantly from those of young adults. There is inadequate experimental evidence to evaluate this assumption critically. Additional complicating factors, particularly in relation to interpreting protein intake data, are the nutritional and metabolic interactions that occur between the dietary intake of major energy-yielding substrates and protein utilization; it is difficult to assess the efficiency of protein utilization from mixtures of proteins consumed with the various meals during the day. Because a significant proportion of the subjects studied by Lonergan et al. (1975) consumed less than the recommended amount of energy, overall protein utilization possibly was reduced. Hence, the protein intake data shown in Table I would tend to underestimate the protein deficiency. Alternatively, the current recommended intakes for energy may be too high, but estimates of individual energy requirements are difficult to assess. Also, it has to be assumed that the relative capacities of different proteins to meet the nutritional needs of the elderly are the same as for young adults. This, too, is uncertain.

The foregoing clearly indicates that a better understanding of protein and amino acid metabolism and requirements of elderly subjects is necessary before an adequate definition of protein nutrition in the aged can be given. In this chapter, we explore some aspects of body protein and amino acid metabolism in the aged human subject and integrate this knowledge with a brief review of the current information on the protein requirements of elderly individuals. Two recent reviews by Young et al. (1976a,b) on protein metabolism and nutrition in the elderly also serve as bases for the following discussion. We do not intend to consider in detail studies that employed experimental animal models, unless they are especially pertinent to the interpretation of the results obtained in studies of human beings. Amino acid requirements also will be omitted; however, the reader is referred to earlier reviews of this topic (Watkin, 1964, 1966; Munro, 1972; Irwin and Hegsted, 1971a; Young et al., 1976a).

TABLE I

Percentage of Elderly Subjects in Edinburgh, Scotland, Whose Daily Intake of Various Nutrients was Less Than That Recommended by DHSS (1969)[1]

Nutrient	Men		Women	
	Percent of subjects	Recommended intake[2]	Percent of subjects	Recommended intake[2]
Energy	53.7	2100 kcal	74.0	1900 kcal
Total protein	14.8	53 g	32.9	48 g
Iron	40.8	10 mg	83.5	10 mg
Calcium	--	500 mg	8.2	500 mg
Vitamin D	72.3	2.5 μg	86.3	2.5 μg

[1]Summarized from Lonergan et al. (1975). Population sample involved 54 men and 67 women between the ages of 75 and 90.
[2]Recommended intakes are based on those of the United Kingdom Department of Health and Social Security (DHSS) (1969).

AMINO ACID METABOLISM AND AGING WITH REFERENCE TO PLASMA AMINO ACIDS

A major function of dietary protein is to provide the substrate necessary for the maintenance of tissue and organ protein synthesis in the adult. This substrate consists of the so-called essential amino acids and a source of nonessential (nonspecific) nitrogen, which is needed for the synthesis of the nonessential (dispensable) amino acids. Amino acids also participate in the synthesis of the purine and pyrimidine moieties of nucleic acids, and in the formation of neurotransmitters and other metabolically-active molecules, such as porphyrins, carnosine, creatine and the peptide hormones. These roles are physiologically important, but presumably account for a small proportion of daily amino acid utilization.

Figure 1 gives a general scheme of amino acid metabolism, which suggests that the requirements and metabolism of amino acids may be influenced by age-related factors, including

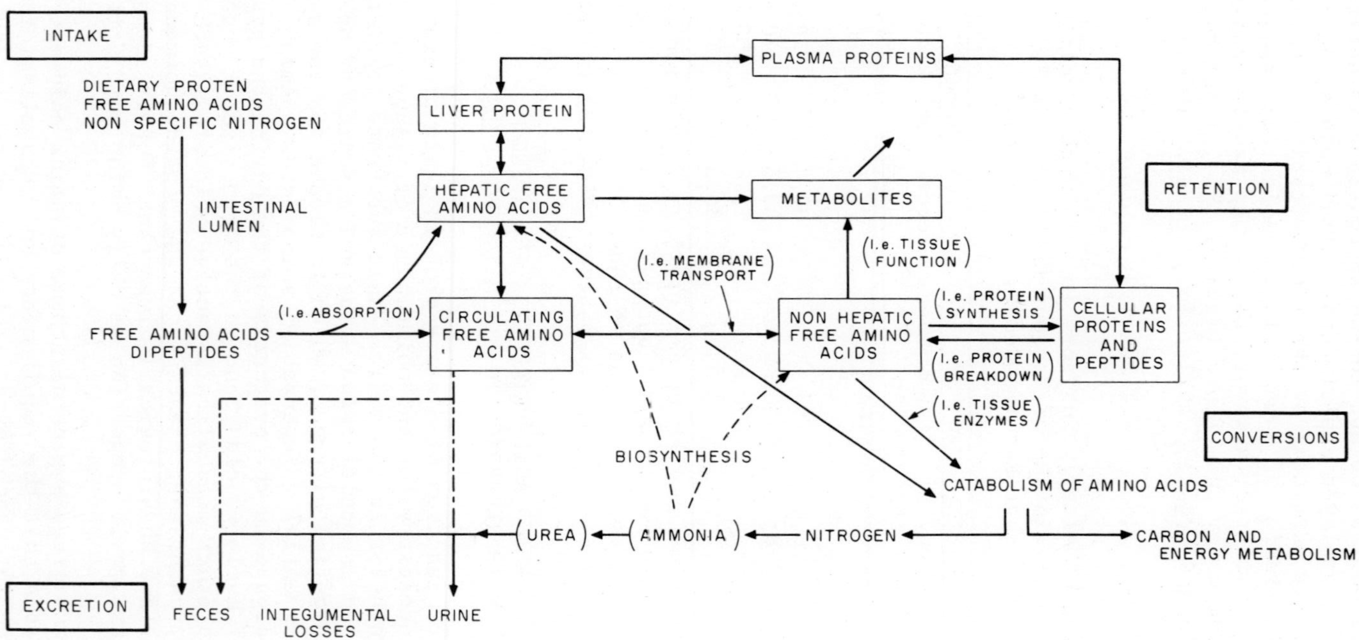

Fig. 1 A general scheme of amino acid metabolism, indicating points at which aging might affect amino acid utilization.

intestinal and cellular membrane transport, tissue enzyme activity, and the protein metabolic status of cells and organs. Although there is extensive information on amino acid metabolism in experimental animals, practical and ethical considerations seriously limit the availability of data on the metabolism of individual amino acids in aging human subjects. However, blood plasma can be readily obtained, and a few studies of plasma amino acids have been carried out in older people. Although many factors regulate the concentration of amino acids in plasma, studies of these levels in various physiological and pathological states have improved our understanding of human protein and amino acid metabolism. Furthermore, the level and pattern of plasma amino acids have important influences on food intake, regulation (e.g., Rogers and Leung, 1973) and central nervous system function (e.g., Wurtman and Fernstrom, 1975). Therefore, it is worthwhile to review data on plasma amino acid levels in elderly subjects.

Two early studies on the amino acid concentrations in blood plasma of older subjects led to different findings. Ackerman and Kheim (1964) compared plasma amino acid levels in young and old men and women and concluded that the levels of six essential amino acids -- valine, methionine, leucine, isoleucine, phenylalanine and lysine -- were lower in the elderly (mean age, 69 years) than in young adults (mean age, 28 and 32 years for men and women, respectively). On the other hand, the only difference found by Wehr and Lewis (1966) was a significantly higher concentration of ornithine in the elderly than in young subjects.

We have recently carried out a series of studies designed to examine the relationships between plasma amino acid levels, amino acid intakes and requirements in human beings of various ages (see Young et al., 1976a, for review). These studies provide an opportunity to compare plasma amino acid patterns in young adults and elderly people.

Because the branched-chain amino acids may inhibit degradation and stimulate synthesis of muscle protein (Buse and Reid, 1975; Fulks et al., 1975) and because they are metabolized preferentially in this tissue (Young, 1970; Sketcher et al., 1974; Yamamoto et al., 1974), we have examined the concentration of these amino acids in blood plasma of young adults and elderly subjects. Table II shows the data we have obtained to date and reveals no important differences in the plasma levels of branched-chain amino acids in a fasting state for the two groups studied. Because more extensive surveys of plasma free amino acids have indicated some sex-related differences (Armstrong and Stave,

1973a, b), the results of the comparison shown in Table II must be interpreted with caution until a more thorough investigation, involving both sexes, has been carried out in elderly people.

TABLE II

Concentrations[1] of Branched-chain Amino Acids in Blood Plasma of Young Adult and Elderly Subjects Consuming an Adequate Free-choice Diet

Amino Acid	Young Men[2]	Elderly Women[3]
Leucine	14.7 ± 1.6	14.1 ± 3.1
Isoleucine	8.2 ± 1.2	6.9 ± 1.5
Valine	24.9 ± 2.7	24.9 ± 3.4
Leucine:Valine Ratio	0.59 ± 0.05	0.57 ± 0.09

[1]Mean ± SD; results are expressed as μmoles per 100 ml. Samples were drawn after a 10-hr overnight fast. (Unpublished data of Perera, Scrimshaw and Young.)
[2]Data are from 19 healthy young men, ages 22 ± 4 years.
[3]Data are from 11 healthy elderly women, ages 69 ± 2 years.

The influence of diet on the branched-chain amino acids provides another means of assessing their metabolism in old age. Furthermore, metabolic interactions occur among these amino acids that depend, in part, on their dietary supply. As shown in figure 2, a reduction in the intake of leucine in young men results in a decrease in plasma leucine and an increase in the concentration of the other two branched-chain amino acids, isoleucine and valine. Although the mechanisms involved are not known, Hambraeus _et al_. (1976) have suggested that the level and availability of dietary leucine regulates the uptake and utilization of the other two branched-chain amino acids. Elderly subjects also show a rise in plasma isoleucine and valine concentrations when the dietary leucine intake is reduced (Table III) and these changes are comparable to those observed in young men (Özalp _et al_., 1972). Therefore, it may be tentatively concluded that branched-chain amino acid metabolism is qualitatively similar in young adults and the elderly. However, measurement of amino acid levels in plasma does not indicate possible differences in the flux and/or fate of amino acids within body tissues and organs. Studies on this phase of amino acid metabolism could be carried out with ^{13}C- and ^{15}N-labeled amino acids in order to confirm and extend our conclusions.

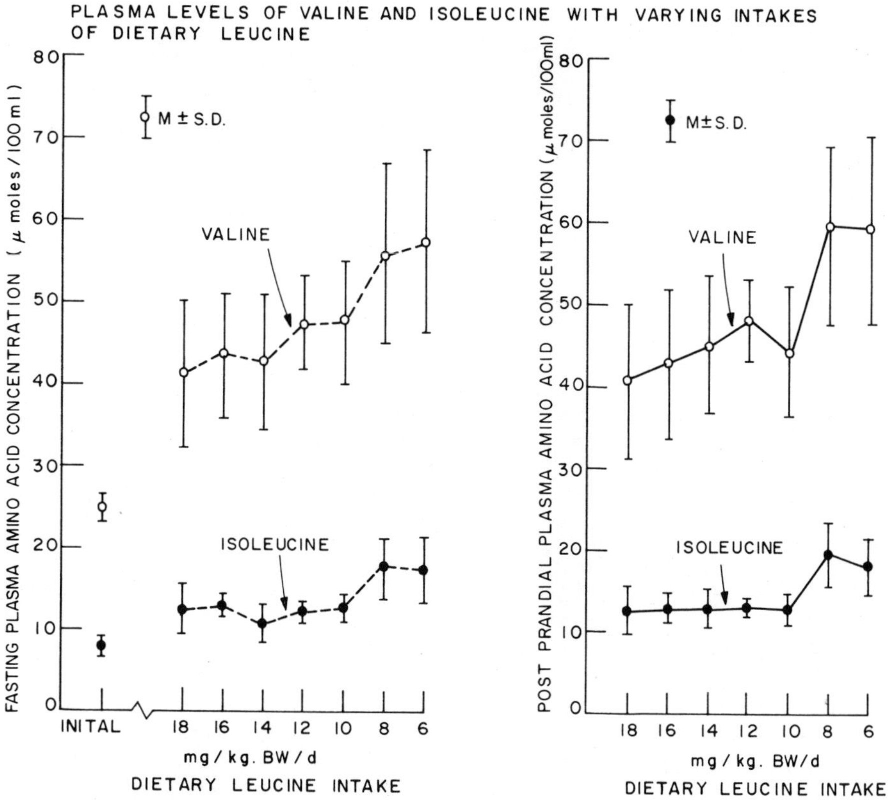

Fig. 2 Changes in plasma free valine and isoleucine in response to graded reductions in leucine intake in young men. The diets were based on synthetic L-amino acid mixtures (e.g., Tontisirin et al., 1974). Fasting and postprandial samples were drawn at 8 AM, after an overnight fast, and at ~11:30 AM, just prior to lunch. (Unpublished data of Perera, Scrimshaw and Young.)

TABLE III

Effect of Reduced Leucine Intake on the Concentration of Branched-chain Amino Acids in Plasma of Young Men and Elderly Women[1]

Amino Acid	Young Men		Elderly Women	
	Normal[2]	Reduced Intake	Normal[2]	Reduced Intake[3]
Leucine	14.2 ± 1.1[4]	11.7 ± 0.7	13.7 ± 1.5	10.4 ± 0.9
Isoleucine	7.7 ± 0.4	12.2 ± 0.3	6.8 ± 1.3	9.2 ± 1.0
Valine	24.3 ± 1.3	41.3 ± 9.8	24.9 ± 0.9	38.1 ± 0.5
Leucine: Valine	0.57± 0.03	0.30± 0.07	0.56± 0.08	0.27± 0.04

[1]Four subjects were in each group. Data are expressed as μmoles per 100 ml. (Unpublished data of Perera, Scrimshaw and Young.)
[2]Samples were taken after a 10-hr overnight fast during a free-choice diet period.
[3]Samples were taken after 7 or 10 days on a diet providing 16 mg of leucine per kg of body weight per day. Diet was similar to that described by Tontisirin et al. (1974).
[4]Mean ± SD.

Plasma amino acid levels are affected by the amount of protein and amino acids in the diet (e.g., Young and Scrimshaw, 1972; McLaughlan, 1974). Therefore, additional information on amino acid metabolism in elderly people can be gained by comparing the effects of alterations in essential amino acid intake on plasma amino acid concentrations in young adult and older subjects. Figure 3 compares the response of plasma tryptophan concentrations to graded decreases in dietary tryptophan intake in three age groups: 1) school-age children with Down's Syndrome, 2) healthy young men, and 3) a group of elderly men and women. The pattern of response was generally similar for all three groups. Therefore, as indicated by changes in plasma levels, tryptophan metabolism is responsive to the adequacy of tryptophan intake and appears to change in parallel ways in both healthy young adults and older people. Additional details about these plasma responses and their relationship to requirements for tryptophan have been given previously (Young et al., 1971; Tontisirin et al., 1972, 1973).

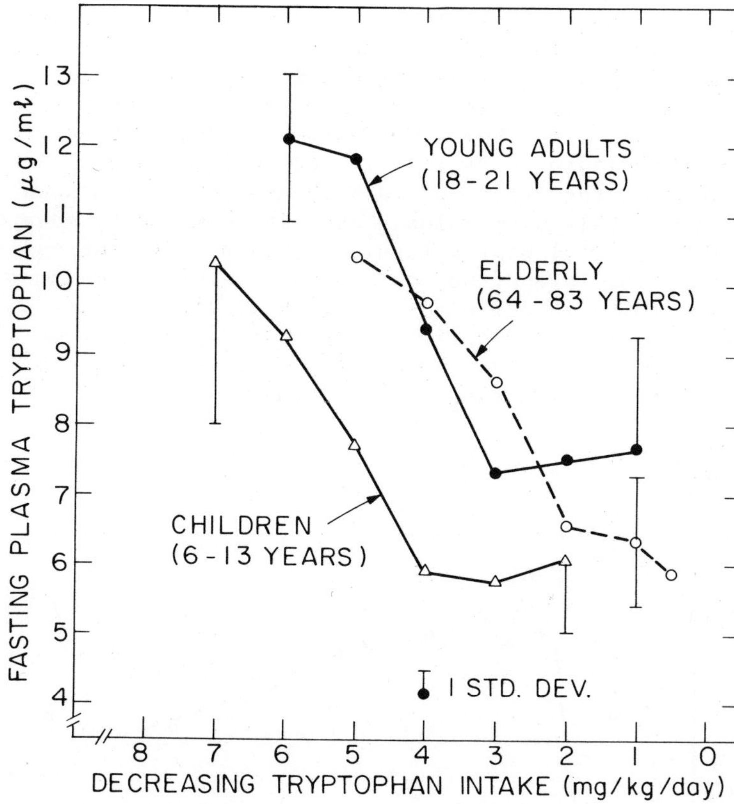

Fig. 3 The response of plasma tryptophan to graded reductions in dietary protein in three age groups. Results are a combination of data from Young *et al*. (1971) and Tontisirin *et al*. (1972, 1973).

BODY PROTEIN METABOLISM

Protein Content of the Whole Body and Skeletal Muscle Mass

The assessment of protein metabolism and needs of the elderly requires knowledge of the body protein mass and whether there are age-related changes in the amount and distribution of body protein.

Both cross-sectional (Fig. 4) and longitudinal studies reveal a progressive decline in total body potassium as aging progresses in humans (Allen *et al*., 1960; Forbes and Reina, 1970). Although its precise physiological significance is uncertain, a loss of body potassium usually implies a decrease in body cell and protein mass. Studies utilizing other approaches to estimate body composition have also indicated a reduction in body cell mass with aging in human beings (Parizkova et al., 1971). From the observations of Korenchevsky (1961) described below, we assume that the change in body potassium indicates a decline in body cell mass with advancing age, although the extent of this change remains unknown. On the basis of this conclusion, Table IV shows that, when calculated from total body potassium, body protein increases rapidly during infancy and childhood, reaching a maximum by about the third decade of life (Allen et al., 1960). Thereafter, body nitrogen declines progressively during the adult years, with the decrease apparently occurring more rapidly in men than in women (Forbes and Reina, 1970).

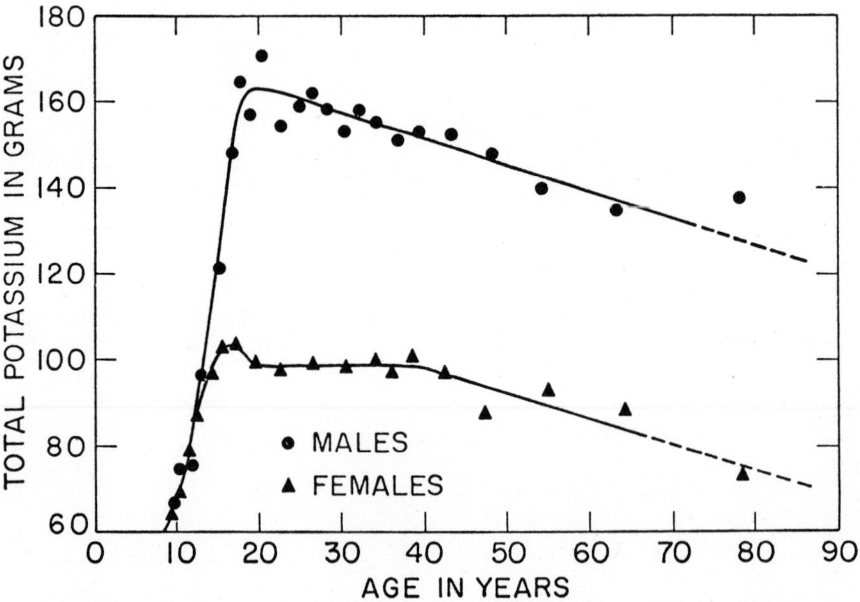

Fig. 4 Total body potassium as a function of age in male and female subjects. Data are based on the study by Allen et al. (1960).

In theory, the lower body nitrogen in the elderly subject may reflect changes in the amount of nitrogen in all, or only in some specific tissues. This problem has not been explored in detail, but atrophy of the skeletal muscles is conspicuous in old age (Gutmann, 1970).

Data on age-related changes in the muscle mass of human beings are limited. Korenchevsky (1961) has summarized data on organ weights obtained postmortem from hospitalized patients and from a small number of accident victims. He concluded that there was close agreement between the two sets of data. As shown in Table V, the percentage of muscle mass apparently declines to a much greater extent than that of liver; the weight of the heart is essentially unchanged as humans age.

TABLE IV

An Estimate of Total Body Nitrogen in Human Males at Various Times of Life

Age Group	Body Nitrogen	
	(g)	(g/kg body wt)
Newborn (full term)[1]	66	19
Infant (1 month)[2]	64	15
Child (8 years)[2]	499	22
Teenager (15 years)[2]	1225	20
Young Adult (25 years)[2]	1339	18
Elderly (65 to 70 years)[2]	1066	15

[1]Data are from Widdowson and Dickerson (1964).
[2]Data for infants were calculated from Novak _et al_. (1970) and for older age groups from Forbes and Reina (1970) and Forbes (1972). Estimates of body nitrogen were made from whole body potassium measurements, assuming that there are 68.1 mEq K per kg of lean body mass and that 3 mEq K is equal to 1 g of nitrogen.

TABLE V

Mean Relative Weights (g/kg Body Weight) of Human Heart, Liver, and Skeletal Muscles as a Function of Age[1]

Age Group	Heart	Liver	Skeletal Muscle
Newborn	6.9	45.3	213
1-5 years	5.0	34.5	175
11-15 years	5.0	26.3	362
21-30 years	5.8	25.4	452
41-50 years	5.7	25.6	402
61-70 years	6.1	21.4	339
> 70 years	7.0	20.3	270
Percent change between the 21- to 30-year-old and > 70-year-old groups	+20.7	-18.2	-40.3

[1]Data were taken, in abbreviated form, from Korenchevsky (1961), who based his data on Roessle and Roulet (1932).

Dynamic Aspects

Whole body protein turnover. Protein synthesis is a major sink for amino acids entering tissue and body fluids through the diet or from tissue protein breakdown. Similarly, protein breakdown in the tissues and organs accounts for a major proportion of the amino acids entering the free amino pools of the body and tissue compartments. Therefore, changes in the intensities and rates of body protein synthesis and breakdown will influence the metabolism and utilization of the individual amino acids.

Thus, the protein and amino acid requirements of the rat decline between weaning and adulthood (*cf.*, Rao *et al.*, 1959; Said and Hegsted, 1970). The turnover of whole body protein decreases with development (Waterlow and Stephen, 1967) in both liver and muscle (Waterlow and Stephen, 1968; Millward *et al.*, 1975). Yousef and Johnson (1970) found that the turnover rate of whole body protein was more rapid in young (150 days or less) than in old rats. However, the significance of these latter observations is uncertain because ^{75}Se-selenomethionine, which was used as a tracer in their studies, is known to be extensively reutilized, causing estimated turnover times to be falsely long (Waterlow *et al.*,

1969).

In humans, protein and energy metabolism are closely related (Brody, 1945; Waterlow, 1968; Munro, 1969) and, as in rats, body protein turnover might be expected to change with old age because basal energy expenditure, expressed per unit of body weight, falls both during growth and development (Kleiber, 1961) and during aging (McGandy et al., 1966).

A review by Waterlow (1969) suggests that the rate of total body N turnover is highest in the newborn (e.g., Nicholson, 1970) and approximately twice as high in children (Picou and Taylor-Roberts, 1969) as in young adults (Steffee et al., 1975).

Sharp et al. (1957) fed diets containing ^{15}N-yeast protein to two older male and to two older female subjects (57-70 years) and to two young adults, one male and one female. They estimated the rates of total body protein synthesis to be 0.28 and 0.20 g of nitrogen per kg of body weight per day, in the young and old subjects, respectively. However, the model (Sprinson and Rittenberg, 1949) used by Sharp et al. (1957) appears to give lower estimates of the rate of body protein synthesis than those used in more recent studies of adults (Waterlow and Stephen, 1967; O'Keefe et al., 1974; Steffee et al., 1975).

Winterer and coworkers (1976) also recently explored dynamic aspects of protein metabolism in healthy subjects, aged 65-91 years, using the ^{15}N-amino acid infusion method proposed by Picou and Taylor-Roberts (1969). Figure 5 shows the time course of ^{15}N-enrichment of urinary urea nitrogen of a representative elderly subject. When ^{15}N-glycine was administered continuously, the time-dependent change in urea ^{15}N-enrichment resembled that observed in young adults receiving a generous level of dietary protein (Steffee et al., 1975). From the plateau level of urea-^{15}N-enrichment, estimates of whole body protein synthesis were made; the results for groups of young adult and elderly subjects are summarized in Table VI. For purposes of comparison, we have included in this table data for neonates and children of about 1 year of age. These values show, in addition to the marked fall in the rate of body protein synthesis during growth and development, that the rates, expressed per unit of body weight, are lower in women than in men. Furthermore, elderly females exhibit lower rates of body protein synthesis than young women ($P < 0.1$), whereas the rates for male subjects were found to be similar in both age groups.

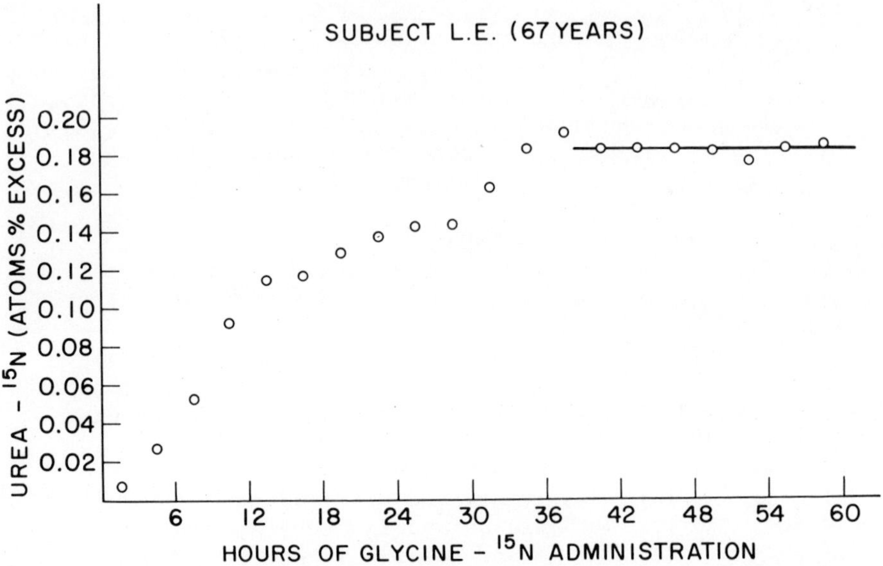

Fig. 5 Time course of enrichment of urinary urea nitrogen with the continuous oral administration of ^{15}N-glycine in a 67-year-old woman. The horizontal line represents the plateau enrichment, from which estimates of whole body protein synthesis and breakdown are derived.

TABLE VI

Whole Body Protein Synthesis in Humans at Various Ages

Group	Age	Number of Studies	Body Protein Synthesis (g/kg body wt/day)
Neonate	1-46 days	10	17.4 ± 7.9
Infant[1]	10-20 months	4	6.9 ± 1.1
Young Adult			
Male	20-25 years	4	3.3 ± 0.3
Female	18-23 years	4	2.6 ± 0.2
Elderly			
Male	65-72 years	4	3.2 ± 0.7
Female	69-91 years	5	2.3 ± 0.4

[1]Taken from the data presented in a study by Picou and Taylor-Roberts(1969); other data were obtained in the authors' laboratories, as described in the text.

To determine whether differences in body composition affect comparisons among the groups, urinary creatinine excretion was determined as an index of muscle mass, and total body potassium, estimated by counting whole body ^{40}K, was used to calculate body cell mass. The rates of whole body protein synthesis and breakdown were then related to these parameters of body composition. The data are shown in figure 6. When expressed per unit creatinine, the rates of total body protein synthesis and breakdown are significantly higher in the elderly than in the young adult subjects. On a body cell mass basis, elderly males showed higher rates than young men. Although this relationship was also apparent for the female subjects, the difference between the two age groups was not statistically significant, possibly because of the low values obtained for one of the elderly female subjects in this study (Winterer et al., 1976).

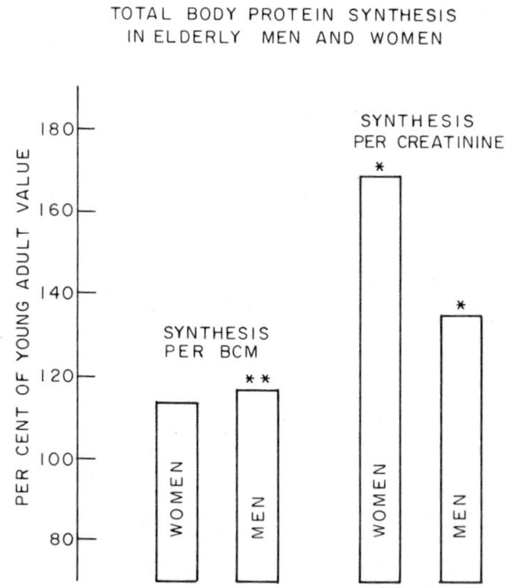

Fig. 6 Comparison of rates of whole body protein synthesis and breakdown, expressed per unit of creatinine excretion and per unit of body cell mass (determined by ^{40}K counting) in elderly and young adult subjects. Data are based on Winterer et al. (1976).

The significantly higher rates of whole body protein synthesis and breakdown, expressed per unit of creatinine, in the elderly than in the young adult subjects suggests an increase in the contribution to whole body protein synthesis and breakdown of the visceral organs, such as the liver and intestines, compared with the skeletal muscle. These results might be anticipated because, as discussed earlier, (a) muscle mass declines with age more than the visceral organs (Korenchevsky, 1961); (b) the fractional rate of protein breakdown is higher in liver and intestines than in skeletal muscle (Millward and Garlick, 1972); (c) there may be a fall in the rate of turnover of muscle protein with advancing age in man, as discussed below. These factors would all tend to decrease the relative importance of muscle, and increase the contribution of the visceral organs in whole body protein turnover.

Muscle protein metabolism. The amount of RNA in cells and tissues is considered to be a general index of protein synthesis in various body organs. Assuming, therefore, that RNA content is an indicator of the intensity of tissue protein synthesis, the relative role of the skeletal musculature in whole body protein metabolism during aging can be assessed further. We have calculated the amount of RNA in the total muscle mass and in the liver of rats at different stages of growth (Young *et al.*, 1976b). When compared with the amount in the liver, the RNA in the skeletal musculature increases steadily throughout normal growth and development. However, after maturity is reached, the relative proportion of body RNA contributed by muscle declines, whereas it again increases in the liver.

In vitro and *in vivo* studies of muscle protein synthesis and turnover in aged experimental animals have been previously reviewed by Young and associates (1976b) and do not need to be considered here. In general, the studies suggest that muscle protein synthesis declines with advancing age. Changes in the level of muscle protein synthesis and breakdown and their contributions to whole body protein turnover in the aged human being have not been explored extensively. However, some crude approximations can be made of the quantitative significance of muscle in whole body protein turnover in adult human subjects. Firstly, Halliday and McKeran (1975) used a ^{15}N-lysine infusion method to estimate rates of whole body and muscle protein synthesis in five adult men, ages 31 to 46 years. Their results are summarized in Table VII and indicate that, for healthy adults, the average rate of muscle protein synthesis or breakdown is 1.9 g/kg of body weight per day. This figure accounts for 53% of the estimated rate of whole body protein synthesis.

Secondly, in their studies of arteriovenous amino acid differences and release across the human forearm, Cahill and coworkers (1972) estimated that muscle protein degradation amounts to approximately 0.5-1 g/kg/day.

TABLE VII

Whole Body and Muscle Protein Synthesis in Healthy Adult Males[1]

Measurement	Protein Synthesis Rate (g/kg body wt/day)
Whole Body	3.50 ± 1.1[2]
Muscle:	
Myofibrillar	0.95 ± 0.4
Sarcoplasmic	0.98 ± 0.3
Total	1.88 ± 0.71
Percent of Whole Body Value	53.0 ± 9.0

[1]Data are based on a study of five adult men, 31-46 years old, by Halliday and McKeran (1975).
[2]Mean ± SD.

Finally, we have combined our data on whole body protein turnover with measurements of 3-methylhistidine excretion to compare muscle protein turnover in young adults and older people. Methylhistidine was used because it is present in the actin of all muscles and the myosin of "white" muscle fibers (see Young _et al._, 1973; Haverberg _et al._, 1975, for brief reviews), and the major proportion of protein-bound 3-methylhistidine is located in skeletal muscle (Haverberg _et al._, 1975). In rats (Young _et al._, 1972) and man (Long _et al._, 1975) the amino acid is quantitatively excreted in the urine and, unlike the common amino acids of body proteins, it is not re-utilized for protein synthesis (Young _et al._, 1972) or metabolized in oxidative pathways (Long _et al._, 1975). These findings are schematically depicted in figure 7, which suggests that the measurement of the daily excretion of 3-methylhistidine should provide an index of muscle protein breakdown in human subjects under various physiological and pathological conditions.

Table VIII summarizes our unpublished results on the urinary excretion of this amino acid in young adults and elderly subjects consuming flesh-free diets. The daily output of 3-methylhistidine is much lower in elderly than in young adults, reflecting the lowered muscle mass in the elderly group. When corrected for differences in creatinine excretion, however, the output of 3-methylhistidine in the elderly is still somewhat below that for young adults. This phenomenon suggests that, per unit of muscle mass, the rate of muscle protein breakdown and synthesis may decline with advancing age.

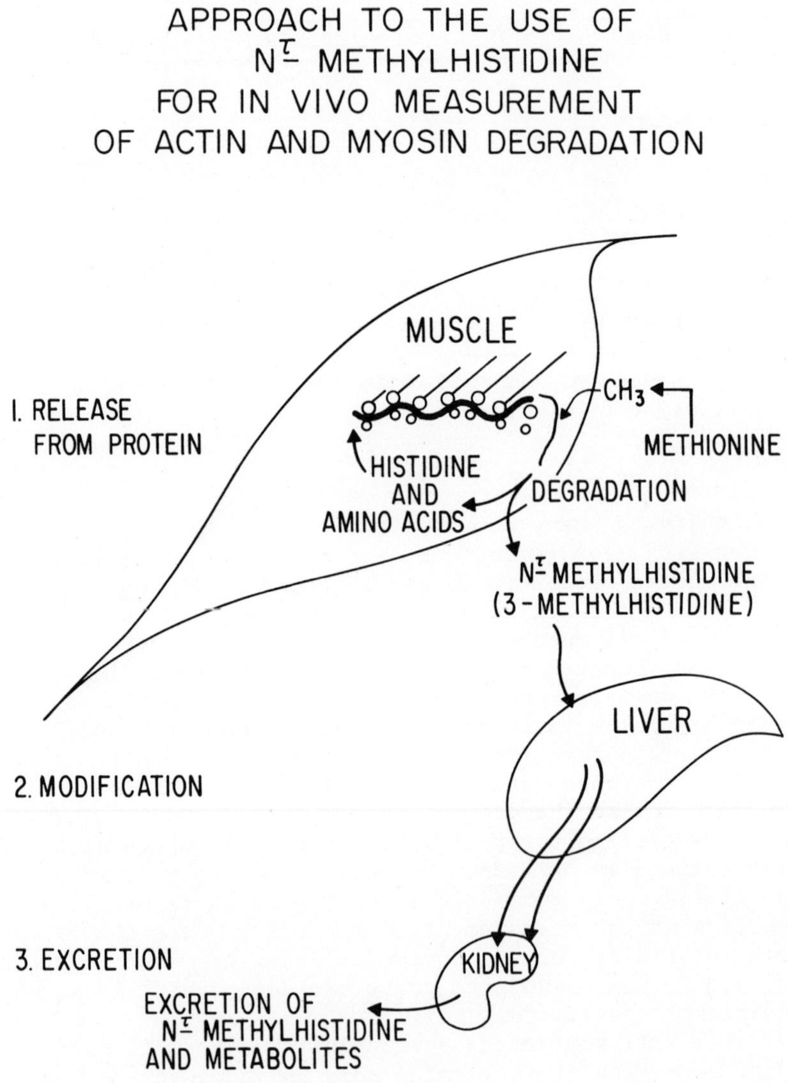

Fig. 7 Schematic outline of 3-methylhistidine ($N^{\underline{t}}$-methylhistidine) in man. Outline is based, in part, on the data of Young *et al.* (1972) and Long *et al.* (1975). Excretion of significant amounts of N-acetyl-3-methylhistidine does not occur in man.

TABLE VIII

Urinary Excretion of 3-Methylhistidine in Adult Subjects Receiving Flesh-free Diets

Group	Number of Subjects	Mean Age (yr)	Body Weight (kg)	Urinary 3-methylhistidine (μmoles)		
				per day	per kg/ day	per g creatinine
Young Men	4	20	72	211 ± 40[1]	3.0 ± 0.4	127 ± 20
Elderly Women	6	77	57	75 ± 20	1.3 ± 0.2	103 ± 10

[1]Mean ± SD (unpublished results).

The output of urinary 3-methylhistidine can also be used to estimate the breakdown of muscle protein and its relationship to whole body protein breakdown. Our studies (Haverberg _et al_., 1975) in adult rats indicate that about 90% of urinary 3-methylhistidine is derived from the breakdown of myofibrillar proteins in skeletal muscle. Furthermore, the limited data available suggest that the concentration of 3-methylhistidine in the mixed proteins of skeletal muscles of human adults (Asatoor and Armstrong, 1967), as well as neonates (Young, V. R., Haverberg, L. N., Pencharz, P. B., and Munro, H. N., unpublished results), is approximately 1.7 μmoles/g mixed proteins. From this value, the amount of muscle protein breakdown can be calculated, if the daily urinary output of the amino acid is known. This assumes that the daily breakdown of myofibrillar and sarcoplasmic proteins is equal. In general terms, the results of Halliday and McKeran (1975) support this assumption. Hence, our estimates of muscle protein breakdown, derived from the urinary 3-methylhistidine data, are summarized in Table IX for young adults and elderly subjects. The mean rates of muscle protein breakdown in young men and elderly women are 1.9 and 0.8 g/kg of body weight per day, respectively, and these estimated are similar to those of Halliday and McKeran (1975) shown earlier in Table VII.

It is important to emphasize that our comparisons of muscle protein turnover are based on preliminary data on 3-methylhistidine excretion and were obtained by cross-sectional study. Additional studies in aged individuals of both sexes would be fruitful in order to explore further aspects of the compartmentation of whole body protein turnover in aging man.

The physiological and health implications of a shift in the distribution of body protein metabolism can only be a matter of speculation at this time. However, muscle plays a significant role in the economy of body nitrogen metabolism and is responsive to alterations in hormonal balance and nutritional state as well as to stressful stimuli such as physical injury or infection (e.g., Young, 1970). It is tempting to speculate that a reduction in the level and intensity of muscle protein metabolism with advancing age might lower the body's capacity for metabolic adaptation to environmental changes, and thus, its ability to overcome unfavorable situations.

Knowledge of the changes in body and tissue protein metabolism in old age improves our understanding of the physiology of human protein metabolism and the factors that affect it. However, it cannot yet be used to predict the quantitative needs for protein and amino acids. It is necessary to determine these requirements directly and, in the following sections, aspects of the protein and amino acid needs of elderly people will be discussed.

TABLE IX

An Estimate of the Rate of Muscle Protein Breakdown, from Urinary 3-Methylhistidine Excretion, and Its Relationship to Whole Body Protein Breakdown in Adults

Group	Number of Subjects	3-Methyl-histidine Excretion	Muscle Protein Breakdown[1]	
			g/kg/day	percent of total body breakdown
		(mg/kg/day)		
Young Men	6	0.50	1.9	70
Elderly Women	6	0.22	0.8	38

[1]Values given are based on the following assumptions:
(a) Mixed protein contains 0.027 g of 3-methylhistidine/100g.
(b) Mean values for whole body protein breakdown rates are 2.7 and 2.1 g/kg/day for young men and elderly women, respectively (unpublished results).

PROTEIN REQUIREMENTS

A number of studies review the protein requirements of humans (e.g., Irwin and Hegsted, 1971b) and of elderly individuals in particular (Watkin, 1957-58, 1964, 1966; Munro, 1972). We have reviewed in detail the approaches used for determining the protein and amino acid requirements of man (Young and Scrimshaw, 1976; Young *et al.*, 1976a), and only selected topics need be covered here.

Protein requirements of adult subjects have been assessed either by the factorial method or by monitoring nitrogen balance response to graded intakes of dietary protein. We have recently discussed the pitfalls and limitations of these methods (Young and Scrimshaw, 1976), but it is worth reviewing some current data as they relate to the protein needs of elderly people.

Factorial Estimation of the Protein Requirement

In using the factorial approach to estimate human protein requirements, the losses of "obligatory" nitrogen through urine and feces are measured and summated with additional corrections for nitrogen losses through the skin and other minor routes. In the case of the growing child, a further allowance is made for the increment in total body nitrogen.

The aim of the method is to determine the total nitrogen lost from the body when the subject receives a protein-free but otherwise adequate diet. This loss, measured after a period of stabilization, is taken to be the obligatory loss, which is thought to represent the minimum nitrogen output consistent with a healthy state. The minimum dietary protein requirement is then computed to be that amount of high-quality protein necessary to balance this endogenous loss.

Obligatory urine and fecal nitrogen losses in adults are measured after a suitable period of stabilization on a protein-free diet. Nitrogen losses through the skin are far more difficult to measure. With a usual dietary protein intake, the cutaneous and other minor nitrogen losses have been estimated to average about 5 mg of nitrogen per kg of body weight in men (Food and Agriculture Organization/WHO, 1973) and about 3.6 mg of nitrogen per kg of body weight in women (Kraut and Müller-Wecker, 1960). Profuse sweating may cause more nitrogen to be lost through the skin, especially in subjects unaccustomed to living and working in hot climates.

The factorial approach proposed by the Food and Agriculture Organization/World Health Organization (FAO/WHO, 1973) Expert Committee for estimating protein requirements and dietary allowances is described in Table X. The minimum obligatory losses are summated and increased by a factor of 1.3 to account for changes in the efficiency of dietary nitrogen utilization over the submaintenance to maintenance range of nitrogen (protein) intake. Because dietary allowances and variations in requirements among individuals must be considered, the mean requirement for maintenance (R_N) is again increased by a factor of 1.3. This adjustment is made under the assumption that the coefficient of variation (CV) in protein requirements among individuals amounts to 15%, and so 30% (i.e., 2 x CV) should cover the needs for nearly all (97.5%) of the population. The details and evidence of these adjustments are described in the report of the 1973 FAO/WHO Committee.

Because no satisfactory data were available until recently on obligatory nitrogen losses for the elderly, Scrimshaw *et al*. (1976) measured these losses in 11 healthy elderly women and compared the findings with those reported for college-age women (Bricker and Smith, 1951) and also with our measurements of obligatory nitrogen losses in young men (Scrimshaw *et al*., 1972).

TABLE X

FAO/WHO (1973) Approach to the Factorial Estimation of Human Protein Requirements and Allowances

1.	Total Obligatory N Losses (O_N) =	Obligatory Urinary N + Obligatory Fecal N + Skin N + Miscellaneous N
2.	Other N Requirements:	Growth (G_N), Pregnancy (P_N), Lactation (L_N)
3.	Total Minimum N Requirements for Maintenance and Growth =	$O_N + G_N$
4.	Nitrogen Requirement Adjusted for Efficiency of N Utilization (R_N) =	$(O_N + G_N) \times 1.3$
5.	Safe Practical Allowance, Adjusted for Individual Variability (SPA) =	$R_N \times 1.3$
6.	Allowance for Pregnancy or Lactation =	$SPA + [(P_N \text{ or } L_N)(1.3)] \times 1.3$

The safe practical allowance for nitrogen is converted to a protein allowance by multiplying by the factor 6.25.

Figure 8 shows the change, with time, in the urinary excretion of nitrogen per unit of body weight among 11 elderly women consuming a protein-free diet. The mean time needed to achieve a stable level of urinary nitrogen loss in elderly and young adults was 4.5 days (Rand, W. M., Young, V. R., and Scrimshaw, N. S., in preparation). The observed urinary and fecal nitrogen losses, together with estimated total nitrogen losses, are expressed in various ways in Table XI. When integumental and miscellaneous nitrogen losses are assumed to be 5 mg per kg of body weight per day, the total mean obligatory nitrogen loss for each of the 11 women was 39.3 mg of nitrogen per kg of body weight per day, with a variation coefficient of 16%.

Table XI also compares these results for elderly women with the data of Bricker and Smith (1951) for young women and with our own data for young men (Scrimshaw *et al.*, 1972). The difference between the nitrogen losses, expressed per unit of body weight, in elderly and young women was not significant. The much higher obligatory nitrogen losses per unit of body weight for young men than for elderly or young women can be accounted for, in part, by their greater body cell mass (BCM) per kg of body weight.

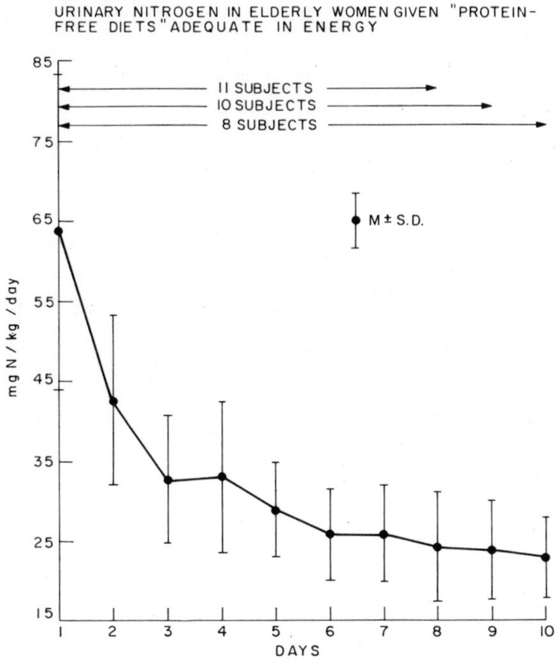

Fig. 8 Change in urinary nitrogen excretion in elderly women during adaptation to a protein-free diet. Data are taken from Scrimshaw *et al.* (1976).

TABLE XI

Obligatory Nitrogen Losses in Elderly Women, Compared With Previous Estimates in Young Women and Young Men [1]

Daily N Losses	Elderly Women [1]	Young Women [2]	Young Men [3]
Urinary:			
grams	1.52 ± 0.29	1.45 ± 0.20	2.69 ± 0.48
mg/kg body wt	24.4 ± 5.2	25.2 ± 3.3	37.2 ± 5.5
mg/basal kcal	1.44 ± 0.14[4]	1.14 ± 0.11	1.77 ± 0.30
g/g creatinine	2.11 ± 0.28	1.49 ± 0.02	1.58 ± 0.22
mg/kg BCM	89.5 ±17.1	62.0 ±10.0[5]	76.8 ±12.5
Fecal:			
grams	0.61 ± 0.16	0.50 ± 0.08	0.63 ± 0.15
mg/kg body wt	9.8 ± 2.7	8.7 ± 2.5	8.8 ± 2.1
mg/basal kcal	0.59 ± 0.17[3]	0.40 ± 0.07	0.42 ± 0.11
Total (Urinary + Fecal):			
grams	2.13 ± 0.36	1.96 ± 0.19	3.33 ± 0.54
mg/kg/body wt	34.2 ± 6.3	33.9 ± 4.2	46.0 ± 6.0
mg/basal kcal	2.03 ± 0.24	1.54 ± 0.14	2.19 ± 0.34
g/g creatinine	2.96 ± 0.32	2.01 ± 0.14	1.94 ± 0.24

[1]Data are from Scrimshaw *et al.* (1976).
[2]Data are from Bricker and Smith (1951).
[3]Data are from Scrimshaw *et al.* (1972).
[4]Data are based on a study of seven subjects.
[5]For comparison, BCM was estimated from data given by Forbes (1974).

Although the studies of Bricker and Smith (1951) did not include body composition measurements, the BCM of their subjects can be approximated from the prediction equations of Forbes (1974); this approach, however, has its limitations (Boddy *et al.*, 1975). Calculated in this way, the urinary nitrogen losses per unit of BCM are higher in the elderly than in the young woman; this difference may be caused by one or more of the following factors: (a) The ^{40}K technique may underestimate BCM in the elderly subjects. We have assumed a constant ratio of body potassium to nitrogen for computing BCM in both age groups, but the ratio may decrease with advancing age (Allen *et al.*, 1960). (b) When given a protein-free diet, elderly subjects may conserve nitrogen less efficiently than younger ones, resulting in a higher output of urinary nitrogen. (c) Changes occur in the turnover and distribution of body protein with advancing age, as discussed earlier, and thus, the output of urinary nitrogen under similar dietary conditions may reflect different metabolic processes between the two age groups. Furthermore, metabolically-active visceral tissues initially lose more nitrogen than muscle tissue when a protein-free diet is consumed (Munro, 1964), but they may be more efficient than muscle in promoting nitrogen reutilization once adaptive metabolic changes have come fully into play. Even when a person eats an adequate diet, at least 70% of the amino nitrogen released during normal tissue protein breakdown is reused; this percentage increases markedly as the tissues adapt to a low-protein or protein-free diet (Waterlow, 1968; Picou and Taylor-Roberts, 1969; Steffee et al., 1975). Thus, age-related changes in the turnover rates of muscle and visceral proteins could modify the effects of age-related changes in tissue mass on urinary nitrogen after adaptation to a protein-free diet.

Under the conditions of a protein-free diet, the creatinine output, per unit of body weight, was lower among the elderly than among the younger individuals. This finding reflects the decrease in muscle mass with aging. Our data indicate that obligatory nitrogen losses per gram of creatinine excreted are higher for elderly women than for either young men or young women. Furthermore, our preliminary studies, discussed above, on the excretion of 3-methylhistidine in the urine suggest that the turnover of muscle protein per unit of muscle mass may be reduced in the elderly. Hence, the higher rate of obligatory nitrogen loss (per unit of creatinine excretion) appears to be caused by a shift in the relative proportions of body protein in the viscera and skeletal muscle and possibly, in part, by a change in the relative turnover rates for protein in the muscular tissues.

By applying the factorial method to the data obtained in this study, we have computed a protein allowance for elderly women. The estimate, shown in Table XII, assumes that healthy elderly subjects metabolize high-quality protein as efficiently as young adults, an assumption implicit in both the FAO/WHO (1973) and the United States Food and Nutrition Board (FNB, 1974) recommendations for dietary protein in adults. The computed "safe" level of intake of 0.42 g of egg or milk protein per kg of body weight per day is less than that proposed for young adults of either sex by the 1973 FAO/WHO Committee (Table XII). It is also less than the protein intake reported to be necessary for the maintenance of nitrogen balance in many elderly subjects, as reviewed in the next section, and direct metabolic studies are needed to evaluate the adequacy of this estimate and to determine more precisely the appropriate safe practical allowance for protein in healthy elderly subjects.

TABLE XII

The Computed "Safe Practical Allowance" of Milk or Egg Protein for Elderly Women as Determined by the FAO/WHO (1973) Factorial Method

Group	Mean Total Obligatory N Loss	Adjusted N Requirement[1]	Safe Level of Intake	
			N	Protein
	(mg/kg/day)	(mg/kg/day)	(mg/kg/day)	(g/kg/day)
Men	54	70	91[2]	0.57
Women	49	64	83[2]	0.52
Elderly Women	39	51	67[3]	0.42

[1]Obligatory N losses are increased by 30% to account for efficiency of N utilization.
[2]Values are adjusted requirement plus 30% to allow for individual variability.
[3]Value is adjusted requirement plus 32% (based on unpublished results of Perera *et al.*).

Nitrogen Balance

The minimum physiological requirement for dietary protein can be determined directly from the nitrogen balance response to graded protein intakes. We have recently discussed these studies (Young *et al.*, 1976a), and Watkin (1957-58) has carefully reviewed this topic and discussed the factors, of which there are many, that may account for the lack of agreement among the various studies. Table XIII lists some of the nitrogen balance studies and the conclusions drawn from them concerning the requirements of elderly subjects. As shown here, some investigators (Kountz *et al.*, 1951) concluded that the need for protein was higher in the elderly than in young adults, whereas others (Watkin, 1957-58; Albanese *et al.*, 1957; Horwitt, 1953) considered that there were no substantial differences between the requirements for protein in young and elderly adults. Conversely, Albanese *et al.* (1952) suggested, on the basis of their early studies, that the protein requirement for elderly women may be lower than that recommended for sedentary young women. It must be recognized also that a number of the studies presented in Table XIII were not based on precise metabolic nitrogen balances, conclusions were made often in conjunction with the then prevailing views on the estimated protein needs of young adults. Also, the level(s) of protein intake tested in the studies did not necessarily determine the minimum intake that would maintain nitrogen equilibrium. Thus, the available data do not allow definitive conclusions to be drawn concerning the minimum needs of older people.

TABLE XIII

Summary of Some Earlier Studies on N Balances and Protein Needs in the Elderly

Estimate and Conclusions	Remarks	Author
N equilibrium in 7 or 8 women studied was 0.7 and 1.0 g of protein/kg/day. (Dietary standards were adequate.)	Healthy women, 52-74 years old, were studied.	Roberts _et_ _al_. (1948)
Good nutritional state was maintained at 54 ± 5 g protein/kg/day.	N balance was assessed from diet records of 20 women, ages 68-88 years.	Albanese _et_ _al_. (1957)
Protein needs of elderly people did not differ from those of younger adults.	Data were taken from a review of studies with older men and women in a mental hospital.	Horwitt (1953)
No evidence was found of qualitative or quantitative changes with age.	N balance was studied in healthy elderly men.	Watkin (1957-1958)
Elderly people require 0.7 g protein/kg/day.	Four poorly nourished men, 69-76 years old, were studied.	Kountz _et_ _al_. (1951)
Protein requirement for elderly women may be 20-30% lower than for young women.	Nine women, 66-94 years old, maintained their health with free-choice intakes.	Albanese _et_ _al_. (1952)

We have recently explored further the minimum protein needs of healthy elderly women through the nitrogen balance approach (Perera, W.D.A., Scrimshaw, N.S., and Young, V.R., unpublished results). Our objective was to determine whether the 1973 FAO/WHO "safe" practical allowance for protein in adults (0.57 g and 0.52 g of egg protein per kg per day for men and women, respectively) was also sufficient to maintain nitrogen equilibrium in the healthy aged individual. Some of the results obtained from six elderly women who received 0.52 g of egg protein per kg per day over relatively prolonged periods are given in Table XIV. As mentioned in the above discussion, this level of protein intake is higher than the safe practical allowance computed by the factorial approach (see Table XII).

TABLE XIV

Nitrogen Balance in Elderly Women Receiving the 1973 FAO/WHO "Safe Practical Allowance" of Egg Protein (0.52 g/kg/day) During Relatively Long Metabloic Balance Periods [1]

Subject	Age	Body Weight	Days of Diet	Nitrogen Balance [2]
	(yr)	(kg)		(g N/day)
1	73	80.0	15 - 21	+1.27
			22 - 31	+0.97
2	84	63.6	8 - 14	-0.73
			15 - 21	-0.65
			22 - 31	-0.24
3	75	79.1	8 - 13	-0.30
			14 - 20	-0.60
			21 - 30	+0.64
4	69	85.2	8 - 14	+1.42
			15 - 21	-1.25
			22 - 31	+0.88
5	82	51.5	8 - 14	+0.22
			15 - 21	+0.49
6	85	51.2	8 - 14	0.0
			15 - 28	-0.05

[1]Data are the unpublished results of Perera, Scrimshaw, and Young.

[2]These values include an allowance of 5 mg N/kg/day for integumental and other unmeasured losses.

From the results shown in Table XIV, only one subject was clearly in positive nitrogen balance after two weeks of study. The others were either in slightly positive or negative balance. These results do not indicate that all the subjects were receiving sufficient protein to maintain a consistent and satisfactory balance of body nitrogen.

Biochemical parameters, including serum albumin and total protein and hemoglobin levels, were also measured in these studies to assess further the adequacy of the 0.52 g of egg protein per kg per day level of intake. For one or more of these parameters, trends toward decreasing values were noted in five subjects whose nitrogen balance data did not clearly indicate that 0.52 g of egg protein per kg per day was an adequate level of protein intake.

Before beginning our studies, we anticipated that the 1973 FAO/WHO "safe" practical allowance for protein would be adequate for healthy elderly people, particularly in view of the lower body cell mass per unit of body weight in this age group as compared with young adults. However, our findings do not support the adequacy of the 1973 FAO/WHO "safe" allowance of egg protein intake for healthy elderly women. Our results may also suggest that the efficiency of utilization of high-quality animal protein in this age group may be less than in young adults. Additional comparative studies are needed to explore this possibility. Our long-term metabolic studies in young adults, which demonstrate the inadequacy of the 1973 FAO/WHO "safe" practical allowance for egg protein in healthy young men (Garza *et al.*, 1976), also indicate the need for a reevaluation of protein requirements in all age groups.

Factors Affecting the Protein Requirement

Appropriate minimum dietary allowances cannot be formulated for population groups, such as the elderly, until individual variations have been studied in a systematic and critical way. Furthermore, it is important to emphasize that our studies have involved healthy individuals.

A number of factors contribute to variations in nutrient requirements. Environmental, host, and agent factors that may affect the utilization and requirements for protein in the elderly are shown in Table XV, and we have considered these in more detail in relation to variability in nutrient needs (Scrimshaw and Young, 1976).

It is well recognized that requirements are less for protein, *per se*, than for essential amino acids, in appropriate proportions, and for a source of nonspecific nitrogen. It is worth noting, in this context, that current estimates of amino acid requirements for adults are based primarily on metabolic balance studies of small numbers of university students, which took place about 20-30 years ago (e.g., Rose, 1957). Differences of over 100% between individuals with the lowest and highest requirements often were observed for some of the essential amino acids. This has been a more or less consistent finding in recent studies (e.g., Hegsted, 1963; Hold and Snyderman, 1965) concerned with estimating individual essential amino acid requirements. This phenomenon makes it difficult to define protein nutrition in terms of essential amino acid and total nitrogen needs, at this time.

TABLE XV

Agent, Host, and Environmental Factors That Influence Dietary Protein Requirements and Nutritional Status in the Elderly

Agent Factors:

1. Level of protein intake
2. Amino acid composition of protein
3. Energy intake
4. Food processing and preparation
5. Other dietary constituents

Host Factors:

1. Age
2. Sex
3. Genetic makeup
4. Pathological states
   a. infection
   b. trauma
   c. neoplasia
5. Psychological state

Environmental Factors:

1. Physical
2. Biological
3. Socioeconomic

In addition to the reported variation in amino acid requirements among individuals participating in any single experiment, the dietary criteria used to judge the requirements have varied both among and within laboratories. This variation makes it impossible to utilize the aggregate data to develop even an approximation of the variation in requirements for any of the essential amino acids in any population group. Furthermore, the practical significance of the published estimates of the minimum requirements for essential amino acids are open to serious question for experimental reasons, which we have discussed previously (Young and Scrimshaw, 1976).

Stress, particularly infection, is a major factor influencing individual requirements for protein and most other nutrients. Any infection, no matter how mild or subclinical, has potentially adverse consequences, the significance of which depends on the previous nutritional status of the individual, the nature, severity, and duration of the infection, as well as the diet during and after the infectious episode.

During mild infections, appetite is reduced, and urinary nitrogen excretion is increased. Other sources of stress, such as physical injury or metabolic disease, increase nitrogen excretion and, therefore, potentially modify protein requirements. The net result is an increase in the amount of protein required to maintain an acceptable nutritional status. Because elderly people are more vulnerable to these factors, it is important to mention their effects on protein metabolism and nutrition. As Watkin (1957-58) has stated: "Socioeconomic factors and presence of disease have far more practical influence than age *per se*, in determining the status of protein nutrition in the aged."

The qualitative effects of some acute infections on dietary nitrogen utilization have been described by Beisel (1966). Unfortunately, the available data are of little value in quantifying the effects of infection on nutrient needs in the elderly. However, it is known that any infection, or other stressful stimuli of physical or psychological origin, produces a tendency toward negative nitrogen balance through the cumulative effect of several different mechanisms. Furthermore, nitrogen is only one of several nutrients that respond to stress with a net loss; potassium and magnesium phosphorus, for example, respond similarly to infection (Beisel *et al.*, 1967), as does zinc metabolism after physical injury (Carr and Wilkinson, 1975).

The anabolic period that follows recovery from infection is characterized by a period of increased nitrogen retention, which is much longer than the catabolic period (Beisel, 1972). In spite of the potential for stressful stimuli and disease states to increase protein and amino acid needs in a majority of elderly people, there are no studies that help to assess the quantitative influence of these factors on nutrient utilization and dietary requirements. It is a complex problem, and there is an urgent need to explore and to define the nutritional and dietary significance of disease states that are common to so many members of the elderly population.

CONCLUSION

This review describes alterations in amino acid and whole body protein metabolism and also considers possible changes in dietary protein needs as a consequence of aging in man. Studies of plasma free amino acid levels do not reveal major differences among young adults and elderly subjects in the response of amino acid metabolism to dietary change. However, there are limitations to this approach, and studies of the quantitative aspects of amino acid utilization will be necessary before an adequate picture can be constructed on this phase of nitrogen metabolism in aging human beings. On the other hand, whole body protein metabolism shows a distinctive age-related shift in distribution, with muscle protein turnover contributing less to total body protein metabolism in the elderly than in the young.

The approaches and methods used for estimating the physiological protein needs in the elderly also are reviewed. Using the 1973 FAO/WHO factorial method, the "safe" practical allowance for high-quality protein is calculated to be 0.42 g per kg of body weight per day for healthy elderly women. The factors affecting the protein requirements of adults are considered together with nitrogen balance studies, and it is concluded that the FAO/WHO "safe" practical allowance underestimates the protein needs of older people. Until more data become available, the safest procedure to follow in planning diets for the elderly would be to adhere to the original United States Food and Nutrition Board estimates of 1 g of protein per kg of body weight per day.

ACKNOWLEDGEMENT

The unpublished results obtained in the authors' laboratories were supported by NIH grants HD 98300, AM 16654, AM 15856, and AM 15892.

REFERENCES

Ackerman, P.G. and Kheim, T. (1964). Clin. Chem. 10, 32.
Albanese, A.A., Higgens, R.A., Vestal, B., Stephanson, L., and Malsch, M. (1952). Geriatrics 7, 109.
Albanese, A.A., Higgens, R.A., Orto, L.A., and Zwattoro, D.N. (1957). Geriatrics 12, 465.
Allen, T.H., Anderson, E.C., and Langham, W.H. (1960). J. Gerontol. 15, 348.
Armstrong, M.D. and Stave, U. (1973a). Metabolism 22, 561.
Armstrong, M.D. and Stave, U. (1973b). Metabolism 22, 571.

Asatoor, A.M. and Armstrong, M.D. (1967). Biochem. Biophys. Res. Commun. 26, 168.
Beaton, G.H. (1972). In "Proceedings of the Western Hemisphere Nutrition Congress, III" (P. L. White, ed.), p. 356, Futura, Mount Kisco, New York.
Beaton, G.H. and Swiss, L.D. (1974). Am. J. Clin. Nutr. 27, 485.
Beisel, W.R. (1966). Fed. Proc. 25, 1682.
Beisel, W.R. (1972). Am. J. Clin. Nutr. 25, 1254.
Beisel, W.R., Sawyer, W.D., Pyll, E.D., and Crazier, D. (1967). Arch. Intern. Med. 67, 744.
Boddy, K., King, P.C., and Carswell, F. (1975). Clin. Sci. Mol. Med. 49, 133.
Bricker, M.L. and Smith, J.M. (1951). J. Nutr. 44, 553.
Brody, S. (1945). "Bioenergetics and Growth". Reinhold, New York.
Buse, M.G. and Reid, S.S. (1975). J. Clin. Invest. 56, 1250.
Cahill, G.F., Jr., Aokc, T.T., and Marless, E.B. (1972). In "Handbook of Physiology" (D. F. Steiner and N. Freinkel, eds.), Vol. 1, p. 563, American Physiology Society, Washington, D. C.
Carr, G. and Wilkinson, A.W. (1975). Clin. Chim. Acta 61, 199.
Department of Health and Social Security. (1969). "Recommended Intakes of Nutrients for the United Kingdom". Report, Public Health, Medical Subject No. 120, Her Majesty's Stationery Office, London.
Food and Agriculture Organization/WHO. (1973). "Energy and Protein Requirements". World Health Organization Report Series No. 522. WHO, Geneva.
Food and Nutrition Board. (1974). "Recommended Dietary Allowances". 8th ed., Revised. National Academy of Sciences, Washington, D. C.
Forbes, G.B. (1972). Growth 36, 325.
Forbes, G.B. (1974). Am. J. Clin. Nutr. 27, 595.
Forbes, G.B. and Reina, J.C. (1970). Metabolism 19, 653.
Fulks, R.M., Li, J.B., and Goldberg, A.L. (1975). J. Biol. Chem. 250, 290.
Garza, C., Scrimshaw, N.S., and Young, V.R. (1976). Am. J. Clin. Nutr. (in press).
Gutmann, E. (1970). Exp. Gerontol. 5, 357.
Halliday, D. and McKeran, R.O. (1975). Clin. Sci. Mol. Med. 49, 581.
Hambraeus, L., Bilmazes, C., Dippel, C., Scrimshaw, N.S., and Young, V.R. (1976). J. Nutr. 106, 230.
Haverberg, L.N., Omstedt, P.T., Munro, H.N., and Young, V.R. (1975). Biochim. Biophys. Acta 405, 67.
Hegsted, D.M. (1963). Fed. Proc. 22, 1424.

Hegsted, D.M. (1972). Ecol. Food Nutr. 1, 225.
Holt, L.E., Jr. and Snyderman, S.E. (1965). Nutr. Abstr. Rev. 35, 1.
Horwitt, M.K. (1953). J. Am. Diet. Assoc. 29, 443.
Irwin, M.I. and Hegsted, D.M. (1971a). J. Nutr. 101, 53.
Irwin, M.I. and Hegsted, D.M. (1971b). J. Nutr. 101, 385.
Kleiber, M. (1961). "The Fire of Life". John Wiley and Sons, New York.
Korenchevsky, V. (1961). "Physiological and Pathological Ageing" (G. H. Bourne, ed.), S. Karger, Basel.
Kountz, W.B., Hofsotter, B.L., and Ackermann, P.C. (1951). J. Gerontol. 6, 20.
Kraut, H. and Müller-Wecker, H. (1960). Hoppe-Seyler's Z. Physiol. Chem. 320, 241.
Lonergan, M.E., Milne, J.S., Maule, M.M., and Williamson, J. (1975). Brit. J. Nutr. 34, 517.
Long, C.O., Haverberg, L.N., Kinney, J.M., Young, V.R., Munro, H.N., and Geiger, J.W. (1975). Metabolism 24, 929.
McGandy, R.B., Barrows, C.H., Jr., Spanias, A., Meredity, A., Stone, J.L., and Norris, A.H. (1966). J. Gerontol. 21, 581.
McLaughlan, J.M. (1974). In "Improvement of Protein Nutriture", p. 89, National Academy of Sciences, Washington, D. C.
Millward, D.J. and Garlick, P.J. (1972). Proc. Nutr. Soc. 31, 257.
Millward, D.J., Garlick, P.J., Steward, R.J.C., Nnanyelugo, D.O., and Waterlow, J.C. (1975). Biochem. J. 150, 235.
Munro, H.N. (1964). In "Mammalian Protein Metabolism" (H. N. Munro and J. B. Allison, eds.), Vol. 1, Chapter 10, Academic Press, New York.
Munro, H.N. (1969). In "Mammalian Protein Metabolism" (H. N. Munro, ed.), Vol. 3, p. 133, Academic Press, New York.
Munro, H.N. (1972). In "Nutrition in Old age" (L. A. Carlson, ed.), p. 32, Swedish Nutrition Foundation, Uppsala.
Nicholson, J.F. (1970). Pediatr. Res. 4, 389.
Novak, L.P., Hamamoto, K., Orves, A.L., and Burke, E.C. (1970). Am. J. Dis. Child. 119, 419.
O'Keefe, S.J.D., Sender, P.M., and James, W.P.T. (1974). Lancet 2, 1035.
Özalp, I., Young, V.R., Nagchaudhury, J., Tontisirin, K., and Scrimshaw, N.S. (1972). J. Nutr. 102, 1147.
Parizkova, J., Eiselt, E., Spryvarova, S., and Wachtlova, M. (1971). J. Appl. Physiol. 31, 323.
Picou, D. and Taylor-Roberts, T. (1969). Clin. Sci. 36, 283.
Rao, R., Metta, V.C., and Johnson, B.C. (1959). J. Nutr. 69, 387.

Roberts, P.H., Kerr, C.H., and Ohlson, M.A. (1948). J. Am. Diet. Assoc. 24, 292.
Roessle, R. and Roulet, F. (1932). In "Pathologie und Klinik in Einzeldarstellungen" (Aschoff et al., eds.), Vol. 5, p. 1, Springer, Berlin. (Cited by Korenchevsky, 1961).
Rogers, Q.R. and Leung, P.M.B. (1973). Fed. Proc. 32, 1709.
Rose, W.C. (1957). Nutr. Abstr. Rev. 27, 631.
Said, A.K. and Hegsted, D.M. (1970). J. Nutr. 100, 1363.
Scrimshaw, N.S. and Young, V.R. (1976). In "Biological and Cultural Sources of Variability in Human Nutrition" (S. Margen, ed.), AVI Publishing Corp., Westport, Conn. (in press).
Scrimshaw, N.S., Taylor, C.E., and Gordon, J.E. (1968). "Interactions of Nutrition and Infection". World Health Organization Monograph Series No. 57. WHO, Geneva.
Scrimshaw, N.S., Hussein, M.A., Murray, E., Rand, W.M., and Young, V.R. (1972). J. Nutr. 102, 1595.
Scrimshaw, N.S., Perera, W.D.A., and Young, V.R. (1976). J. Nutr. (in press).
Sharp, C.S., Lassen, S., Shankman, S., Hazlet, J.W., and Kednis, M.S. (1957). J. Nutr. 63, 155.
Sketcher, R.D., Fern, E.B., and James, W.P.T. (1974). Brit. J. Nutr. 31, 333.
Sprinson, D.B. and Rittenberg, D. (1949). J. Biol. Chem. 180, 715.
Steffee, W.P., Goldsmith, R.S., Pencharz, P.B., Scrimshaw, N.S., and Young, V.R. (1975). Metabolism (in press).
Tontisirin, K., Young, V.R., and Scrimshaw, N.S. (1972). Am. J. Clin. Nutr. 25, 976.
Tontisirin, K., Young, V.R., Miller, M., and Scrimshaw, N.S. (1973). J. Nutr. 103, 1220.
Tontisirin, K., Young, V.R., Rand, W.M., and Scrimshaw, N.S. (1974). J. Nutr. 104, 495.
Waterlow, J.C. (1968). Lancet 2, 1091.
Waterlow, J.C. (1969). In "Mammalian Protein Metabolism" (H. N. Munro, ed.), Vol. 3, p. 325, Academic Press, New York.
Waterlow, J.C. and Stephen, J.M.L. (1967). Clin. Sci. 33, 489.
Waterlow, J.C. and Stephen, J.M.L. (1968). Clin. Sci. 35, 287.
Waterlow, J.C., Garrow, J.S., and Millward, D.J. (1969). Clin. Sci. 36, 489.
Watkin, D.M. (1957-58). Ann. N.Y. Acad. Sci. 69, 902.
Watkin, D.M. (1964). In "Mammalian Protein Metabolism" (H.N. Munro, and J.B. Allison, eds.), Vol. 2, p. 247, Academic Press, New York.

Watkin, D.M. (1966). In "World Review of Nutrition and Dietetics" (G.H. Bourne, ed.), Vol. 6, p. 124, S. Karger, Basel.
Wehr, R.F. and Lewis, G.T. (1966). Proc. Soc. Exp. Biol. Med. 121, 349.
Widdowson, E.M. and Dickerson, J.W.T. (1964). In "Mineral Metabolism" (C. L. Comar and F. Bronner, eds.), Vol. 2, Part A, pp. 1-247, Academic Press, New York.
Winterer, J.C., Steffee, W.P., Perera, W.D.S., Uuay, R., Scrimshaw, N.S., and Young, V.R. (1976). Exp. Gerontol. (in press).
Wurtman, R.J. and Fernstrom, J.D. (1975). Am. J. Clin. Nutr. 28, 638.
Yamamoto, H., Aikowa, T., Motsutaka, H., Okuda, T., and Ishidawa, E. (1974). Am. J. Physiol. 226, 1428.
Young, V.R. (1970). In "Mammalian Protein Metabolism" (H.N. Munro, ed.), Vol. 4, pp. 585-674, Academic Press, New York.
Young, V.R. and Scrimshaw, N.S. (1972). In "Protein and Amino Acid Functions" (E. J. Bigwood, ed.), Vol. 11, p. 541, Pergamon Press, New York.
Young, V.R. and Scrimshaw, N.S. (1976). In "Proteins for Human Consumption" (C. E. Bodwell, ed.), Chapter 2, AVI Publishing Corp., Westport, Conn. (in press).
Young, V.R., Hussein, M.A., Murray, E., and Scrimshaw, N.S. (1971). J. Nutr. 101, 45.
Young, V.R., Alexis, S.D., Baliga, B.S., Munro, H.N., and Muecke, W. (1972). J. Biol. Chem. 247, 3592.
Young, V.R., Haverberg, L.N., Bilmazes, C., and Munro, H.N. (1973). Metabolism 22, 1429.
Young, V.R., Perera, W.D., Winterer, J.S., and Scrimshaw, N.S. (1976a). In "Nutrition and Aging" (M. Winick, ed.), J. Wiley and Sons, New York (in press).
Young, V.R., Winterer, J.S., Munro, H.N., and Scrimshaw, N.S. (1976b). Adv. Exp. Aging Res. 1 (in press).
Yousef, M.K. and Johnson, H.D. (1970). Proc. Soc. Exp. Biol. Med. 133, 1351.

BEHAVIORAL ASPECTS OF NUTRITION AND LONGEVITY IN ANIMALS[1]

Leonard F. Jakubczak, Ph.D.

Veterans Administration Hospital
St. Louis, Missouri 63125

Prospectus

Changes in the environment may modify the duration of life. Diet is one such environmental factor. Feeding behavior is an essential link in nutrition. Since nutrition affects duration of life, free feeding behavior, at least in part, influences aging and disease, and may in turn be influenced by them. The effects of aging on spontaneous activity may contribute to overnutrition and further enhance aging. On the other hand, increased spontaneous activity may retard aging. Because of their critical roles in longevity, the age-related changes in mechanisms underlying short-term and long-term control of feeding and activity deserve further investigation by gerontologists.

Aging

Aging is a process of unfavorable progressive change, usually correlated with the passage of time, becoming apparent after maturity and terminating invariably in death of the individual (Lansing, 1959). Other alternatives to this irreversible decrement model of aging, however, are possible (Schaie, 1965).

Longevity, growth, aging and disease are commonly held to be interrelated (Silberberg and Silberberg, 1955). Accelerated aging is generally thought to shorten the duration of life, and the retardation of aging is considered to prolong life. In the majority of cases life is terminated by intervening diseases, although some deaths cannot be attributed to specific diseases. Finally, the rate of growth, or some correlate of it, may determine the rate of aging and thus the duration of life.

Morbidity

The relationship between morbidity and mortality has

[1]Medical Research Information System Number 0150.

been well demonstrated by Simms (1965). The relationship between the logarithmic probability of onset of lesions (five major diseases added together) and the logarithmic probability of death is linear. Thus a constant percentage change in the lesion probability produces a constant percentage change in probability of death. In other words, the probability of death increases as a power function of the probability of lesion.

However, aging is considered a process involving loss of the ability to live. Degenerative diseases that may or may not lead to death of the individual are considered separate from aging (Lansing, 1959). They may have their origins in mechanisms quite apart from aging, or they may do their damage in a system made vulnerable by aging. A sharp line cannot be drawn between aging and degenerative disease because we lack specific criteria for either.

What factors determine the duration of life in general and in particular, and what is the relative influence of each of these factors in producing death?

Nutrition

On the most general level, life expectancy is determined by the interaction of genetic and environmental factors which both influence the rate of aging and bring on death through disease or, in rare instances, cause life to end in "natural" death (Silberberg and Silberberg, 1955). Changes in the environment may modify the duration of life. Diet is one such environmental factor. Dietary influences may exert their effects on the duration of life by affecting the course of disease as well as the process of aging.

Nutrition is the process of assimilating food for the biochemical process of living. The organism needs to be nourished to perform the normal and essential functions of life such as growth, maintenance, reproduction, lactation and behavior. The fundamental requirements for adequate nutrition include water, energy, carbohydrates, fats, proteins, minerals and vitamins. These are supplied the organism through diet - the customary allowance of food and water taken by an individual from day to day.

Behavior

In complex organisms, the diet has to be taken into the individual by the behavioral processes of eating and drinking. The latter has been neglected in longitudinal nutritional studies (McCay, 1952). In his review of the evolution of food-getting behavior, Bates (1958) concluded that, in general, vertebrates are committed to active, food-seeking behavior, and this is perhaps correlated with their generally large body size which requires considerable food for maintenance. It is also correlated with the structure of the vertebrate nervous system with its centralized brain - a system that allows for plasticity or modifiability of behavior and for an increasing dominance of various kinds of learning and habituation processes in behavior. Thus, food-getting behavior and survival are interrelated.

That food-getting behavior and nutrition are interrelated is suggested by the work of Fernstrom and Wurtman (1971). These investigators found that when a meal rich in carbohydrate is eaten, the brain produces larger quantities of the nerve-impulse transmitter, serotonin. This mechanism may be part of a closed circle in which diet influences food consumption and *vice versa*. My point of view in this paper is that free-feeding behavior influences aging and disease via its nutritional effects and may, in turn, be influenced by aging and disease.

Animals

There are several reasons for using animal subjects in studies of nutrition and aging. First, a great deal is known about age-related changes in the anatomy, the physiology and the behavior of animal subjects. If one wants to test the effects of nutrition on such age-related changes, one should use similar organisms. Second, certain experimental procedures may be carried out with animals that could not be carried out on man because of their danger and discomfort, *e.g.*, arresting growth by means of dietary restriction. Third, because of the relatively short life span of animals and because of the possibility of genetic, nutritional and environmental control and manipulation over the entire life span, research with animals should make an important contribution to the understanding of such determinants of biological and behavioral aging. The working assumption in this area is that the basic mechanisms of aging are similar enough in man and other mammals so that research on the latter will often generalize to man.

Dietary Factors Influencing Longevity

Previous reviews on the relationship between life expectancy, morbidity, and nutrition include those by McCay (1952), Silberberg and Silberberg (1955), Ross (1959), and Comfort (1964).

Early investigations indicated that moderate dietary restriction during certain periods of life have a beneficial effect on longevity (Silberberg and Silberberg, 1955). A high level of dietary fat had, generally, adverse effects on life expectancy. The effects were in certain respects the opposite of those exhibited by underfeeding. The current review indicates that longevity depends on diet, its caloric value and quality, mode and duration of feeding, and age at which a diet is introduced; increases in longevity are correlated with postponement of onsets of diseases to older ages; and early dietary preferences are related to disease and longevity.

Quantity

Severe restriction of calories retards growth but increases longevity. Groups of weanling rats were reared by McCay *et al.* (1943) on a single, restricted diet sufficient in all other constituents but deficient in calories, and their growth slightly retarded. After periods of growth retardation up to 1000 days, the restriction of calorie intake was terminated and the rats were allowed to eat the source of additional calories *ad libitum*, with resulting more rapid growth restored. The rats then grew rapidly almost to adult size and lived longer than the unretarded groups. The long survival was accompanied by a decrease in the incidence of pulmonary disease and tumors.

These findings were confirmed and extended by Berg (1960) and Berg and Simms (1960). Levels of food restriction were used which prevented accumulation of an excess of body fat and yet provided for good skeletal growth. When food intake was thus restricted (single diet), longevity was extended (Simms, 1965) and onset of disease was delayed (Berg and Simms, 1960). Thus longevity can be extended without necessarily retarding growth.

Quantity, Quality of Diet and Mode of Feeding

Longevity is influenced not only by the quantity, but also by the quality of diet and the mode of its feeding. Ross (1961) varied the components of the diet of rats separately and allowed some rats free access to these diets but restricted others. The findings suggest that, under conditions of restriction, whether spontaneous or administered, enhancement of life span may be accomplished by the reduction in intake of total dietary components. Under unrestricted conditions the relationship of the dietary constituents to one another (*e.g.*, protein/carbohydrate) assumes a large role

(Ross, 1961).

The mode of feeding influences the effects of each particular diet on longevity and disease. Under conditions of restricted diet, the emphasis is on the nutritional aspects of the diet as an independent variable. The investigator exerts relatively direct control over the nutrition (*e.g.*, Ross, 1961) and can make deductions about its effects on some dependent variable - *i.e.*, morbidity, longevity, biochemistry, etc. Under *ad libitum* conditions of feeding, the effects of nutrition on such dependent variables are *secondary* to the effects of variation in the dietary components, as well as to other factors, such as mechanisms controlling food intake. Variations in amounts of food eaten must be taken into account in evaluating dietary influences on longevity. They focus in on the mechanisms that control the amounts of food eaten and whether they are themselves affected by diseases and aging.

Returning to Ross (1961), semisynthetic diets resulted in longer life expectancies when rats were fed on a restricted than on an unrestricted basis. The only exception to this observation was the diet low in protein and high in carbohydrate (8% and 83%, respectively) which when fed *ad libitum* was equally as effective in enhancing life expectancy as when fed on a restricted basis. Under unrestricted conditions, the total intake of food was higher for rats on the other three diets. Hence this *self-imposed* limitation in food consumption which is generally seen in rats fed diets with levels low in protein and high in carbohydrate (Hamilton, 1965) may account for the relatively longer life expectancy. Such effects, however, must be presumed as secondary to the effects of variations in relative proportions of the dietary constituents upon mechanisms regulating food intake (Ross *et al.*, 1970).

Nevertheless, when the diets are given on a restricted basis, the superiority of low protein-high carbohydrate diet on an unrestricted basis is lost, since even longer life expectancies are produced by feeding on the three other diets.

The quality of the restricted diet seems to have had some differential effect on life expectancy. Restriction of protein alone produced little increase in longevity; restriction of carbohydrate produced some gain, but less than when protein, calorie intake and carbohydrate were all restricted in one diet. The increase in longevity resulting from diet restriction is correlated with a displacement of incidence of kidney disease and tumors to later chronological age (Bras and Ross, 1964; Ross and Bras, 1965). This delay is inversely correlated with caloric intake - *i.e.*, the lower the caloric intake the greater the delay in appearance of pathology. This caloric effect may be mediated by rates of weight gain and maximal weight earlier in life. It seems that the more rapid the weight gain and the higher the maximal weight, the higher the probability that a tumor will develop (Ross *et al.*, 1970).

Further experimentation confirmed that the quality of diet as well as calories and mode of feeding influence longevity. The protein/calorie ratio of a diet under *ad libitum* and restricted isocaloric conditions of feeding modify the risk of increasing spontaneous tumors in the male rat. The direction and magnitude of the influence, which differs with *mode of feeding*, is dependent on the tissue origin, type and malignancy of the tumor (Ross and Bras, 1973). Nevertheless, in both *ad libitum* and restricted dietary series, life expectancy increased as the portion of dietary protein increased. The restricted rats lived longer than the *ad libitum* rats. Separate, direct correlations, representing individual differences among animals, were obtained between the average daily amount of protein consumed and life expectancy of each diet group. These results showed how much chronic protein undernutrition and protein overnutrition under isocaloric conditions modify the tumor-type spectrum and mortality of the rats. This diversity of response seems to negate an earlier view that the nutritional effects are mediated through a single common underlying mechanism (Ross and Bras, 1965, 1971). Ross and Bras (1973) feel that these changes in predisposition appear to be commensurate with the effects of defects in the functional activities of both the endocrine and cell-mediated immune systems. Thus the effects of nutrition on longevity may be mediated in part at least by the endocrine and immune systems. Walford (1969) believes that the latter system is of prime importance.

Age

Age at which diet is introduced seems to be critical in determining the direction and extent of the effects of dietary restriction on longevity. Extreme undernutrition of the mammalian organism during early development can affect ultimate body weight and cause various abnormalities in metabolism and functional capacities (Roeder and Chow, 1972). The alterations that accompanied *prenatal* undernourishment of rats and mice included stunted growth, deficient renal tubular function, retarded neuromotor development, and impaired *learning* capacity. When the period of undernourishment extended through both pre- and early postnatal life, *i.e.*, until weaning, the effects were similar but of much greater magnitude. Many of the characteristics of the survivors during early life indicated delayed development and, therefore, perhaps a reduced rate of aging. However, during adulthood and senescence these experimental animals resembled chronologically *older* ones on the basis of several criteria such as response to stress and rate of development of age-associated biochemical changes. This apparent *acceleration* of aging may be related to increased food intake relative to body weight throughout postweaning life.

At the other end of the life span, McCay *et al*. (1941) showed that no further increase in longevity could be brought about by restricting rats beyond the first year of life. Barrows and Roeder (1965) reported that rats subjected to reduced dietary intake during the latter part of life did not live longer than *ad libitum*-fed control rats.

In view of these considerations, longevity studies were undertaken to assess the influence upon length of life of both the level of food intake and the age of the rat when an experimental dietary regimen was instituted (Ross, 1972). Length of life was found to be influenced by the dietary experience early in life, *i.e*., post-weaning. A period of restriction of food intake from 21 to 70 days only, even though followed by *ad libitum* feedings, resulted in a decrease in tumor risk and an increase in length of life (Ross and Bras,1971; Ross,1972). The effects of *ad libitum* feeding early in life were overcome, in part, by the regimen of restriction subsequently imposed.

The level of restriction most conducive to an increase in length of life was found to change with age. The rats that were severely restricted in their intake of food throughout *post-weaning* life lived the longest. When the same level of restriction was imposed at later ages, life expectancy progressively decreased; in older rats the duration of life was drastically curtailed. Length of life of older and heavier rats, however, could be extended by restriction of food intake, when degree of restriction was less severe (Ross, 1972). These results raise the possibility that the nutritional status of the young, which is most conducive to an increase in life expectancy, may be of the type that adversely influences behavioral development probably by affecting the central nervous system (Kaplan, 1972). On the other hand, the life-shortening effects of a full feeding regimen early in life can, to some extent, be overcome by changing the dietary regimen after the critical periods have been passed (Ross, 1972).

Self-Selection

Longevity and diseases of age seem to be related to dietary preferences, especially early in life. In most studies, diets of fixed composition are offered either *ad libitum* or in limited amounts for arbitrarily assigned periods. Under *ad libitum* conditions, however, except for the amount of food consumed, the animals have no choice but to eat the diet provided; under restricted feeding conditions, even this option is denied them.

Recently, Ross and Bras (1974) provided each rat fed on a self-selection basis three complete isocaloric diets in separate containers instead of individual components. This allowed the rats free choice of the diet components. The choices differed only in the casein and sucrose content. To determine the influence of each of the diets separately, other rats were fed *ad libitum* in the conventional manner. Far more spontaneous tumors and more cases of kidney, heart, and prostate disease occurred among the *self-selection* rats than among the rats fed the same diets singly. The age-related diseases included glomerulonephrosis, myocardial fibrosis, and prostatitis. Further correlational analysis of the data from the group given a choice of diet (Ross and Bras, 1975) indicated that rats that chose to consume large amounts of food were more likely to be short-lived than rats whose intake was smaller. Furthermore, the protein content of the diet selected by long-lived rats remained relatively uniform throughout the greater part of life. By contrast, short-lived rats showed a progression of changes in preference. Caloric-density preferences also seem to change with age in a short-lived strain of rat but not in a long-lived strain (Jakubczak, 1973a). However, the ability to select essential nutrients seems to decline gradually with age in rats (McCay and Eaton, 1947).

Ross and Bras (1974) interpret the individual differences in mortality and morbidity as the direct consequence of the specific selections made by the individual rat in satisfying its unique metabolic needs. However, factors that lead to disease in later life may also influence the mechanisms mediating dietary choice. How the preferences for such selections came about is not known. Is the animal equipped with prewired recognition systems for each of the many substances for which it can have a need, or does it learn preferences for the tastes of only those foods associated with recovery from the needs it happened to have experienced (Rozin and Kalat, 1971)? How do the "needs" come about? Further work needs to be done to clarify these issues.

Thus, in general, aging and age-related disease are

affected by nutrition which in turn is affected, at least in part, by feeding behavior:

"Since dietary composition influences appetite, the relative degree of 'internal restriction' must be taken into account in evaluating dietary influence upon life span" (Ross, 1961).

"...the impressive increase in the risk of developing tumors or of other diseases of age must be viewed as the direct consequence of the specific selection made by the individual in satisfying its unique metabolic 'needs'" (Ross and Bras, 1974).

"...the level of dietary protein under *ad libitum* conditions can also be considered to influence the tumorgenesis ...such effects, however, must be presumed as secondary to the effects of variation in relative proportions of the dietary constituents upon *mechanisms regulating food intake*" (Ross and Bras, 1970, my italics).

If the mechanisms regulating food intake are so critical in affecting age-specific disease and longevity during free feeding, what do we know about them during aging? Little!

Food Intake

Investigation of the effects of aging on the mechanisms that control food intake, body weight and activity is important since, it appears that aging is associated with less effective satiety mechanisms with respect to eating, leading to both greater obesity and finickiness (Kennedy, 1950). A similar view is presented by Verzar (1963). The caloric surplus represented by such obesity may reflect failure of the behavioral and physiological mechanisms by which energy balance is normally controlled (Mayer and Thomas, 1967; LeMagnen *et al*., 1973). Not only in man, but in rats and mice as well, increased age brings about an increase in amount and variability of body fat (Korenchevsky, 1961; Lesser *et al*., 1970). This suggests that naturally occurring and experimental obesity in animals may be models for obesity in man.

The study of the contribution of *either* the behavioral or the metabolic effect or of both to the regulation of energy provides a means for elucidating the nature of the involved central systems and their relationships (LeMagnen, 1971). Food intake may be considered an animal response that is a component of several not necessarily compatible systems of physiological regulation (Hamilton, 1965). *Feeding is a central link in the control of energy balance of the body and nutrition*.

Relatively little is known about the influence of aging on the mechanisms that control food intake and activity. The capacity of these mechanisms to respond to starvation, to changes in caloric value of their food, and to ambient temperature remains intact over a large span of the rat's lifetime (Jakubczak, 1970, 1973c, 1976). However, in older animals, palatibility factors, such as taste and texture, influence this capacity and lead to over- or under-eating (Jakubczak, 1970). These age differences were influenced by the genetic makeup of the animal (Jakubczak, 1973b). The results were consistent with those of Kennedy (1950) and Nisbett et al. (1975) and extended them to older age groups. Are there other aspects of the control of food intake and body weight that change with age?

A distinction should be made between long-term characteristics of feeding as measured in body weight and grams of food per day, and the short-term reactions such as the initiation and cessation of single meals and the actual rate of eating (Hamilton, 1965). The free daily intake of food is a product of meal sizes and meal frequency. By measuring separately the two components of the daily accumulative intake it might be possible to identify different factors involved in the control of these two parameters and to look for their relative contribution to the daily regulation (LeMagnen, 1971). Panskepp (1973), however, suggests that ratios of meal size to inter-meal intervals might be more informative.

There seem to be age-related decrements in the mechanisms that mediate meal size and frequency. Studies indicate that there are age differences in the day-night pattern of amount of food intake (Jakubczak, 1975), and that these differences are primarily due to increased meal size, especially during the daylight hours (Fig. 1). These data suggest age-related decrements in the development of satiety during a meal, but also in its dissipation since the increased meal size was not followed by a decreased inter-meal interval! Such a failure would result in a positive energy balance, leading to and/or maintaining obesity (LeMagnen et al., 1973; Kenney and Mook, 1974).

Factors that control meal size, meal frequency, and activity patterns are now briefly reviewed, and related to the state of gerontological knowledge. Although basic research in these areas is very active, and thus its conclusions and models tentative, they may be considered heuristic to gerontological research (Birren, 1959).

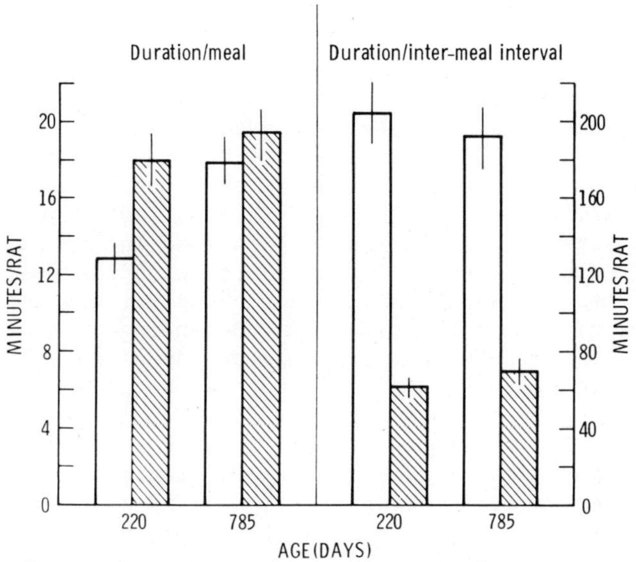

Fig. 1 Means and standard error of the means of meal durations and inter-meal intervals of rats as a function of age and lighting conditions (time of day). Note different scales. White bars = light (0600-1800 hrs.); cross-hatched bars = dark (1800-0600 hrs.).

Meal Size

Meal size seems to be determined by orogastric actions of the food (Snowdon, 1970; LeMagnen, 1971; Davis and Campbell, 1973), gut hormones (Smith *et al.*, 1974), and conditioned satiety (Booth, 1972). The initial facilitation of eating depends upon orosensory actions of the food as well as possible activating effect of an empty stomach. The deceleration of eating rate during the latter part of the meal seems to be due to inhibiting effects of foods present in the stomach. Furthermore, the range within which meal sizes vary is mediated centrally via the vagus nerve in response to nutritive deficits or surfeits (Snowdon, 1970). The peripherally induced satiety is transient since it depends upon the emptying time of the stomach which in turn depends upon the volume of the meal and its nutritive/osmotic properties (Snowdon, 1970). The satiety which occurs at the termination of a spontaneous meal also may be due to the intestinal hormone cholecystokinin (CCK) (Smith *et al.*, 1974). Finally, oral control of meal size can be conditioned (Booth, 1972). Thus oral qualities of a familiar food may enable an animal to anticipate the food's caloric value or the duration of its satiety effect (LeMagnen, 1971; Garcia et al., 1974).

Orogastric factors certainly are implicated in age-related differences in food intake as suggested by Kennedy (1950). Young and old rats responded equally to the dilution of the caloric density of food with water by increasing total intake, thus regulating the number of calories eaten and body weight (Jakubczak, 1970). However, addition of quinine to the food attenuated this increase in food intake to a greater degree in old rats than in young rats, with the result that the old rats did not maintain their body weights as well as the young rats. In the same vein, depending on the strain, old rats prefer calorically dense, greasy diets either to an equal degree or to a lesser degree than do young rats (Jakubczak, 1973a). However, taste thresholds are higher with increasing age in rats (Goodrick, 1969). The seeming inconsistency between age-related decrements in taste sensitivity observed by Goodrick (1969) and the age-related increments in finickiness which Kennedy (1950) and Jakubczak (1970) observed needs clarification.

Little is known of age-related changes in gastric factors. The intensity, duration, and frequency of stomach contractions are less in old than in young hungry dogs (Ivy and Grossman, 1952). Information on gastric motility and emptying is lacking (Ceokas, 1969). The effects of removal of stomach contents, gastric emptying, gastric loads, and vagotomy on meal size and meal frequency as a function of age need to be studied.

Even less is known about the relationship between age and conditioned satiety in animals. Classical conditioning is more difficult with increasing age (Jakubczak, 1973d). Perhaps the older rat is relatively insensitive to the internal signs of his caloric state and the caloric effects of a meal, or cannot associate these when novel food is used, or cannot "recall" these when familiar foods are used. Conditioned satiety as a function of age needs investigation to clarify the roles played by conditioning factors in the age-related decrement in satiety.

Meal Frequency

Meal frequency is controlled by glucostatic mechanisms which are modulated by lipostatic factors (LeMagnen et al., 1973) and/or by rate of stomach emptying (Snowdon, 1970). If in fact the old rat eats a meal of greater volume, it would then be expected to delay onset of the next meal (LeMagnen, 1971), but does not. Consequently, the failure to compensate for increased meal size may be due to age-related decrements in glucostatic, lipostatic, or gastric emptying mechanisms.

The glucostatic theory is a leading hypothesis for the explanation of the short-term control of food intake (Mayer and Thomas, 1967; Novin et al., 1973). Central as well as peripheral glucoreceptors signal "satiety" when glucose utilization is elevated. Glucose utilization, however, appears to decrease with age in humans (Silverstone et al., 1957), as well as animals (Klimas, 1968; Gommers, 1971). Such an age-related decrease in glucose utilization may decrease the "satiety" signal that follows a meal. This signal distortion may result in an error of short-term control of food intake leading to obesity.

Recent work by LeMagnen et al. (1973) suggests that a physiological, fat storage-fat release, diurnal cycle plays an important role in the daily control of food intake. Both the glucostatic control of food intake and the maintenance of a constant body weight seem dependent on the control of the diurnal reversibility of fat synthesis and release mechanisms. Impairment of the control of this movement of fats, particularly the mobilization in the daytime of fats stored in the night, seems to lead inevitably to 24-hour hyperphagia and to obesity. Is this what happens with increasing age to some degree? There is an age-dependent decrement of lipolysis in rats (Jelinkova and Stuchlíková, 1968). This may reduce the daylight lipolysis and also reduce the inter-meal interval. "The so-called nutritional obesity and the fattening in old age appear as exceptions to, or as a disruption of lipostatic regulation" (LeMagnen et al., 1973). This conjecture with respect to old age is to date without empirical basis.

An age-related decrease in hypothalamic functioning has been postulated to account for age-related decrements in hormonal functioning (Dilman, 1971; Everitt, 1973), autonomic nervous control (Froklis, 1968), homeostasis (Verzar, 1963), satiety (Kennedy, 1950), and activity, sexual behavior, and placidity (Nisbett et al., 1975). In turn, these decrements in hypothalamic functioning may be due to age-related loss of cells in the hypothalamic area or areas influencing the hypothalamus (Verzar, 1963). Consequently, the age-related decrements in the controls of meal size and meal frequency may be due to age-related decrements in the functioning of hypothalamic areas. On the other hand, changes in the ventromedial and lateral hypothalamus with age may also involve long-term changes in set-point around which the levels of body fat are regulated (Keesey and Powley, 1975).

Activity

Decreases in energy output via lowered activity levels also contribute to the age-related increases in obesity (Mayer and Thomas, 1967). Like slowness of response, age-related decrements in amounts of activity may be a universal characteristic of aging in animals, man included (Jakubczak, 1973d). With increasing age beyond sexual maturity, the levels of various forms of activity decrease in animals ranging from spiders to man. These various forms of general activity are more difficult to energize but easier to inhibit with increasing age. These decreases in activity are not accompanied by decreases in food and contribute to a surplus of calories and thus obesity. There seems to be a partial decoupling of the adjustment between food intake and activity. How this decoupling comes about is not known (Mayer, 1967) but its elucidation has tremendous implications for controlling the age-related increases in obesity. Mayer has proposed that the decoupling between food intake and activity is a consequence of evolutionary selection in which survival is enhanced by the ability to store energy in intervals of idleness.

The age-related decrement in daily activity of the rat as measured by an activity wheel, is due to decrements in frequency and duration of bursts of running, as well as speed (Jakubczak, 1973b). Thus, with increasing age, the rat runs at slower speeds, for a shorter time, and pauses longer. This may be due to age-related decrements in speed of responding, resistance to fatigue and recovery from it, or to age-related increases in levels of free fatty acids and decreases in the rate of their metabolism (Collier and Hirsch, 1971). These age-related decreases in activity also may be due, in part, to age-related <u>increases</u> in the effectiveness of inhibiting centers of the brain or to age-related decreases in the effectiveness of activation centers, or both (Campbell <u>et al</u>., 1969). Since vagotomized rats run more during food deprivation than sham-operated control rats, chronic stimuli from the stomach may somehow depress wheel-running during starvation (Messing and Campbell, 1971). It is not known whether there are age-related increases in such chronic inhibitory stimuli from the stomach either during food deprivation or during <u>ad libitum</u> feeding.

Generalized excitatory and inhibitory systems in the brain regulate overall levels of arousal (Campbell <u>et al</u>., 1969). The main excitatory center is thought to be the brainstem reticular formation. Acting in opposition to this excitatory region are certain forebrain structures which serve to modulate reticular excitability. The biochemical substrates of the arousal areas in the hindbrain and the inhibitory centers in the forebrain are distinct, with the former primarily adrenergic and the latter predominantly cholinergic. There is considerable support for the view that the early stages of development are characterized by unchecked reticular excitability leading to correspondingly high levels of behavioral arousal (Moorcroft *et al.*, 1971). Then as maturation of the telencephelon proceeds, the later developing inhibitory centers gradually assume greater control over the reticular excitability resulting in a decrease in behavioral arousal and the ultimate assumption of the low levels of spontaneous activity characteristic of the adult rat. Thus, the age-related decrements in behavioral excitability may be due in part to age-related increases in effectiveness of inhibitory centers.

Age-related decrements in the excitatory centers may also be involved in the age-decrement in activity. Amphetamine increases activity, as measured by photobeam interruptions, to a greater degree in young than old rats, while phentolamine, an adrenergic blocking agent, decreases this form of activity to a lesser extent in young than old rats (Farner, 1960, 1961). Thus age-related decreases in activity may be due, in part, to age-related increases in effectiveness of inhibitory centers, or to age-related decreases in the effectiveness of excitatory centers, or both.

Activity During Dietary Restriction

Casual observation of the deprived rats during longevity studies indicated that they were more active in their cages than were *ad libitum* fed rats. This phenomenon was observed by McCay (1952), Berg (1960), and Ross (1959) and suggests that the beneficial effects of diet restriction on longevity might be mediated, at least in part, by the increased spontaneous exercise experienced by the restricted animals.

Exercise seems to play a beneficial role on longevity. Middle-aged rats restricted to low levels of caloric intake increased their longevity when forced to exercise (McCay *et al.*, 1941), as did middle-aged male sated mice from a highly active strain when allowed to run in activity wheels (Goodrick, 1974). Female mice, however, failed to show an improvement (Goodrick, 1974). Forced exercise throughout life also increased the longevity of rats as compared to non-exercised controls (Retzlaff *et al.*, 1966). The forced and free exercise may have decreased adiposity, thus increasing longevity since access to activity wheels decreases food intake and adiposity in young rats (Collier, 1970; Leshner, 1971). However, the effect seems to depend on the age of the animal and its activity level (Jakubczak, 1969; but see Collier *et al.*, 1972).

However, access to activity wheels from weaning *decreased*

longevity of sated rats (Slonaker, 1912). Access to such wheels early in life has profound affects on the physiology of sated rats (Riss *et al.*, 1959) as well as the hungry rat (Pare, 1975). Perhaps under the *ad libitum* conditions used by Slonaker (1912) access to an activity wheel resulted in an increased energy expenditure (Riss *et al.*, 1959), decreased food intake (Collier, 1970), increased probability of an activity-stress ulcer (Pare, 1975), and a decreased life expectancy.

These studies indicate that exercise is beneficial for longevity, at least under certain conditions. Is there an increase in the home-cage activity and thus exercise of the food-restricted rat during longevity studies? If there is, then the increased longevity among food-restricted rats may, in part, at least be due to their increased exercise. After 8 months of restricted feeding, the physical activity of food-restricted rats showed a *reduction* in the total random movements estimated in a suspension type cage as compared with *ad libitum* fed rats of the same age (Olewine *et al.*, 1964). In contrast, the activity of the food-deprived rats, as measured by activity wheels, increased somewhat. Although, in general, food deprivation leads to a change in activity, the extent and direction of this change is a function of apparatus used to measure the activity (Strong, 1957; Finger, 1972). Strong (1957) found that hunger primarily increased activity of gross locomotor nature and decreases fine, essentially non-locomotor activity. Perhaps the device used by Olewine *et al.* (1964) was primarily sensitive to such fine non-locomotor measurements. On the other hand, the decrease in random activity may not be just an artifact, but may reflect an adaptive energy conserving stratagem on the part of the severely food-deprived rats in an apparatus that is not conducive to continued activity (Campbell, 1964; Morrison, 1968). If what happens in the suspension cage reflects what happens in the home cage, then increased exercise during food deprivation does not contribute significantly to the increased longevity.

Summary

What factors determine the duration of life and what is the relative influence of each of these factors?

Changes in the environment modify the duration of life. Diet is one such environmental factor. Longevity depends on diet, its caloric value and quality, mode of feeding, and age at which each such variable is introduced. Early dietary preferences are related to the onset of disease and longevity. Increased longevity is directly related to postponement of the onset of different diseases to older ages.

Feeding behavior is an essential link in nutrition. Since nutrition affects duration of life, free feeding behavior, at least in part, influences aging and disease, and may in turn be influenced by them.

Activity also affects aging and disease and is affected by them. Age-related decreases in energy output via lowered activity levels contribute to the age-related increases in obesity and thus shortened longevity. On the other hand, increased spontaneous activity may retard aging and increase longevity.

Because of their critical roles in longevity, the age-related changes in mechanisms underlying short-term and long-term control of feeding and activity deserve further investigation by gerontologists. The roles of gastric, glucostatic, lipostatic, thermostatic, neural and conditioning factors in these age-related changes need elucidation.

These interrelations among longevity, aging, disease, activity and feeding are indicated in figure 2. Such a scheme places nutrition in a broad organismic context and may serve pedagogical and heuristic purposes.

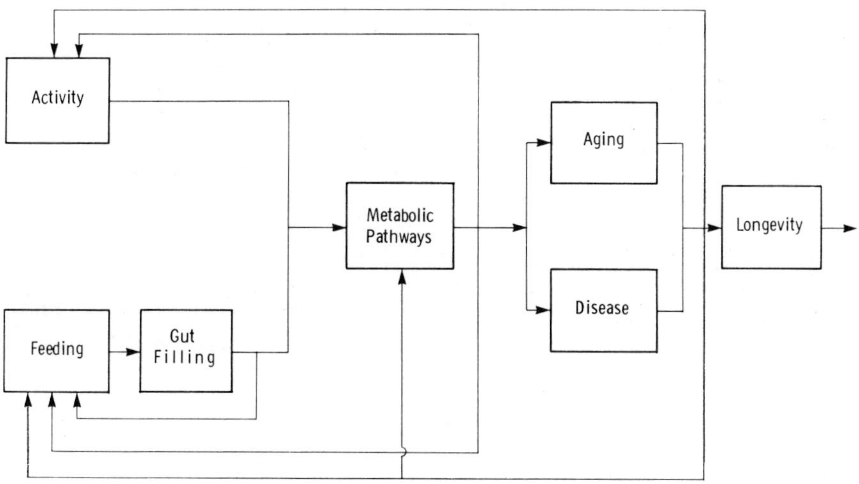

Fig. 2 The interrelationships among longevity, aging, disease, activity, and feeding. Feeding and activity affect aging and disease and are in turn affected by them.

REFERENCES

Barrows, C. H. and Roeder, L. M. (1965). J. Gerontol. 20, 69.
Bates, M. (1958). In "Behavior and Evolution" (A. Roe and G. G. Simpson, eds.), pp. 206-223, Yale University Press, New Haven.
Berg, B. N. (1960). J. Nutr. 71, 242.
Berg, B. N. and Simms, H. S. (1960). J. Nutr. 71, 255.
Birren, J. E. (1959). In "Handbook of Aging and the Individual" (J. E. Birren, ed.), pg. 16, University of Chicago Press, Chicago.
Booth, D. A. (1972). J. Comp. Physiol. Psychol. 81, 457.
Bras, G. and Ross, M. H. (1964). Toxicol. Appl. Pharmacol. 6, 247.
Campbell, B. A. (1964). In "Thirst" (M. J. Wayner, ed.), pp. 317-334, MacMillan, New York.
Campbell, B. A., Lytle, L. D., and Fibiger, H. C. (1969). Science 166, 637.
Ceokas, A. (1969). Am. J. Surg. 117, 881.
Collier, G. (1970). Trans. N.Y. Acad. Sci. 32, 557.
Collier, G. and Hirsch, E. (1971). J. Comp. Physiol. Psychol. 77, 155.
Collier, G., Hirsch, E., and Heshner, A. I. (1972). Physiol. Behavior 8, 881.
Comfort, A. (1964). "Ageing: The Biology of Senescence". Holt, New York.
Davis, J. D. and Campbell, C. S. (1973). J. Comp. Physiol. Psychol. 83, 379.
Dilman, V. M. (1971). Lancet 1, 1211.
Everitt, A. V. (1973). Exp. Gerontol. 8, 265.
Farner, D. (1960). Gerontologia 4, 144.
Farner, D. (1961). Gerontologia 5, 35.
Fernstrom, J. D. and Wurtman, R. J. (1971). Science 174, 1023.
Finger, F. W. (1972). In "Methods in Psychobiology" (R. D. Myers, ed.), Vol. 2, pp. 1-19, Academic Press, New York.
Froklis, V. (1968). Exp. Gerontol. 3, 113.
Garcia, J., Hankins, W., and Risiniak, K. (1974). Science 185, 824.
Gommers, A. (1971). Gerontologia 17, 228.
Goodrick, C. L. (1969). Genetic Psychol. 115, 121.
Goodrick, C. L. (1974). J. Gerontol. 29, 129.
Hamilton, C. L. (1965). In "Physiological Controls and Regulations" (W. S. Yamamoto and J. R. Brobeck, eds.), pp. 274-294, W. B. Saunders, Philadelphia.
Ivy, A. C. and Grossman, M. I. (1952). In "Cowdry's Problems of Ageing" (A. I. Lansing, ed.), pp. 481-526, Williams and Wilkins, Baltimore.

Jakubczak, L. F. (1969). Am. J. Physiol. 216, 1081.
Jakubczak, L. F. (1970). The Gerontologist 10, 27.
Jakubczak, L. F. (1973a). Bull. Psychonomic Soc. 1, 395.
Jakubczak, L. F. (1973b). Animal Learning and Behavior 1, 13.
Jakubczak, L. F. (1973c). Bull. Psychonomic Soc. 1, 304.
Jakubczak, L. F. (1973d). In "The Psychology of Adult Development and Aging" (C. Eisdorfer and M. Lawton, eds.) pp. 98-111, Amer. Psychol. Assn., Washington, D. C.
Jakubczak, L. F. (1975). Bull. Psychonomic Soc. 6, 491.
Jakubczak, L. F. (1976). Physiol. Behavior (in press).
Jelinkova, M. and Stuchlíková, E. (1968). Exp. Gerontol. 3, 193.
Kaplan, B. J. (1972). Psychol. Bull. 78, 321.
Keesey, R. E. and Powley, R. T. (1975). Am. Sci. 63, 558.
Kennedy, G. (1950). Proc. Royal Soc. London 137, 535.
Kenney, N. J. and Mook, D. (1974). J. Comp. Physiol. Psychol. 87, 302.
Klimas, J. (1968). J. Gerontol. 23, 31.
Korenchevsky, V. (1961). "Physiological and Pathological Aging". Hafner, New York.
Lansing, A. I. (1959). In "Handbook of Aging and the Individual" (J. E. Birren, ed.), pp. 119-135, University of Chicago Press, Chicago.
LeMagnen, J. (1971). In "Progress in Physiological Psychology" (E. Stellar and J. Sprague, eds.), pp. 204-262, Academic Press, New York.
LeMagnen, J., Devos, M., Guadilliere, J., Louis-Sylvestre, J., and Tallon, S. (1973). J. Comp. Physiol. Psychol. 84, 1.
Leshner, A. I. (1971). Physiol. Behavior 6, 551.
Lesser, G., Deutsch, S., and Markofsky, J. (1970). J. Gerontol. 25, 108.
Mayer, J. (1967). In "Handbook of Physiology, Section 6, Alimentary Canal" (C. F. Code, ed.), pp. 3-9, Vol. I, American Physiological Society, Washington, D. C.
Mayer, J. and Thomas, D. (1967). Science 156, 328.
McCay, C. M. (1952). In "Cowdry's Problems of Ageing" (A. I. Lansing, ed.), pp. 139-202, Williams and Wilkins, Baltimore.
McCay, C. M. and Eaton, E. (1947). J. Nutr. 34, 351.
McCay, C. M., Maynard, L. A., Sperling, G., and Osgood, H. S. (1941). J. Nutr. 21, 45.
McCay, C. M., Sperling, G., and Barnes, L. L. (1943). Arch. Biochem. 2, 469.
Messing, R. B. and Campbell, B. A. (1971). J. Comp. Physiol. Psychol. 77, 403.
Moorcroft, W., Lytle, L., and Campbell, B. (1971). J. Comp. Physiol. Psychol. 75, 59.

Morrison, S. D. (1968). J. Physiol. 197, 305.
Nisbett, R. E., Braver, A., Jusela, G., and Kezur, D. (1975). J. Comp. Physiol. Psychol. 88, 735.
Novin, D., Vander Weele, D., and Rezek, M. (1973). Science 181, 858.
Olewine, D. A., Barrows, C. H., and Shock, N. W. (1964). J. Gerontol. 19, 230.
Panskepp, J. (1973). J. Comp. Physiol. Psychol. 82, 78.
Pare, W. P. (1975). Am. J. Digest. Dis. 20, 262.
Retzlaff, E., Fontaine, J., and Futura, W. (1966). Geriatrics 21, 171
Riss, W., Burstein, S. D., Johnson, R. T. and Lutz, A. (1959). J. Comp. Physiol. Psychol. 52, 618.
Roeder, L. M. and Chow, B. F. (1972). Am. J. Clin. Nutr. 25, 812.
Ross, M. H. (1959). Fed. Proc. 18, 1190.
Ross, M. H. (1961). J. Nutr. 75, 197.
Ross, M. H. (1972). Am. J. Clin. Nutr. 25, 834.
Ross, M. H. and Bras, G. (1965). J. Nutr. 87, 245.
Ross, M. H. and Bras, G. (1971). J. Natl. Cancer Inst. 47, 1095.
Ross, M. H. and Bras, G. (1973). J. Nutr. 103, 944.
Ross, M. H. and Bras, G. (1974). Nature 250, 263.
Ross, M. H. and Bras, G. (1975). Science 190, 165.
Ross, M. H., Bras, G., and Ragbeer, M. S. (1970). J. Nutr. 100, 177.
Rozin, P. and Kalat, J. W. (1971). Psychol. Rev. 78, 459.
Schaie, K. W. (1965). Psychol. Bull. 64, 92.
Silberberg, M. and Silberberg, R. (1955). Physiol. Rev. 35, 347.
Silverstone, F., Brandfonbrener, M., Shock, N., and Yiengst, M. (1957). J. Clin. Invest. 36, 504.
Simms, H. (1965). In "The Aging and Levels of Biological Organization" (A. N. Brues and G. A. Sacher, eds.), pp. 87-122, University of Chicago Press, Chicago.
Slonaker, J. (1912). J. Animal Behavior 2, 20.
Smith, G., Gibbs, J., and Young, R. (1974). Fed. Proc. 33, 1146.
Snowdon, C. (1970). J. Comp. Physiol. Psychol. 71, 68.
Strong, P. N. (1957). J. Comp. Physiol. Psychol. 50, 596.
Verzar, F. (1963). "Lectures in Experimental Gerontology". Charles C Thomas, Springfield, Illinois.
Walford, R. L. (1969). "The Immunologic Theory of Aging". Williams and Wilkins, Baltimore.

THE POSSIBLE ROLE OF VITAMINS IN THE AGING PROCESS[1]

Olaf Mickelsen, Ph.D.[2]

Department of Food Science and Human Nutrition
Michigan State University
East Lansing, Michigan 48824

There are a number of fundamental or practical considerations which should be recognized before one ventures too far into a discussion of theoretical factors that may be important in aging. For those who have worked with both laboratory animals and human subjects, it may be obvious that there are anomalies within both of these groups. These anomalies mitigate the significance of research findings especially when an attempt is made to translate such findings from the laboratory to human reality. There are many advantages in using laboratory animals as experimental models. They do have their place in research but, too frequently, the results secured thereby are made to appear completely relevant to human beings without any indication of the limitations of the observations.

Limitations of Laboratory Animal Studies

One of the areas where laboratory animal studies have contributed immensely to human health and welfare is in the field of nutrition. There is no doubt that progress in elucidating the amino acids, fatty acids, vitamins and minerals required by man was possible within a span of about 50 years only because the groundwork for those advances was laid by painstaking research with laboratory animals. Without the information obtained from animal research, we would still be groping with what would otherwise be a horrendous problem. However, the real contribution of such animal research to human nutrition has been only to suggest that certain nutrients may be needed in man's diet. When those suggestions have

---

[1]Published as Journal Article No.7667 by the Michigan Agricultural Experiment Station.

[2]Jointly with Eleanor D. Schlenker, Ph.D., Department of Home Economics, Agricultural Experiment Station, University of Vermont, Burlington, Vermont.

been followed by appropriate human studies, it became evident that not all observations with laboratory animals could be applied directly to man. This was true from both the qualitative and quantitative standpoints.

The white rat, for various reasons, has been used more extensively than any other animal in nutrition research. Yet, the differences between it and man are too frequently glossed over when some startling laboratory observation is reported. Furthermore, in many popular reports, there is a glaring failure to qualify clearly and honestly the results secured with laboratory animals and the application thereof to the taxpayer who supports so much of biomedical research. Similarly, too many scientific reviews are written in such a way that the reader cannot adequately differentiate between the results of animal studies and those made with human subjects. Results in the two arenas are so intertwined in many reports, that the overall impression is that the conclusions pertain equally to both animals and man.

The limitations of animal studies, especially from the quantitative standpoint, are well illustrated by the attempts to determine whether lysine is present in white flour at such a low level that it restricts the biological value of its protein for man. There is no question about the inability of the protein in white flour to support growth in the rat and that the addition of lysine to such a ration markedly improves that growth. The limitations of such animal research became evident when a graduate student attempted to feed rats her native Iranian bread adequately supplemented with the essential nutrients other than protein (Bolourchi, 1963). At the conclusion of her work, she found, as one would anticipate, that the rats did not grow unless fairly large amounts of skim milk powder or legumes were added to the Iranian bread diet. Calculations of the essential amino acid intakes of her animals confirmed her observation that, for the rat, reduced levels of lysine and a number of other amino acids in the bread limited growth. However, similar calculations indicated that if an Iranian farmer, consuming 2500 kcal per day, were to secure 70 percent of his caloric intake from white flour, his intake of lysine would more than meet his requirement. Some years earlier, Hegsted (1962), on the basis of such calculations, suggested that both adults and children could secure a sufficient amount of all essential amino acids from wheat products if they provided 80 percent of the caloric requirements. Until 1964, no one had attempted to determine whether normal young men could secure an adequate intake of all the essential amino acids from wheat products. Our study indicated that it was possible for normal young men to attain and maintain nitrogen equilibrium for 50 days when 90 to 95 percent of their protein intake came from wheat, primarily white flour. There was no animal protein in those diets (Bolourchi et al., 1968).

A possible explanation for the quantitative differences between results secured with laboratory animals and human subjects involves, among other things, the difference in species-specific growth rates (Vaghefi et al., 1974). At weaning, the laboratory rat can double its body weight in about five days; the human infant, under ideal conditions, doubles its body weight in at least six to eight weeks. That difference in growth rates means that the dietary ration for the rat must be much more concentrated in essential nutrients than that for the human infant. This is very apparent when one considers the composition of rat and human milk (Yang and Mickelsen, 1974). If one were to reason, as so many do, that rat growth is the arbiter of the biological value of foods intended for human use, then a good argument could be made for the inadequacy of breast milk for the human infant. This would be contrary to the experience of over many thousands of years which indicates that the human infant does as well, if not better, when fed breast milk than when fed even the most sophisticated formula. Considerations similar to these should make us wary of accepting results of animal studies until they have been verified with human subjects.

Problems of Human Subject Studies

Results of human studies also indicate a number of anomalies which should elicit some concern. Most of these appear to be ignored by many investigators. One of these relates to the differential life expectancy of males and females. Women outlive men despite the fact that they reportedly have twice the amount of body fat as men do (Mickelsen, 1958; Ljunggren, 1965; Rockstein, 1974). This is contrary to the results of many studies with laboratory animals which indicate that, for both sexes, as the percentage of body fat increases, the life span is shortened (McCay et al., 1939, 1943). Even insurance statistics (Society of Actuaries, 1959) suggest that those men who are underweight live longer than those who are overweight (and presumably have more body fat).

If we look at mortality from the standpoint of prior nutritional experience, again, one arrives at an impasse. This is evident when we consider the reports which suggest that throughout childhood and especially in adolescence there is a greater incidence of nutritional disturbances and a poorer nutritional intake among girls than among boys (Mickelsen, 1971). The voracious appetite of boys insures, in most cases, a more adequate intake of the essential nutrients. The greater food intake of the male continues into adulthood (Buzina, 1968). Thus, on that basis, one could argue that better nutritional status, as judged by food intake, should insure a longer life among men than women. Obviously, there are many factors other than nutrition and body fat which have contributed to the differential mortality of men and women.

Hawthorne and Placebo Effects

Two additional problems associated with studies of human subjects that are frequently overlooked are the "Hawthorne" and "placebo" effects. In some ways, these two effects are related. The Hawthorne effect occurs when a subject in a study experiences an improvement in his well-being that, primarily, is a result of his participation in the study. In other words, when an individual volunteers for a study, he may very well benefit from that experience and the improvement may not necessarily be a result of the variable under study. Almost every longitudinal study which involved men as subjects for cardiovascular investigations reported a lower than anticipated mortality experience. Actually, this observation has been so consistent that one might propose that a simple means of avoiding an early cardiovascular accident is to volunteer as a subject for such a study. Gerontological studies are beginning to experience a similar phenomenon as evidenced in the Duke study (Palmore, 1971) where mortality among the subjects has been lower than expected. This phenomenon was also observed to occur for a group of male Civil Service retirees studied initially in Washington by Granick and Patterson (1971). They observed "a significantly greater than expected survival rate and a high level of emotional health" among their subjects.

Many factors may be responsible for the greater longevity of such human "guinea pigs". These subjects may represent that fraction of men who, under any circumstance, would be in the long-lived category. This is a possibility since so many studies are started with "healthy" subjects. Among them, one would anticipate greater survival than among the general population. Proper compensation for the Hawthorne effect is an urgent need in all studies involving human subjects. Thus, the need exists to develop means of evaluating the person who volunteers for a study and his motive in volunteering. Such evaluation should include an estimate of the psychological makeup of that individual and a means of interpreting the results of such psychological tests. The test should provide some indication of the individual's previous "life style" and how that might be altered during the study period. Any change in the subject's way of life that might result from his participation in the study may have profound effects on the results.

This leads to a consideration of the "placebo" effect, which is a positive response to what the British call a "dummy" pill. It is sometimes difficult to differentiate between the effect of the experimental variable under study (e.g., food, nutrient, pill, etc.) and that of the placebo. An illustration of the placebo effect was observed in the reduction in colds among the University of Minnesota students who, prior to World War II, were involved in evaluating vitamin C as a preventive for that malady. When the study was concluded, Cowan and his colleagues (1942) observed a significant reduction in the incidence of colds among the students who consumed fairly large amounts of vitamin C throughout the coldest part of one school year. However, when the experience of the "placebo" group was examined, a reduction comparable to that of the vitamin C group was observed. When Dr. Cowan presented the results of that study at a medical meeting, the discussion brought out the fact that the subjects in the "placebo" group by virtue of the fact that they were part of a study probably, unconsciously, exercised greater care in their overall health practices than they would otherwise have done. This, in turn, may have produced the reduced incidence of colds observed among the students in the "placebo" group.

More specifically related to our topic is the so-called "booster" effect reportedly observed among older individuals receiving vitamin B_{12} injections. No statistics are available on the number of older people who routinely received such therapy and who claimed highly beneficial effects therefrom (Felstein, 1973). There is some theoretical basis for such therapy; that involves the reduction, with age, in serum vitamin B_{12} levels in healthy individuals, as reported by Chow and Yeh (1963) and a number of other investigators. Presumably, similar changes occur in the serum level of vitamin B_6. The latter change, however, was based not on analyses of the serum for pyridoxine but of the enzyme SGOT (serum glutamic oxalic transaminase). Chow and Yeh (1963) reported that, "Available data lead to the conclusion that regression of vitamin B_{12} and B_6 in sera with aging is well established". The explanation for these reductions in serum vitamin levels is not completely understood despite some reports of a reduced intrinsic factor production by the secretory cells in the stomachs of older people (Hyams, 1973). More importantly, whether an improvement in overall well-being of an aged individual will result from therapy with supplementation of either of these vitamins is open to question.

Despite the absence of adequate scientific data in this area, many aged individuals will continue to receive some benefit from therapy with these and other dietary supplements. Whether such responses are an illustration of the "Hawthorne" or "placebo" effect will be difficult to determine. Furthermore, who is to deny such therapy to those older people who maintain they secure great benefits, be they psychological or physiological or both, from injections of vitamin B_{12}.

Dental Condition and Nutrient Intake

One final word of caution, for those working with older people, involves the relation between dental condition and nutrient intake. That poor condition of the teeth axiomatically means a poor nutrient intake has been accepted by some investigators (Söremark and Nilsson, 1972; Shank, 1975). However, support for this conclusion, although it appears rational, was not observed by Davidson and coworkers (1962) who stated that, "No correlations between nutrient intake and oral status were found among a group of 104 men and women, two-thirds of whom were over seventy years of age". Similar observations were made by Bates and coworkers (1971). Among 282 males and 422 females 65 years of age and older in South Wales, there was no relation between the nutritional state of the subjects and their oral condition. The nutritional state was assessed by height, weight, skin-fold thickness, packed cell volume, serum folic acid and serum vitamin B_{12} levels. The level of hemoglobin and packed cell volume were significantly related to the oral condition but the biological significance of those correlations was not apparent in the report.

Vitamin Requirements of Older People

Of more direct relevance to the problem of forestalling premature aging is the question of the role that nutrient intake might play in such a process. According to the statements of many nutritionists and the pronouncements of the Food and Nutrition Board (1974), the requirements of older people are no different from those of younger adults with the possible exception of caloric intake which should decrease as an individual ages. Actually, there is very little experimental evidence to support this statement. Most of the controlled studies have dealt with the vitamins and a large share of that was done by Horwitt and his colleagues at Elgin (Horwitt, 1953). They observed essentially the same response to various levels of vitamin intake in men who were over 70 years as in those of about 35 years of age. Most of Horwitt's studies were of such a long period that if any differences existed between the two groups, they should have been apparent in the experimental period.

From a theoretical standpoint, one could argue that the requirement of older people for many nutrients should be lower than that of younger people. For some of the vitamin B complex, this is based on the fact that the requirements of these vitamins are related to the caloric intake. With advancing age, the need for calories decreases and consequently one might anticipate that the need of the body for vitamins should likewise diminish. Furthermore, there is some evidence (Forbes and Reina, 1970) that the number of active cells in the bodies of older people is reduced. Since the actively-metabolizing cells of the body are the main determinants of nutrient requirements, any reductions in their numbers should result in a corresponding reduction in the body's needs.

The preceding should not be interpreted to mean that all older people can be maintained in good health at the level of nutrient intake which is adequate for a much younger person. With advancing years, various disturbances of the gastrointestinal tract or more overt forms of illness afflict the body. These secondary conditions may have a marked effect on the older individual's nutritional requirements, or, at least, make the older person think that some of his physical ailments have a dietary origin.

The disturbances to which older people are prone, be they either real or imaginary, frequently resulted in altered dietary habits. Frequently, these individuals increase their intake of vitamins. Whether such increased nutrient intake has any effect on the subject's health or longevity has not been conclusively established. There are, however, a number of reports which suggest that beneficial effects redound to those older individuals who have increased their intake of some nutrients. Related thereto is the evidence which is beginning to emerge from a number of fields of research that the nature of the diet may influence the condition of the skeleton. The remainder of this paper will be devoted to an evaluation of the reports relating to these claims.

Reported Benefits of High Vitamin Intakes by Older People

One of the early suggestions that higher vitamin intakes conferred a benefit upon older individuals was the study of Chope and Dray (1951) and by Chope (1954) among the older inhabitants of San Mateo County, California. Of the 577 individuals over 50 years of age first seen in 1948-1949, 49 had died by the fall of 1952. The initial examination involved a thorough study of the dietary intake of each subject, blood levels of various nutrients, and an extensive medical examination with special attention to any signs or symptoms that might have a nutritional connotation (Gillum and Morgan, 1955). On the basis of the dietary information secured in 1948-1949, the mortality data were compared with nutrient intakes. Chope (1954) concluded that among these older people,

"There seemed to be relationships between mortality and intake of vitamin A, niacin and ascorbic acid".

For vitamin A, there were 158 subjects whose intake was less than 5000 I.U. per day. Among the individuals in that group, there were 22 deaths, or a mortality rate of 13.9 percent. Among the 160 subjects whose daily intake was 5000 to 7999 I.U., there were 11 deaths, or a 6.9 percent mortality. For the 211 individuals whose intake was 8000 or more I.U. per day, there were 9 deaths or a 4.3 percent mortality. Even when all subjects were combined, for those whose intake was above 5000 I.U. per day, the mortality in that group was 5.4 percent, which is lower than the 13.9 percent in the group ingesting less than 5000 I.U. per day.

For niacin, the reduction in mortality with increasing intake was definite but not as dramatic as that for vitamin A. The data for vitamin C were more impressive. Among the 130 older people who consumed diets which provided less than 50 mg of vitamin C per day, there were 24 deaths, for a mortality rate of 18.5 percent. For the 251 subjects ingesting 50 - 109 mg daily, there were 9 deaths, for a mortality rate of 3.6 percent. Among the 148 whose intake was 110 mg and over, there were 9 deaths or 6.1 percent mortality. Again, when all subjects ingesting 50 mg or more vitamin C per day are pooled, the mortality rate was 4.5 percent, which is far less than the 18.5 percent among those consuming less than 50 mg per day.

These data are similar to those we observed in a longitudinal study of 100 women from whom dietary records were first secured in 1948 (Schlenker, 1976); those women were chosen on the basis of census tracts in the Lansing area. At the time of the first examination (1948), the women were 40 years or older. Between 1948 and 1972, 60 of the women died. The dietary records in 1948 for those who subsequently died were lower in vitamin C and protein than for those who survived. The average protein intake was 50.8 ± 14.2 g protein per day for the women who died, while those who were alive in 1972 had had an intake in 1948 of 58.4 ± 17.9 g ($P \leq 0.05$). For vitamin C, the intakes in 1948 were 51 ± 40 mg, for those who died, vs 73 ± 40 mg ($P \leq 0.05$), for those who survived, at least up to 1972. These values include only vitamin C intake from foods since the information collected in 1948 does not permit an estimate of supplementary vitamin intakes. Although the difference in vitamin C intake was significant at the 5 percent level, the plasma vitamin C concentrations determined in 1948 did not differ; the level for the deceased women was 0.87 ± 0.42 per 100 ml, while for the survivors, it was 1.00 ± 0.44 mg per 100 ml.

At first glance, it might appear that the differential

mortality of the two groups of women in the Lansing study might be explained on the basis of their ages at the time of the initial examination. In 1948, the women who died prior to 1972 averaged 67.4 years, while those who survived averaged 52.1 years. However, the mean age at the time of death for the 60 women who died prior to 1972 was 67.4, while that of the survivors was 74.8 years in 1972. This difference in age is significant ($P \leq .05$). That age at the time of the initial examination may not be the only factor involved in this mortality difference is suggested by the fact that those women who survived until 1972 maintained or increased their vitamin C intake as evidenced by a comparison of dietary intakes in 1948 and 1972. Over that period of time, there was an increase in average vitamin C intake, by the survivors, from 73 to 93 mg per day ($P \leq 0.5$).

There is adequate information to indicate that there is a low vitamin C content in the diets of older people, expecially among those who are institutionalized. That is probably also true of the older individuals who rely on food brought into their living quarters by an organization such as "Meals on Wheels". A study in Great Britain of the vitamin C content of such food indicated that the destruction of the vitamin may exceed 50 percent. By analysis, that was the fate of the vitamin C in the foods tested during the two to three hours elapsing from its preparation until delivery to the recipient (Davies et al., 1973).

During the last few decades, a number of suggestions have appeared which imply that the intakes of low or "inadequate" nutrients, among which vitamin C is frequently listed, may be associated with a number of distrubances which are often found among older people. These include such complaints as "unexplained tiredness, backache, persistent headache, joint pains", etc. These complaints were found by Kelley and coworkers (1957) among those 200 older women whose intakes of vitamins A and C were only 40 percent of the Recommended Dietary Allowances (RDA). (Unfortunately, the absolute amounts were not listed and the levels of these vitamins in the RDA have undergone some changes in subsequent editions.) Mortality among these women was also related to reported nutrient intake. Among the 200 women examined in 1948 and again in 1955, the mortality rate was higher for those "who reported intakes of less than 40 percent of recommended quantities of one or more nutrient (sic) than among those with higher intakes of nutrients". Unfortunately, these data are presented in such abbreviated form that it is impossible to properly interpret them.

Reports of older people with swollen gums, "sheet hemorrhages" and other signs suggestive of vitamin deficiencies prompted a study by Taylor (1968) of the efficacy of vitamin supplements to older hospital patients in Farnborough, England. Of the hospital patients, 80 "were selected, not because of their clinical signs, but because I (Taylor) thought they would survive for the one year planned for the trial, and because they were willing and able to co-operate". Half of these subjects were given a pill daily for one year which contained: 15 mg thiamine, 15 mg riboflavin, 50 mg nicotinamide, 10 mg pyridoxine and 200 mg ascorbic acid. The other half, the control group, received "dummy tablets" as a placebo. Over the year, the group receiving the vitamin tablets showed an improvement in "the classical signs of malnutrition" with a return to normal. Accompanying that "was a striking improvement in the general physical and mental condition". This change among the vitamin supplemented individuals was in marked contrast to the subjects in the placebo group where "clinical signs did not improve and in many cases deteriorated". The English investigators continued to observe these older people for six to nine months at the end of the one year of vitamin supplementation. According to Taylor (1968), who performed the clinical evaluation himself, during that subsequent six to nine month period when no supplemental vitamins were provided, "signs of nutritional deficiencies reappeared in many previously treated cases".

Admittedly, there are criticisms that can be leveled at the Farnborough study. Many of them were brought out by the discussants at the symposium where the report was presented. Despite the comments made at the meeting, Professor A.C. Frazer (1968) stated "the Farnborough survey is a most creditable and exciting effort".

Subsequent to that study, Dymock and Brocklehurst (1973) gave 126 "geriatric patients" with various afflictions a daily supplement of one of the vitamins used in the Farnborough study. Over a period of one year, these single vitamin supplements had no effect on such physical signs as cheilosis, angular stomatitis, condition of tongue or increase in hemoglobin level. Although this might vitiate the Farnborough results, there is the possibility that the single vitamin supplements were not as effective as the combined therapy, or, more likely, the small number of subjects in each group (18) and the high mortality (4 to 10 per group) may have obscured any beneficial effects.

In a similar manner, another report from England suggests that the survival time of geriatric patients admitted to a hospital was related to the level of vitamin C in their blood (Wilson et al., 1972). For the 32 patients who entered the hospital with less than 12 μg vitamin C per 10^8 leucocytes and platelets, the mortality rate during the next four weeks was 47 percent. The mortality rate progressively decreased to 10 percent with increasing vitamin C levels for the 49 patients who had over 25 μg per 10^8 leucocytes and platelets. Although the authors indicate that the chronic diseases of old age were distributed about equally in the groups, there was no indication as to whether any factor such as fever influenced the observed vitamin levels. As has been recognized for many years, even a small increase in body temperature is associated with a prompt and dramatic reduction in serum vitamin C levels (Keys and Mickelsen, 1944).

The same group of investigators (Wilson et al., 1973) attempted a therapeutic trial with vitamin C supplements. In that study, 98 men and 173 women received daily 200 mg vitamin C; an equal number received placeboes. After both four and six weeks of supplementation, there was no difference in mortality of either group. However, those patients who entered the hospital with leucocyte and platelet levels of vitamin C above 15 μg per 10^8 WBC, had a lower mortality through 100 days than those with levels below 15 μg.

On the basis of Recommended Dietary Allowances accepted in the United States, many older people, especially those in other countries, should be grossly deficient in vitamin C and on the basis of the previously discussed work, should have a much shorter survival period than those in this country. A report from Finland of a dietary survey of 135 men and women with average ages of 71 and 74 years, respectively, indicated that 81 of these received 30 mg or less of vitamin C per day. The plasma vitamin C levels, although low by our standards, were surprisingly high for the amount of the vitamin reportedly present in their diet (Roine et al., 1974). These individuals "were in good health for their age". The older people in Finland might be one group that should be studied to determine whether there is any beneficial effect on well-being and longevity from an increased vitamin C intake.

Osteoporosis

Osteoporosis is one of the more common and treacherous complications associated with aging. Although estimates of the prevalence of osteoporosis is at best a guess, there appears general agreement that the percentage of individuals afflicted with it increases with age. According to Garn (1970), X-ray evidence of osteoporosis increases from 7 percent among 50-year old women to 100 percent among those 80 years of age or older. There is also agreement that osteoporosis is more common among aging women than men (Nordin, 1971; Albanese et al., 1974; Albanese, 1975).

There is no universally accepted explanation for the underlying cause of osteoporosis. That some factor such as diet may be implicated in its development is suggested by the report that osteoporosis is probably ten times more prevalent among the whites in South Africa than among the Bantus (Solomon, 1968). A similar differential incidence exists among whites and blacks in the United States (Vincent and Urist, 1961; Gyepes et al., 1962).

A possible explanation for the racial difference in osteoporosis may be the greater mineralization of the bones of blacks. That was brought out by the work of Trotter and her colleagues (1960). They found the long bones of 20 white American males to be significantly less dense than comparable bones from 20 age-matched American blacks from the same geographic region. The bones of 20 black females were of the same density as those of the white males. Comparable bones from age-matched white females were less dense than either the black females or white males. For all four groups, the decrease in bone density with the age of the individual at time of death followed the same slope. The density was estimated by Trotter et al. (1960) by weighing the whole bones in air and measuring their volume by millet seed displacement.

The similarity of the slopes for changes in density with age for the four preceding groups suggests that the rate of mineral loss from the bone is the same for men and women as well as for blacks and whites. Others, using X-ray techniques, have observed that the cortical bone mass shows a progressive reduction as an individual ages (Garn, 1970). The time when osteoclastic activity of bone becomes greater than osteoblastic activity is not precisely known. Some investigators (Garn, 1970) believe the change occurs shortly after age 40, whereas others (Meunier et al., 1973) maintain that "rarefaction of bone begins from 20 years of age...". There is evidence that bone dissolution is a phenomenon common to adults both in the United States and in Central America. The latter is based on a study of hand X-rays of 4200 people in Guatemala and El Salvadore who ranged in age from 40 to 90 years (Garn et al., 1967).

The same rate of bone loss was observed on cross-sectional studies of groups of adults as well as a longitudinal study of 34 men and 53 women in southwestern Ohio whose hands were X-rayed over a period of 15 years for the males and 23 years for the females (Garn et al., 1967). On that basis and supported by other data, Garn (1970) has proposed that bone loss is a universal concomitant of aging. This means that, since the rate of bone loss appears to occur at a uniform rate once it has started, the factor determining whether an individual develops osteoporosis will be the size and perhaps the degree of skeletal mineralization during early adulthood.

It has been proposed that the most effective and perhaps the only cure for osteoporosis is prevention. That is based on the report of a number of investigators (Garn et al.,1967;

Smith, 1967; Hegsted, 1967; Frost, 1973) that no change, or at most, only a minimal alteration can be made in the rate of bone loss once that process has been initiated. Since the condition of the skeleton in early adulthood assumes such importance in determining that person's susceptibility to osteoporosis in later life, it should be beneficial for individuals basking in the full bloom of life to do everything possible to enhance the mineralization of their bones. How to accomplish that has not been clearly defined. There are a number of suggestions that bone density can be enhanced early in life by such factors as the fluoride content of the water (Bernstein et al., 1966) and the nature of the diet.

That the nature of the diet may influence mineralization of the bones was suggested by Walker et al. (1970). They found, on the basis of X-ray studies, that Bantu women 70 or more years old had bones that were as densely mineralized as those of the Caucasian women in South Africa. The calcium intake of the Bantu women was reported to be 200 to 400 mg per day, while that of the Caucasians was 800 to 900 mg. This difference in calcium intake was accentuated by the more frequent pregnancies and longer lactation periods among the Bantus resulting in a greater drain of body calcium. Nevertheless, despite the low calcium intake and the greater loss of calcium associated with reproduction, the Bantu women have only a tenth of femoral neck fractures of white women (Solomon, 1968).

One dietary component that is receiving some attention in relation to the calcium content of the body is protein. The work of Linkswiler and coworkers (1974) has demonstrated that as dietary protein levels are increased, there must be a corresponding increase in calcium intake to maintain equilibrium. These investigators point out that many nutritionists have suggested that higher levels of dietary protein improved calcium absorption, but the increased protein intake also accentuates urinary calcium loss. They found that for normal young men, equilibrium was possible with an intake of 400 mg per day of calcium, when the diet provided 42 g protein. An increase in dietary protein to 95 and 142 g resulted in a reduction in the amount of calcium retained by the subjects and the development of a negative calcium balance. These investigators point out that a daily loss from the body of 100 mg calcium observed with the highest protein intake, could, over a period of 10 to 20 years, produce a "significant dissolution of bone...".

Chu et al. (1975) secured results similar to the preceding insofar as urinary calcium losses were concerned. Their normal male subjects increased urinary calcium excretion as the dietary protein level was raised. The latter was associated with a slightly greater increase in calcium absorption as indicated by fecal calcium levels. Although their work emphasizes the importance of considering dietary protein levels in studies of calcium metabolism, they did not observe the marked negative calcium balances reported by Linkswiler and colleagues (1974).

The one dietary factor that does not appear to have been considered by either of the two previous groups of investigators is the acid-base changes that may have occurred in their subjects as a result of the dietary manipulations. That this, at least in the extreme situation, may be important has been recognized for many years (for references, see Wachman and Bernstein, 1968). These workers have known that the supplementation of a diet with an acidifying agent such as ammonium chloride produced a loss of calcium from the bones. In contrast thereto, an alkalinizing agent such as sodium bicarbonate had the opposite effect. This concept was resurrected by Barzel and Bernstein (Anon., 1969), who reported the feeding of an alkali-ash diet supplemented daily with 1 g sodium and potassium phosphate to 40 osteoporetic patients. The rationale for this therapy appears to have been the suggestion that "Osteoporosis may be caused, at least in part, by acid overloading resulting from a meat-rich diet". Unfortunately, these investigators present no research data in support of that hypothesis.

Barzel and Jowsey (1969) reported that when adult rats were offered solutions containing either ammonium chloride or a mixture of sodium and potassium bicarbonate to drink, the composition of their bones was affected. From that work, they concluded that "acid or alkali ingestion affects bone as a tissue, including the inorganic and organic phases of bone". An extension of that work was made to "immobilized healthy adult volunteers" who received 220 mg of calcium per day in their diets (Barzel, 1971). The negative calcium balances were improved in those subjects receiving sodium and potassium bicarbonate in capsular form. For those subjects, there was a decreased loss of calcium in both the stool and urine whereas placeboes, given to other subjects, had no effect on the calcium balance.

The suggestion of Wachman and Bernstein (1968) that a vegetarian diet might be "worthwhile to consider" for "decreasing the rate of bone attrition" has been explored by Ellis _et al_. (1972). On that basis, they hypothesized that "one would expect to observe a greater degree of bone dissolution in a diet that contains meat (a primary source of acid ash) than in a vegetarian diet". To test that, they secured hand X-rays from 8 men and 17 women ovolactovegetarians ranging in age from 53 to 79 years. Age- and sex-matched individuals who were omnivores were also studied. The density of the bones "was significantly greater in the vegetarians than in the omnivores". That was true for all age groups with the differences being of such magnitude that the bone density of the 70 to 79 year old vegetarians was similar to that of the 50 to 59 year old omnivores. This study appears to be of limited value due to a serious methodological error. That was discovered by Meema (1973), who on the basis of "enquiries with the authors" learned from the radiologist (Holesh) in the British study "that the bone density values reported in the article are not those of bone density but of photographic density...". Accordingly, conclusions just the reverse of those reported by Ellis _et al_. (1972) should be obtained when the radiographic readings are correctly evaluated. Meema (1973) also criticized the study for the small and unequal numbers of subjects in the two groups. Another limitation is the lack of information as to the length of time the subjects followed their respective dietary regimens.

These observations suggest that work is urgently needed to explore the dietary factors that may be related to the development of osteoporosis. Such investigations should include not only a consideration of the calcium, fluoride and vitamin intakes but also the level and nature of the dietary protein. An attempt should be made to quantitate these nutrients in the diet during that period of life when active bone formation was taking place. Such studies may be most readily performed by comparing vegetarians and omnivores in the same geographic area, thus minimizing the influence of environmental factors. If that were done, some attempt should be made to determine when the individual became a vegetarian and the steadfastness with which the prescribed regimen was followed.

It is intriguing that, in one area of nutritional gerontology, there appears suggestive evidence that a high intake of such a nutrient as vitamin C may bestow a variety of health benefits, whereas the development of osteoporosis may be ameliorated, if not prevented, by a reduction in the level of dietary protein intake and a possible change in the kinds of protein which have been advocated for so long by so many.

SUMMARY

Individuals who have acknowledged that the aging process is affecting them are concerned about anything that will prevent or, at least, slow down the deterioration which they experience or imagine. For many of those people, diet appears to be a major means of ameliorating the alterations in their health and performance.

Evidence from a number of sources suggests that the nutrient intake of older people is not influenced by their dental condition. Despite the absence of teeth, many older people manage to consume a reasonably good diet with the result that, except for those individuals in special circumstances, the incidence of malnutrition is no greater among them than among those with more adequate dental facilities.

Although there is still some interest in evaluating the effects of nutrient deficiencies on the health of older people, considerable emphasis is being directed towards studies of larger than "normal" intakes on the health of these people. One of these areas involves vitamin C. The results of a number of studies imply that a higher than normal intake of that vitamin appears to reduce the aches and pains to which older people are prone, to lower mortality when the aged are ill and to increase their longevity.

In contrast to the dietary level of vitamin C, a possible deleterious effect is being associated with high protein intake, especially during late adolescence and early adulthood. At those periods, high protein intake may restrict the deposition and/or retention of minerals in bones and thus lead to the development of osteoporosis at a later date. Not only may the level of the protein in the diet be important in influencing the development of osteoporosis, but so may the nature of the protein. The latter is based largely on the suggestion that the African Bantu, with his sturdy bones, consumes a diet restricted in animal protein. Such a diet which is largely vegetarian produces an alkaline condition in the body which enhances the deposition and/or retention of bone minerals.

Dietary factors may be important during that period of development when the individual's bones are increasing in density. The role of dietary factors is becoming important since the studies suggesting that diet insures strong bones in an individual's old age involved nutrient levels well within the usual range of intake. Such work suggests that the nature of the dietary protein may be as important or more so than its quantity in determining the degree of bone mineralization in early adulthood and, correspondingly, the nature and severity of the skeletal problems in old age. The latter appear to be related to the degree of bone mineralization present in the fourth decade of an individual's life. Thereafter, bone loss occurs at a uniform rate among all individuals (Garn, 1975). Additional studies of human subjects are urgently needed since so much of the previous nutrition education has emphasized the health importance of high intakes of the animal proteins which are now being implicated in the etiology of osteoporosis. A concerted effort should be made to determine whether the factors discussed in this report are important in influencing the degree of mineralization of bones. If they do determine the density of the bones at age 30 to 40 years, will that influence to a marked degree an individual's susceptibility to develop osteoporosis at a later age?

A major problem facing the investigator who hopes to secure valid results in this area is the characterization of his subjects. Experimental investigators overcome that problem by using animals that have a relatively uniform genetic background. Sufficient numbers are used to minimize the variability among the animals. These possibilities are not always available to the investigator working with human subjects. Since investigations of older people are the only means whereby many of the problems in gerontology can be solved, it is imperative that adequate means be used in describing the subjects. The instrument for that purpose should be one that will be accepted and used by most investigators doing human studies. Furthermore, it should be of such a nature that its results can be readily and easily presented as a valid description of the subjects involved in the study.

REFERENCES

Albanese, A. A. (1975). Food Nutr. News, National Live Stock and Meat Board, Vol. 47, No. 1.

Albanese, A. A., Lorenz, E. J., Jr., Edelson, A. H., Wein, E. H., and Orto, L. A. (1974). "Problems of Bone Health in the Elderly". Presented at National Dairy Council Food Writers' Conference, June 3-4.

Anon. (1969). Med. World News, Feb. 21, p. 18.

Barzel, U. S. (1971). Israel J. Med. Sci. 7, 499.

Barzel, U. S. and Jowsey, J. (1969). Clin. Sci. 36, 517.

Bates, J. F., Elwood, P. C., and Foster, W. (1971). Gerontol. Clin. 13, 227.

Bernstein, D. S., Sadowsky, N., Hegsted, D. M., Guri, C. C., and Stare, F. J. (1966). J. Am. Med. Assoc. 198, 499.

Bolourchi, S. D. (1963). "The Biological Value and Composition of Different Breads from Various Countries". M.S. Thesis, Michigan State University.

Bolourchi, S. D., Friedemann,C. M., and Mickelsen, O. (1968). Am. J. Clin. Nutr. 21, 827.

Buzina, R. (1968). In "Vitamins in the Elderly" (A. N. Exton-Smith and D. L. Scott, eds.), pp. 5-11, John Wright & Sons, Bristol.

Chope, H. D. (1954). Calif. Med. 81, 335.

Chope, H. D. and Dray, S. (1951). Calif. Med. 74, 105.

Chow, B. F. and Yeh, S. D. J. (1963). In "Clinical Principles and Drugs in the Aging" (J. T. Freeman, ed.), p. 219, Charles C Thomas, Springfield, Illinois.

Chu, J. Y., Margen, S., and Costa, F. M. (1975). Am. J. Clin. Nutr. 28, 1028.

Cowan, D. W., Diehl, H. S., and Baker, A. B. (1942). J. Am. Med. Assoc. 120, 1268.

Davidson, C. S., Livermore, J., Anderson, P., and Kaufman, S. (1962). Am. J. Clin. Nutr. 10, 181.

Davies, L., Hastrop, K., and Bender, A. E. (1973). Mod. Geriat. 3, 390.

Dymock, S. M. and Brocklehurst, J. C. (1973). Age Ageing 2, 172.

Ellis, F. R., Holesh, S., and Ellis, J. W. (1972). Am. J. Clin. Nutr. 25, 555.

Felstein, I. (1973). "Living to be a Hundred". David & Charles Newton Abbot, Devon, England.

Food and Nutrition Board, National Research Council (1974). "Recommended Dietary Allowances", 8th Rev. Ed., Nat. Acad. Sci., Washington, D. C.

Forbes, G. B. and Reina, J. C. (1970). Metabolism 19, 653.

Frazer, A. C. (1968). In "Vitamins in the Elderly" (A. N. Exton-Smith and D. L. Scott, eds.), p. 84, John Wright & Sons, Bristol.

Frost, H. M. (1973). Clin. Endocrinol. Metabolism 2, 257.

Garn, S. M. (1970). "The Earlier Gain and the Later Loss of Cortical Bone in Nutritional Perspective". Charles C Thomas, Springfield, Illinois.

Garn, S. M. (1975). In "Physiology and Pathology of Human Aging" (R. Goldman and M. Rockstein, eds.), p. 39, Academic Press, New York.

Garn, S. M., Rohmann, C. G., and Wagner, B. (1967). Fed. Proc. 26, 1729.

Gillum, H. L. and Morgan, A. F. (1955). J. Nutr. 55, 265.

Granick, S. and Patterson, R. D. (1971). In "Human Aging II An Eleven-Year Followup Biomedical and Behavioral Study" (S. Granick and R. D. Patterson, eds.), p. 1, National Institute of Mental Health, DHEW Pub. No. (HSM) 71-9037.

Gyepes, M., Mellins, H. Z., and Katz, I. (1962). J. Am. Med. Assoc. 181, 1073.

Hegsted, D. M. (1962). In "Role of Wheat in World's Food Supply" (R. T. Prescott, ed.), Report of a Conference, pp. 96-103, Western Regional Research Laboratory, Albany, California.

Hegsted, D. M. (1967). Fed. Proc. 26, 1747.

Horwitt, M. K. (1953). J. Am. Diet. Assoc. 29, 443.

Hyams, D. E. (1973). In "Textbook of Geriatric Medicine and

Gerontology" (J. C. Brocklehurst, ed.), p. 555, Churchill Livingstone, Edinburgh.
Kelley, L., Ohlson, M. A., and Harper, L. J. (1957). J. Am. Diet. Assoc. 33, 466.
Keys, A. and Mickelsen, O. (1944). Fed. Proc. 3, 207.
Linkswiler, H. M., Joyce, C. L., and Anand, C. R. (1974). Trans. N. Y. Acad. Sci. Ser. II, 36, 333.
Ljunggren, H. (1965). In "Human Body Composition" (J. Brozek, ed.), pp. 129-138, Pergamon Press, Oxford.
McCay, C. M., Ellis, G. M., Barnes, L. L., Smith, C. A. H., and Sperling, G. (1939). J. Nutr. 18, 15.
McCay, C. M., Sperling, G., and Barnes, L. L. (1943). Arch. Biochem. 2, 469.
Meema, H. E. (1973). Am. J. Clin. Nutr. 26, 687.
Meunier, P., Courpron, P., Edouard, C., Bernard, J., Bringuier, J., and Vignon, G. (1973). Clin. Endocrinol. Metabolism 2, 238.
Mickelsen, O. (1958). Public Health Rep. 73, 295.
Mickelsen, O. (1971). J. Periodont. 42, 460.
Nordin, B. E. C. (1971). Brit. Med. J. 1, 571.
Palmore, E. (1971). Postgrad. Med. 50, 160.
Rockstein, M. (1974). In "Theoretical Aspects of Aging" (M. Rockstein, M. L. Sussman, J. Chesky, eds.), p. 1, Academic Press, New York.
Roine, P., Koivula, L., Pekkarinen, M., and Rissanen, A. (1974). Int. J. Vitam. Nutr. Res. 44, 95.
Schlenker, E. D. (1976). "The Nutritional Status of Older Women". Ph.D. Thesis, Michigan State University.
Shank, R. E. (1975). In "Epidemiology of Aging" (A. M. Ostfeld and D. C. Gibson, eds.), pp. 202, 204, National Institute for Child Health and Human Development, DHEW Pub. No. (NIH) 75-711.
Smith, R. W. J. (1967). Fed. Proc. 26, 1737.
Society of Actuaries (1959). "Build and Blood Pressure Study", Vol. 1, Chicago, Illinois.
Solomon, L. (1968). J. Bone Jt. Surg. 50B, 2.
Soremark, R. and Nilsson, B. (1972). In "Nutrition in Old Age" (L. A. Carlson, ed.), 10th Symposium, Swedish Nutrition Foundation, p. 155, Almquist & Wiksell, Uppsala, Sweden.
Taylor, G. F. (1968). In "Vitamins in the Elderly" (A. N. Exton-Smith and D. L. Scott, eds.), pp. 51-56, John Wright & Sons, Bristol.
Trotter, M., Broman, G. E., and Peterson, R. R. (1960). J. Bone Jt. Surg. 42A, 50.
Vaghefi, S. B., Makdani, D. D., and Mickelsen, O. (1974). Am. J. Clin. Nutr. 27, 1231.

Vincent, P. J. and Urist, M. R. (1961). Clin. Orthoped. 19, 245.

Wachman, A. and Bernstein, D. S. (1968). Lancet 1, 1958.

Walker, A. R. P., Walker, B. F., Richardson, B. D., and Christ, H. H. (1970). Am. J. Clin. Nutr. 23, 243.

Wilson, T. S., Weeks, M. M., Mukherjee, S. K., Murrell, J. S., and Andrews, C. T. (1972). Gerontol. Clin. 14, 17.

Wilson, T. S., Datta, S. B., Murrell, J. S., and Andrews, C. T. (1973). Age Ageing 2, 163.

Yang, M. G. and Mickelsen, O. (1974). In "Methods of Animal Experimentation" (W. I. Gay, ed.), Vol. 5, p. 1, Academic Press, New York.

AGING AND ATHEROSCLEROSIS: INTERACTIONS WITH DIET, HEREDITY, AND ASSOCIATED RISK FACTORS[1]

William R. Hazzard[2]

University of Washington
School of Medicine
Seattle, Washington

Atherosclerosis is a disease of extraordinary complexity. Whereas atherogenesis begins in childhood, it is rarely expressed until middle or old age through one or more of its clinical manifestations: coronary occlusion, stroke, peripheral vascular ischemia, or other relative or total occlusion of large arteries. Increasing evidence (Ross and Glomset, 1974) suggests an intricate interplay of many factors at the tissue and cellular level in the atherogenic process: (1) mechanical, chemical, or immunological trauma to the endothelium of the arterial intima; (2) platelet aggregates which form at sites of endothelial loss; these in turn release a chemical factor which, like low density lipoproteins and insulin, promotes the replication of arterial smooth muscle cells; (3) these cells migrate through the internal elastic lamina, where they constitute the principal cellular component in the atherosclerotic plaque and elaborate extracellular substances including collagen and glycosaminoglycans; (4) in the presence of high ambient low density lipoprotein concentrations these cells incorporate and store excessive amounts of cholesterol esters, and this sequence is perpetuated in a vicious cycle ultimately resulting in the formation of a complicated atherosclerotic plaque.

---

[1]Investigation was supported by Contract NHLI-71-2157. Dr. Hazzard is currently Investigator, Howard Hughes Medical Institute; Associate Professor of Medicine, University of Washington; and Director, Northwest Lipid Research Clinic at Harborview Medical Center, Seattle.

[2]Jointly with Robert H. Knopp, Associate Professor of Medicine, University of Washington; and Deputy Director, Northwest Lipid Research Clinic at Harborview Medical Center, Seattle.

Each of these factors is in turn controlled by multiple influences, including heredity and nutritional status. Hence, an analysis of the nutritional basis of atherosclerosis in an aging population must broadly consider all major risk factors and the interaction of diet, both quality and quantity, with the hereditary predisposition to hyperlipidemia and premature atherosclerosis.

Particularly germane to the central role of aging in the atherosclerotic process is a consideration of the prominence of the various atherosclerotic risk factors in middle vs. old age. A corollary to this issue is the important question of whether dietary manipulation can prevent atherosclerotic disease in these age groups.

Therefore, this article will consider the following issues:

(1) The prognostic role of major risk factors, individually and in combination, in predicting coronary heart disease incidence in middle-aged populations;

(2) A translation of such population-based data to the potential benefit of risk factor reduction in the individual patient as a function of age and sex;

(3) The relative roles of genetic and non-genetic forms of hyperlipidemia in premature atherosclerosis;

(4) Nutritional influences on hyperlipidemia and coronary heart disease; and

(5) The state of knowledge regarding the efficacy of dietary intervention in preventing the complications of atherosclerosis in middle and old age.

EPIDEMIOLOGICAL STUDIES

Given these complex interrelationships and the infinite variety of their quantitative roles in the atherogenic process over the lifetime of an individual, the degree to which atherosclerotic disease can be predicted among adult populations in impressive. Pioneered by the well known Framingham study, prospective epidemiological investigations have consistently identified several important risk factors, prognostic indices of future cardiovascular events. Several of these studies have shared a similar design and execution, allowing grouping of their data in a national cooperative Pooling Project (Stamler and Epstein, 1972). The base population for the figures presented herein was derived from five studies which included 7,594 white males aged 30-59, free of signs of any definite coronary heart disease at entry. In figures 1 through 3 the three variables were first treated singly. Regarding serum cholesterol, in agreement with most U.S. prospective studies, the risk of developing premature coronary heart disease was found to increase continuously with the serum cholesterol concentration. This relationship was most evident for the first major coronary event. However, since in this age group coronary heart disease (CHD) is the single most important cause of death, total mortality could also be related to the serum cholesterol level. For the first major coronary event there was a nearly 4-fold increase in risk between those with cholesterol levels less than 175 mg percent relative to those with cholesterol concentrations exceeding 300 mg percent. Nearly half of the new events occurred in those men with cholesterol levels exceeding 250 mg percent, the upper third of the population under study. Individuals in this group had nearly twice the ten-year coronary heart disease risk as those below this cholesterol level.

Similar findings were evident in the relationships between diastolic blood pressure and between cigarette smoking and first major coronary event, sudden death, all coronary heart disease deaths, and all deaths. As with the serum cholesterol level, the degree of diastolic hypertension and the degree of cigarette smoking each carried their separate continuous risks; the higher the blood pressure the higher the risk, the heavier the cigarette smoking the greater the risk. Thus, for each of these three major quantitative variables there is a steady increment in risk as the level of the particular risk factor increases. Only for cigarette smoking was there evidence for a cutpoint of biological significance, below which the subgroups were relatively immune to premature atherosclerosis. Thus, with the exception of cigarette smoking (for which there is no biological requirement), the terms "normal" and "abnormal" are inappropriate. Simply put, "the lower the better".

However, clinical practice requires that arbitrary cutpoints be set to assist in therapeutic decision-making. Nevertheless, realizing that the gradient of risk exists below as well as above the 250 mg percent cutpoint, an individual and his physician may decide to embark on a cholesterol-lowering regimen at a cholesterol level which others might consider "normal".

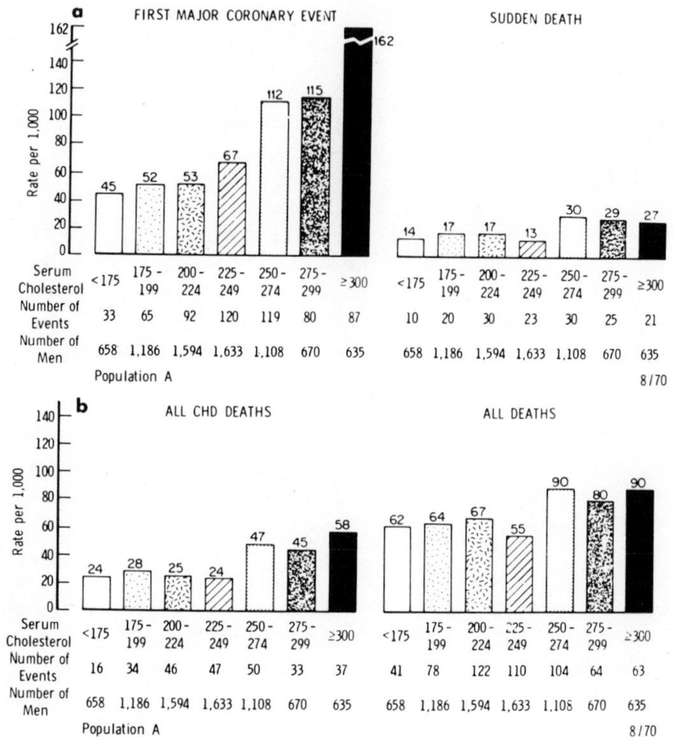

Fig. 1 National cooperative Pooling Project: serum cholesterol level at entry and 10-year age-adjusted rates per 1,000 men for: first major coronary event, sudden death (1a); any coronary death (CHD), death from all causes (1b). First major coronary event includes nonfatal myocardial infarction (MI), fatal MI, sudden death due to CHD; U. S. white males age 30-59 at entry; all rates age-adjusted by 10-year age groups to the U. S. white male population, 1960. (From Stamler and Epstein, 1972.)

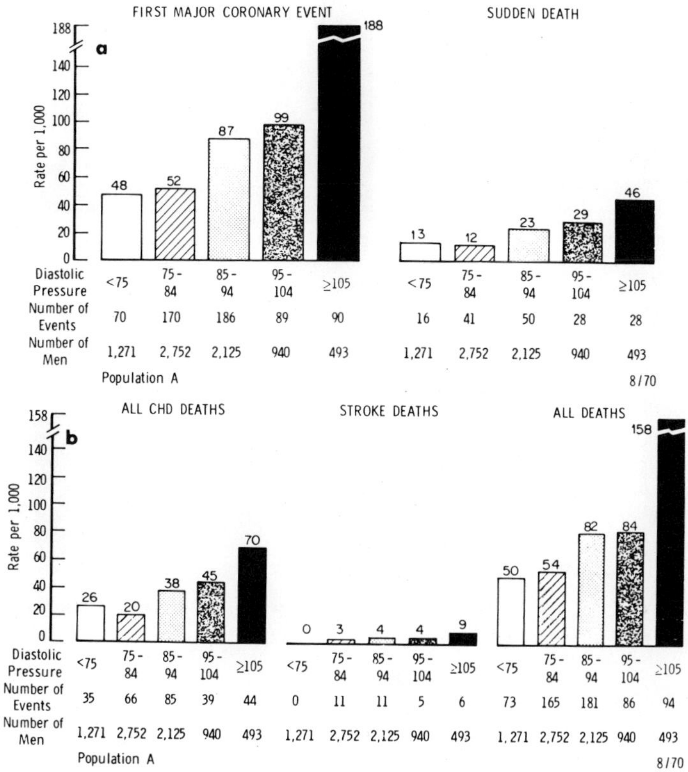

Fig. 2 National cooperative Pooling Project; diastolic blood pressure level at entry and 10-year age-adjusted rates per 1,000 men for: first major coronary event and sudden death (2a); any coronary death (CHD), stroke death, death from all causes (2b). First major coronary event includes nonfatal MI, fatal MI, sudden death due to CHD; U. S. white males age 30-59 at entry; all rates age-adjusted by 10-year age groups to the U. S. white male population, 1960. (From Stamler and Epstein, 1972.)

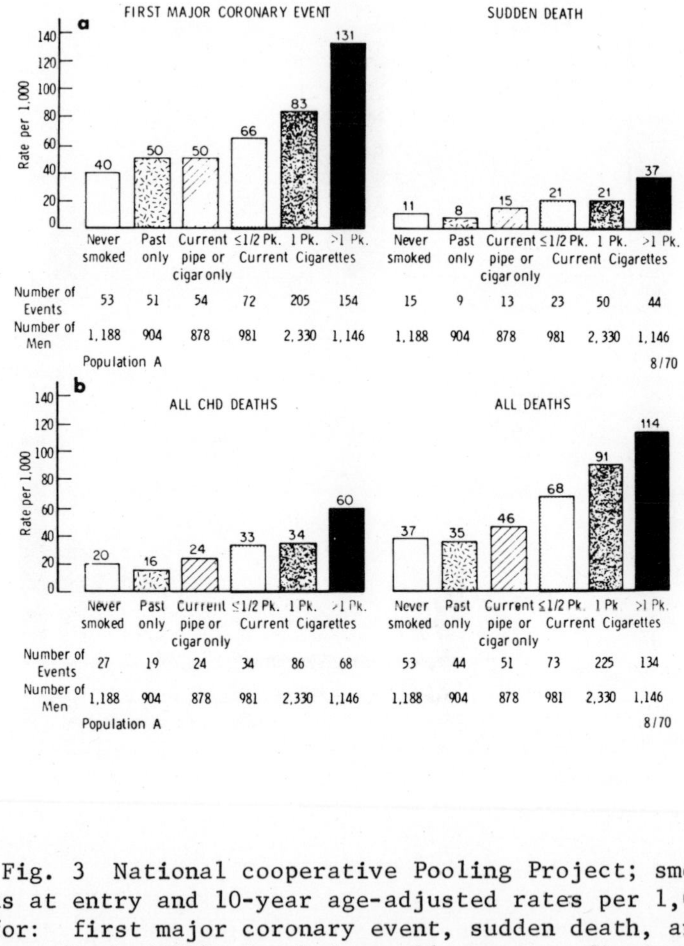

Fig. 3 National cooperative Pooling Project; smoking status at entry and 10-year age-adjusted rates per 1,000 men for: first major coronary event, sudden death, any coronary death (CHD), death from all causes: first major coronary event includes nonfatal MI, fatal MI, sudden death due to CHD; U. S. white males age 30-59 at entry; all rates age-adjusted by 10-year age groups to the U. S. white male population, 1960. Graphs present smoking status at entry and the 10-year age-adjusted rates, irrespective of other risk factors.
(From Stamler and Epstein, 1972.)

Even more impressive are the figures which detail the interaction among these three major risk factors (Fig. 4). Thus, where hypercholesterolemia is considered a risk factor at a level exceeding 250 mg percent, hypertension at a diastolic pressure exceeding 90 mm Hg, and cigarette smoking with the current use of any cigarettes at all; any one of these three factors more than doubled the risk of a first major coronary event. Two concurrent factors again doubled this risk; the presence of all three once again doubled this risk, for an 8-fold gradient between those with all three risk factors relative to those with none. A similar gradient is evident for sudden death, all coronary heart disease deaths and, in this group of relatively young males, total mortality, in which a 5-fold risk ratio was evident between those with all three versus those with none of these risk factors.

It is difficult to underestimate the implications of these results for the health of adult Western populations. The majority of middle-aged white males is clearly in a relatively high risk category; in the Pooling Project only 17% were classified as free of all three risk factors. The rest had one or more: 45% had one, 30% two, and 8% all three. The 38% with two or more risk factors experienced a disproportionate incidence of coronary heart disease events: 58% of first major coronary events, 62% of sudden deaths, 57% of coronary deaths, and 55% of all deaths.

INDIVIDUALIZED RISK FACTOR ANALYSIS

Thus, through measurement of plasma cholesterol and blood pressure and ascertainment of smoking history a rather precise estimate of the risk of future coronary events can be made for <u>groups</u> of adult Americans. How does this translate to the clinical circumstance in which <u>individual</u> estimates of risk are attempted; <u>i.e.</u>, where "n=1"?

Since the variance in these associations is considerable among populations, prognostication for the individual subject is an imprecise art. Nevertheless, average risks can be readily computed from, for instance, the Framingham data and used as the basis for designing therapeutic regimens. Such estimates have recently been calculated by Whyte (1975) from analysis of the Framingham experience. These risks can be broken down by cholesterol level, age, sex and association with other measured risk factors including cigarette smoking, left-ventricular hypertrophy, hypertension and glucose intolerance. They are then expressed in terms of the potential benefit of lowering cholesterol by a given amount. Thus, for

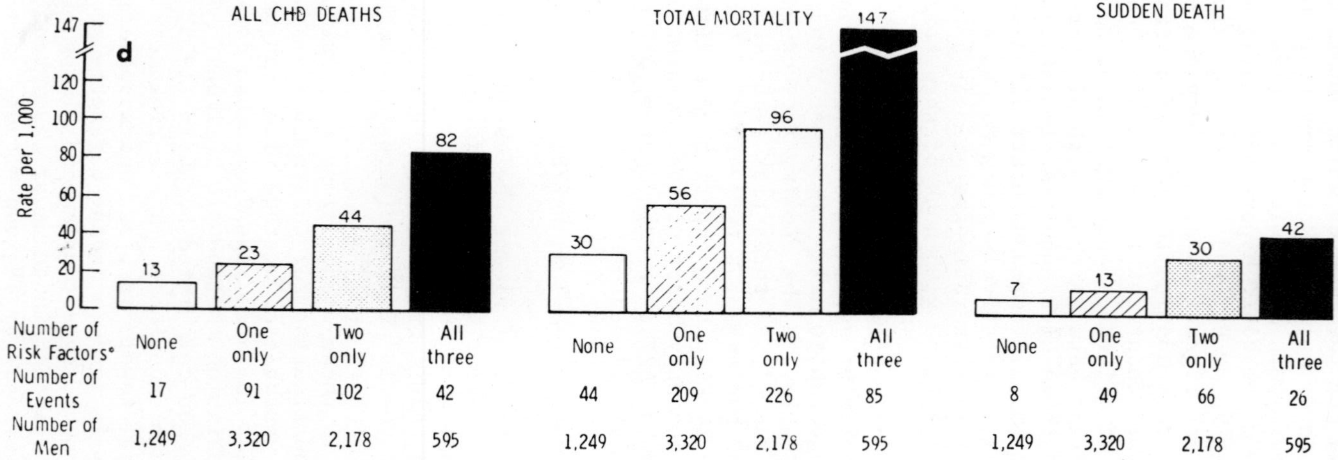

*Cutting Points: Serum Cholesterol ≥250 mg./dl.; Diastolic BP ≥ 90 mm. Hg;
Any use of Cigarettes at entry; Population A 8/70

Fig. 4 National cooperative Pooling Project; hypercholesterolemia, hypertension, cigarette smoking and 10-year age-adjusted rates per 1,000 men for: any coronary death, death from all causes, and sudden death; U.S. white males age 30-59 at entry; all rates age-adjusted by 10-year age groups to the U.S. white male population, 1960. (From Stamler and Epstein, 1972.)

instance, at a cholesterol of 310 mg percent the risk of developing overt coronary heart disease during the ensuing 20 years is 14% among 35-year-old men who are non-smokers, have a systolic blood pressure of less than 120 mm Hg, and manifest no electrocardiographic abnormality (Table I).

TABLE I

Probability of Developing Coronary Heart Disease (CHD) in 20 Years for Young Men Who Otherwise Have Low or High Risk Characteristics: And the Potential Benefit From Lowering the Plasma-Cholesterol.[2]

Plasma-Cholesterol (mg/100 ml)	Probability (%)	
	Low Risk[1]	High Risk[1]
310	14	57
260	8	41
210	5	28
Potential benefit		
310 → 260	6 (43%)	16 (28%)
260 → 210	3 (38%)	13 (32%)
310 → 210	9 (64%)	29 (54%)

[1]Low risk = non-smoker, systolic blood pressure 120 mm Hg, no ECG abnormality. High risk = cigarette smoker, systolic blood pressure 165 mm Hg, left-ventricular hypertrophy.
[2](From Whyte, 1975.)

This risk is reduced to 5% in the same man if his cholesterol is 210 mg percent. Thus, his potential benefit from a reduction in cholesterol from 310 to 210 is a decrease from 14% to 5% or a 64% reduction in incidence of disease. In the 35-year-old man at high risk (Table I), a similar cholesterol reduction reduces his risk of experiencing overt coronary heart disease over 20 years from 57% to 28% (a 54% reduction). Note that the potential benefit of cholesterol reduction to the high risk individual is greater than to the low risk man in absolute terms but smaller in relative terms. Similar individualized risks can be calculated risk-factor-by-risk-factor as in Table II.

Of particular relevance in regard to the role of aging, it should be noted that the potential benefit of cholesterol lowering decreases progressively with increasing age in both sexes. This is reflected in figures 5 through 7. Thus,

TABLE II

Probability (Per 1000) of Developing Coronary Heart Disease (CHD) in 20 Years by Sex, Starting Age, Cigarette Smoking, Left-Ventricular Hypertrophy, Hypertension (Systolic Blood Pressure), Glucose Intolerance, and Plasma-Cholesterol.[1]

Smoking			-	+	-	-	+	+	-	+	-	+
Left-ventricular hypertrophy			-	-	+	-	+	-	+	+	-	+
Hypertension			-	-	-	+	-	+	+	+	-	+
Glucose intolerance			-	-	-	-	-	-	-	-	+	+
SEX	AGE	CHOLESTEROL (mg/100 ml)	PROBABILITY (PER 1000) OF DEVELOPING CHD IN 20 YEARS									
M	35	310	135	208	277	220	402	326	418	571	172	661
		260	84	133	180	141	274	216	286	414	110	449
		210	51	84	114	89	180	139	189	285	68	354
	45	310	225	335	430	352	585	495	604	757	284	831
		260	169	257	336	270	478	394	496	654	216	741
		210	126	196	261	206	382	307	397	549	162	640
	55	310	239	352	448	370	604	515	623	774	..	..
		260	209	311	400	327	552	464	571	727	..	..
		210	182	276	359	289	510	418	522	681	..	..
F	45	310	91	96	156	164	164	172	268	282	122	361
		260	67	72	119	124	126	131	212	222	94	288
		210	51	55	92	96	98	101	165	173	70	226
	55	310	149	157	248	261	261	274	408	426	..	..
		260	118	125	200	212	211	222	340	355	..	..
		210	94	99	161	170	170	180	281	293	..	..

[1](From Whyte, 1975.)

increased age, even more than the coexistence of other risk factors, dampens the potential effect of cholesterol lowering in reducing the incidence of coronary disease. Therefore, both population data and individualized estimates of potential benefit of cholesterol lowering strongly suggest that therapeutic intervention designed to lower blood lipid levels must be instituted early in life in order to yield its maximum and predicted benefit.

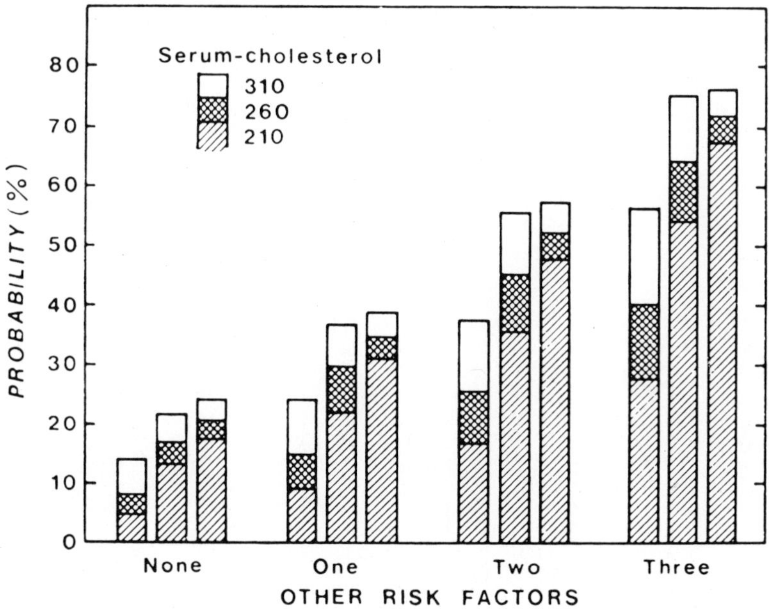

Fig. 5 Estimated probability of developing coronary heart disease in 20 years for men starting at 3 different ages (35, 45, 55 years, left- to right-hand bars of each group of 3, respectively) according to their initial plasma cholesterol and presence or absence of other measured risk factors (see Table I). (From Whyte, 1975.)

It is to be emphasized that such estimates of potential benefit are based upon the most optimistic assumption; namely, that at the time of examination, antecedent hypercholesterolemia (or cigarette smoking or hypertension) has not produced irreparable damage; i.e., that the lowering of an individual's cholesterol level from, for instance, 310 to 210 mg percent instantly reduces his risk of future events to that of a person who has been at the 210 mg percent range all along.

However, this assumption is almost certain to prove unrealistic and therein may lie the major reason for the largely inconclusive and confusing results of dietary intervention trials reported to date. Even in primates rendered dramatically hypercholesterolemic through cholesterol feeding (who experienced an accelerated course in the development of overt atherosclerosis), a three-year lag in regression of lesions following restitution of normal diet and cholesterol levels has been demonstrated (Armstrong _et al._, 1970).

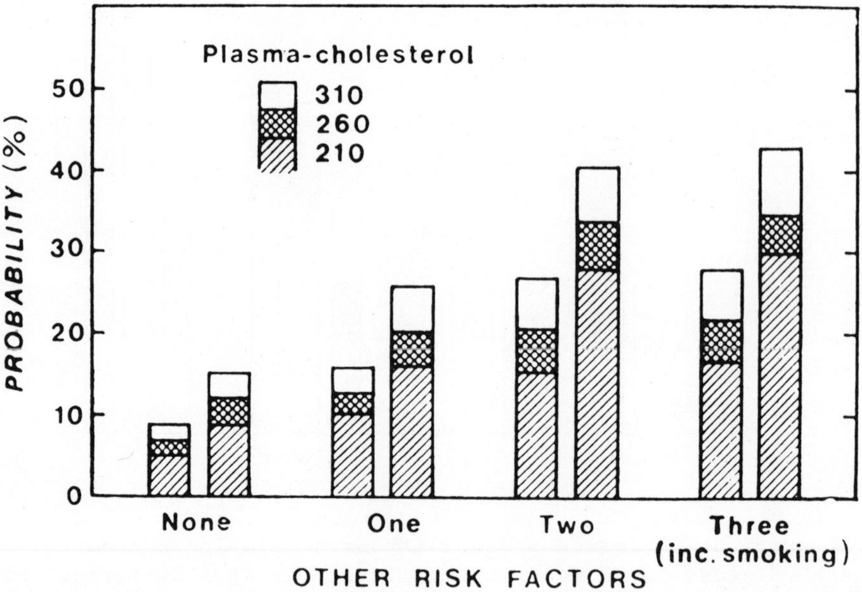

Fig. 6 Estimated probability of developing coronary heart disease in 20 years for women starting at 35 or 45 years (left-hand bar of each pair) or 55 years (right-hand bar) according to their initial plasma cholesterol and presence or absence of other measured risk factors (see Table I). (From Whyte, 1975.)

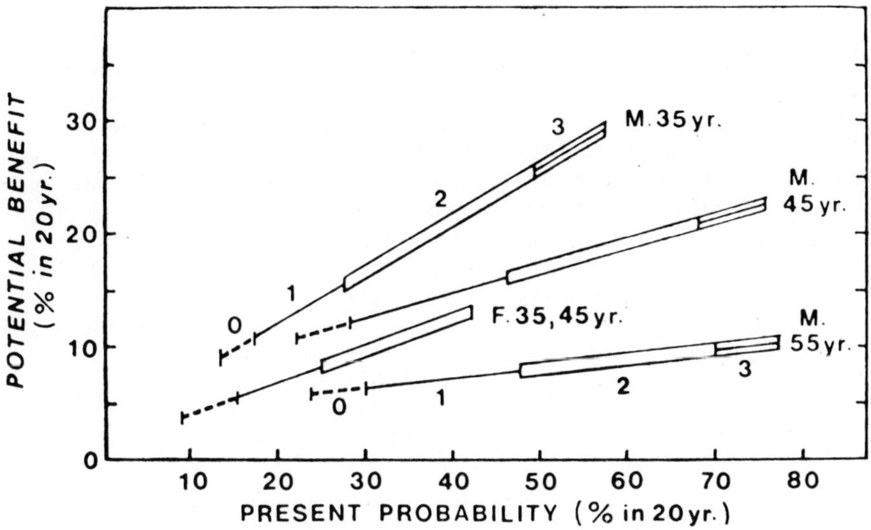

Fig. 7 Potential benefit, shown as the decrease in probability of developing coronary heart disease over the succeeding 20 years, to be gained from lowering the plasma cholesterol from 310 to 210 mg/100 ml, according to the number of associated risk factor (arabic numerals above the lines) (see Table I) for men (M) and women (F). (From Whyte, 1975.)

INTERVENTION TRIALS

There is an essential difference between epidemiological associations, which imply but do not prove a causal relationship, between a given risk factor and the incidence of coronary heart disease, and the demonstration that intervention designed to lower those risk factors indeed reduces the incidence of that disease. This customarily requires a convincing demonstration of benefit in a well designed and conducted, double-blind, randomized, prospective clinical intervention trial. Regarding cigarette smoking, it appears unlikely that such a trial will ever be conducted, nor is it rationally necessary. Nevertheless, longitudinal observation of those who have stopped smoking versus those who continue to smoke [as present in the data from the Pooling Project and work of Reid (1972), figure 8], as well as the results of anticigarette smoking campaigns in secondary coronary disease prevention clinics (Wilhelmsson et al., 1975), strongly suggest that the cessation of cigarette smoking yields major benefits. Even in this circumstance, however, the stopping of cigarette smoking is of less obvious benefit among older than in younger persons in the middle age range (Reid, 1972). Note in figure 8 that among the older subset there may even have occurred an immediate rise in disease incidence following the discontinuation of smoking, which was overcome with time. Other studies specifically restricted to the elderly suggest that the cessation of cigarette smoking appears to afford no substantial benefit and, surprisingly, among women may even have a deleterious impact (Seltzer, 1975). Nevertheless, given the lack of demonstrable benefit from cigarette smoking and the relative ease of intervention against this risk factor (it being of an "all-or-none" variety), the consensus against cigarette smoking among the medical and public health communities is clear.

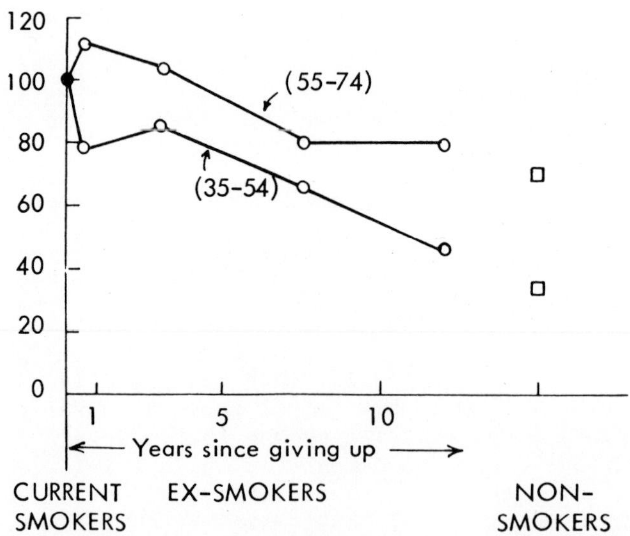

Fig. 8 Relative risk of death from coronary heart disease in male current smokers (1.00), ex-smokers, and non-smokers. (From Reid, 1972, as derived from data in Hammond, 1966.)

With respect to hypertension, it required the demonstration of substantial benefit of treatment among severely hypertensive patients in the randomized clinical trial conducted by the Veterans Administration Cooperative Group (1970) to change patient and physician behavior. Despite the absence of evidence in that trial that the incidence of coronary heart disease *per se* could be reduced through lowering of high blood pressure, the impressive decline in non-coronary disease (from 55% to 18% 5-year incidence rates) among the severely hypertensive subjects in that trial has led to a dramatic increase in the detection and treatment of hypertension in America.

Unfortunately, similar data and consensus do not exist regarding the advisability of lipid-lowering to reduce the incidence of atherosclerotic cardiovascular disease. As discussed below, the lack of clear evidence from previous trials, both dietary and pharmacologic, can be retrospectively rationalized and assigned to errors in design or lack of knowledge of the natural history of the atherosclerotic process. However, until a prospective intervention trial convincingly demonstrates benefit from lipid-lowering, it is unlikely that physicians and the general public will be motivated to change their dietary habits to the degree which would, according to epidemiological evidence, be required to effect a major reduction in coronary heart disease incidence.

In the following discussion we shall delineate those hereditary and nutritional factors which combine to produce the hyperlipidemia so prevalent in Western society. We shall also summarize the results of four dietary intervention trials, all of which, when combined with knowledge of the natural history of hyperlipidemia and atherosclerosis, suggest that hypolipidemic intervention should be instituted among the young and middle aged, not the aged.

THE NATURAL HISTORY OF ATHEROSCLEROTIC CARDIOVASCULAR DISEASE

As schematically depicted in figure 9, coronary heart disease is seen as the end stage of a life-long process. Diet and heredity, aggravated by obesity, produce stage 1, hypercholesterolemia. This, given time and often the coexistence of other risk factors such as hypertension, leads to asymptomatic atherosclerosis. Cigarette smoking, stress and physical activity superimposed on (and possibly perpetuating) this atherosclerosis results in clinical coronary heart disease. Thus, in order to understand the stages of silent atherosclerosis and coronary heart disease, we must first examine the interaction of diet and heredity in the production of hypercholesterolemia.

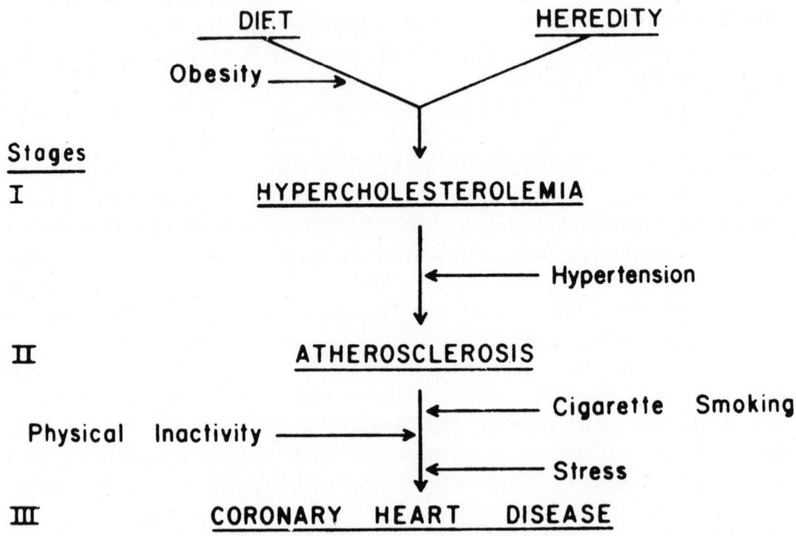

Fig. 9 The conceptualized stages and critical factors in the development of coronary heart disease. (From Connor and Connor, 1972.)

GENETICS OF HYPERLIPIDEMIA AND CORONARY HEART DISEASE

Since age, sex, and diet are all known to affect plasma lipid levels, any attempt to delineate the genetics of hyperlipidemia in coronary heart disease must utilize methods which neutralize these effects. One of the first such studies to employ such techniques took place in Seattle between November, 1970 and October, 1971 (Goldstein et al., 1973a), during which time all patients admitted to the Coronary Care Units of thirteen metropolitan Seattle hospitals were examined to determine whether a definite myocardial infarction had occurred. Of 2,793 such records examined, those of 1,166 patients fulfilled exacting criteria for infarction. From these 1,166, 500 3-month survivors were selected for analysis of the distribution of their overnight fasting cholesterol and triglyceride levels compared to that of a control population. The criteria for selecting these 500 survivors are outlined in figure 10, in which the lower early mortality of younger versus older survivors and our emphasis upon ascertainment of lipid levels of all 3-month survivors under age 60 is evident. The control subjects for this study were comprised of 550 adult women and 400 adult men selected from the non-blood relatives of the survivors (spouses of the survivors and their blood relatives). Since these individuals shared the same environment (including diet) as the survivors and their blood relatives, it was of interest to determine whether lipid levels of spouse pairs could be correlated. Since among 441 such pairs there was no significant correlation for either cholesterol (r = -0.023) or triglyceride (r = 0.098), it appeared reasonable to conclude that any differences in lipid levels between coronary survivors and their spouses were not due to environmental factors.

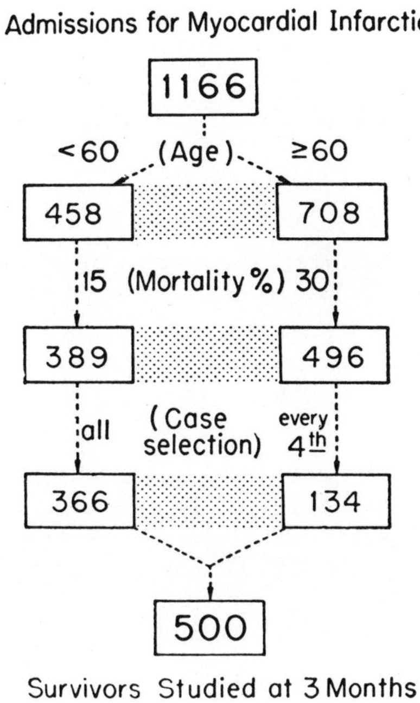

Fig. 10 Method of selection of 500 survivors of acute myocardial infarction for lipid studies.
(From Goldstein *et al.*, 1972.)

When the lipid levels of the 950 controls were plotted as a function of age (Fig. 11), both cholesterol and triglyceride were shown to increase with age with a statistically significant linear correlation among both males and females.

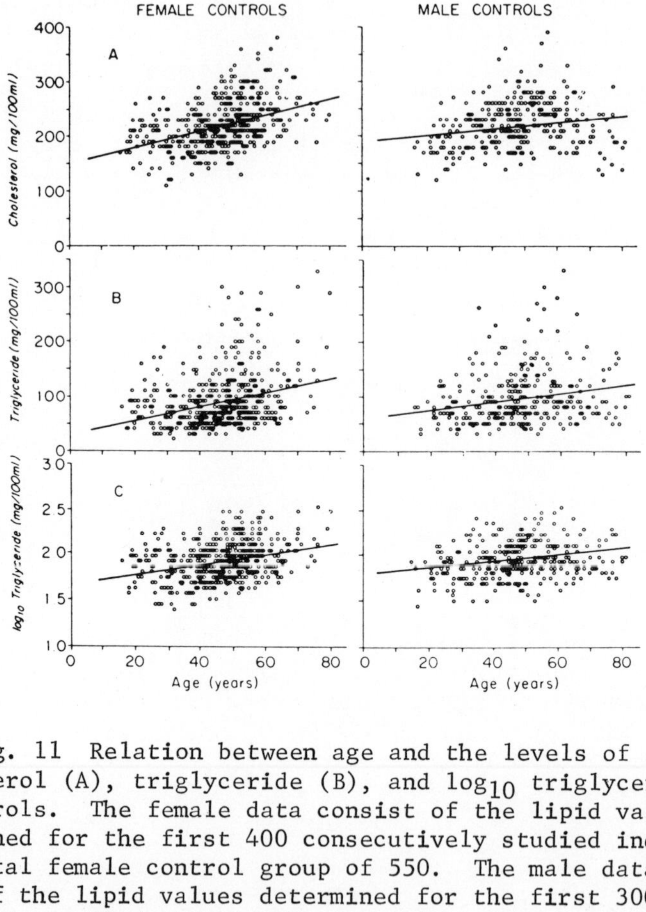

Fig. 11 Relation between age and the levels of plasma cholesterol (A), triglyceride (B), and $\log_{10}$ triglyceride (C) in controls. The female data consist of the lipid values determined for the first 400 consecutively studied individuals of a total female control group of 550. The male data consists of the lipid values determined for the first 300 consecutively studied individuals of a total male control group of 400. The triglyceride values of four controls (301, 450, 680, 850 mg/100 ml), although included in the calculation of the regression equations, are not shown in panels B and C. (From Goldstein <u>et al</u>., 1973a.)

The coefficients of these linear regressions were then used to age- and sex-correct the lipid levels. This was done recognizing that the paucity of high levels among elderly male controls could be criticized as a misapplication of linear regression in a function which was not truly linearly related to age. However, the alternative explanation, namely that the lack of high lipid levels among elderly male controls reflected the premature cardiovascular death of the hyperlipidemic men, was used to justify this linear approach. For cholesterol, the coefficient of linear regression in women was 1.540 mg percent per year, whereas in men it was 0.610. The Y intercept was lower for women, 155 mg percent, than for men, 193 mg percent. The two lines intersected at age 45. A similar relationship was seen for triglyceride with a coefficient of linear regression of 1.294 mg percent per year for women and 0.759 for men. The Y intercept was 35 for women and 63 for men. The two lines again intersected in the middle of the fifth decade. Thus, the slopes of these lines could be used to effect both an age- and sex-correction by multiplying the difference between an individual subject's age and 45 years by the respective coefficient and correcting the values for cholesterol and triglyceride by the number obtained. Thus, it was concluded that utilization of this sex- and age-correction could eliminate the effect of both factors upon the lipid levels observed in coronary survivors relative to the control population.

When the age- and sex-corrected cholesterol and triglyceride values of the 950 controls were plotted (Fig. 12), a normal distribution for cholesterol was obtained with a mean of 218 mg percent and a 95th percentile of 285. For triglyceride, which was skewed to the right in the non-log-transformed histogram, these values were 83 and 165, respectively. For the purposes of this study, hyperlipidemia was arbitrarily defined to exist when the age- and sex-adjusted cholesterol and/or triglyceride levels exceeded these 95th percentile values.

When the lipid distributions of the 500 3-month coronary survivors were superimposed upon those of the 950 controls (Fig. 13), a total of 31% of the 500 were hyperlipidemic. Of these, 7.6% had hypercholesterolemia alone, 15.6% hypertriglyceridemia alone, and 7.8% both hypercholesterolemia and hypertriglyceridemia. It is of note that the surplus of high levels among coronary survivors was not confined to those above the 95th percentiles but that there was a deficit of those below the 50th percentile for both cholesterol and triglyceride relative to the control population and a surplus between the 50th and 95th percentiles. However, at the highest percentiles the ratio of numbers of coronary survivors versus numbers of those in the control population was grossly exaggerated. Thus, at the 99th percentile, for instance, there was a 6.8-fold surplus of survivors with hypercholesterolemia and a 14.3-fold surplus of those with hypertriglyceridemia.

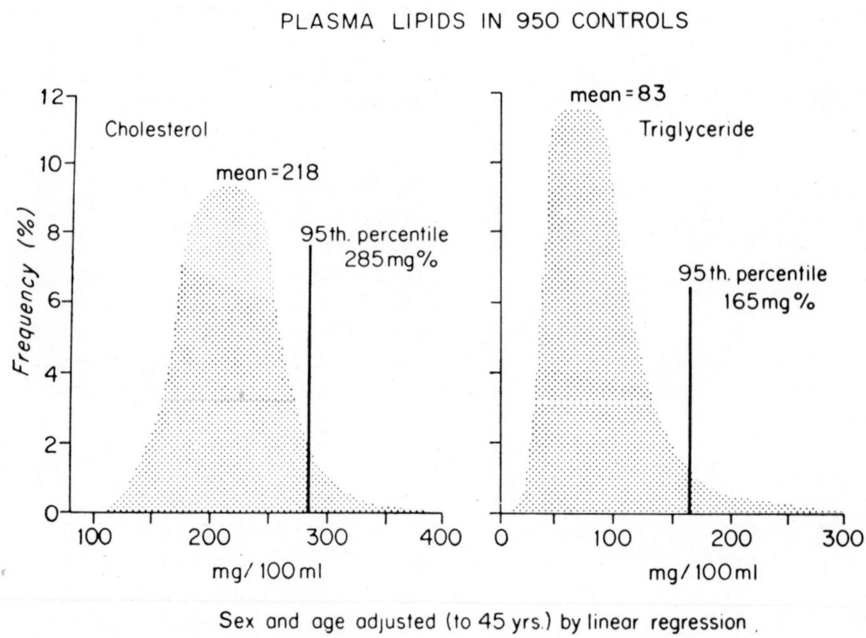

Fig. 12 Distribution of plasma lipids in spouse controls. Adjustments for differences in age and sex between individuals were carried out by the following formula: Adjusted lipid value = (observed lipid value - mean lipid value of appropriate age and sex) + mean lipid value at age 45 years of approrpiate sex.
(From Goldstein et al., 1973a.)

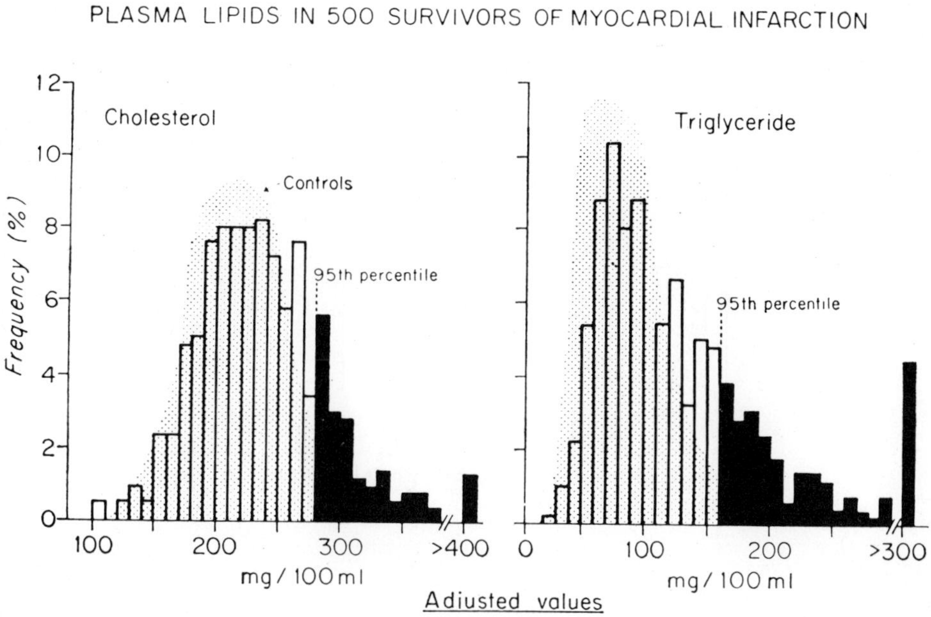

Fig. 13 Comparison of the distribution of plasma lipids in controls and in survivors of myocardial infarction. (From Goldstein et al., 1972.)

It was also of interest to determine the effect of age upon the relationship between hyperlipidemia and coronary disease in these survivors. As can be seen in figure 14, this relationship was most evident in younger survivors, declining in stepwise fashion with increasing age until, above age 70, there was no enrichment of hyperlipidemia among the male coronary survivors relative to the male controls. However, among females, despite a decline in this relationship with each decade, at all ages there was a surplus of hyperlipidemic survivors relative to hyperlipidemic female controls. Given the relative protection which their sex affords, it may thus be easier to detect the role of hyperlipidemia as a risk to coronary disease in women.

These basic descriptive data, which confirm the same relationships observed in other epidemiological studies, served to tie this study to clear-cut epidemiologic investigations during the subsequent analysis of the familial distribution of lipid levels among the hyperlipidemic survivors.

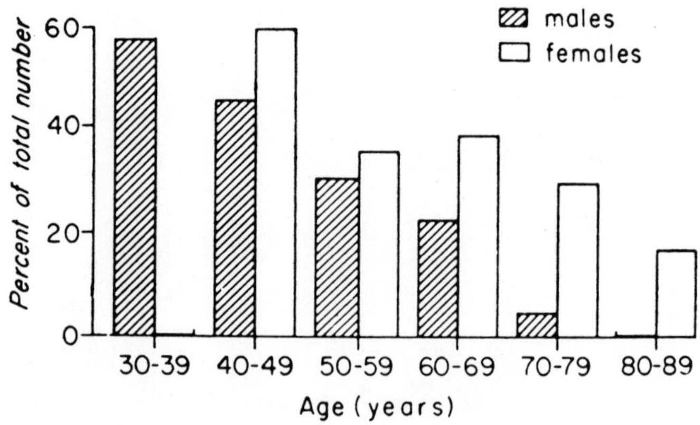

Fig. 14 Relation between frequency of hyperlipidemia and age and sex of survivors.
(From Goldstein et al., 1973a.)

Of the 500 survivors, those with hyperlipidemia (157 in number) served as propositi for in-depth family studies. In these investigations, overnight fasting cholesterol and triglyceride levels of all first-degree relatives were sought, with 95% ascertainment. Additional second-degree and selected third-degree relatives were also similarly studied.

As extensively justified elsewhere (Goldstein et al., 1973b), these studies disclosed the presence of three, separate, clear-cut, monogenic disorders of lipid transport among the hyperlipidemic survivors. The first was the classical disorder called familial hypercholesterolemia. Affecting 16 survivors, this resulted in a marked elevation of cholesterol alone in survivors and affected relatives. As depicted in figure 15, the frequency distribution of adjusted lipid levels in 132 relatives of these 16 survivors revealed a bimodal distribution for cholesterol levels, one mode corresponding to the normal distribution and a second clearly separated from it with a mean level of 299 mg percent. Although certain individuals with this disorder had mild elevations of triglyceride as well, this rarely exceeded half their cholesterol concentration, and the triglyceride distribution in the relatives was superimposable upon that for the controls. Seven of these families contained individuals with known tendinous xanthomas, commonly considered pathognomonic for this disease.

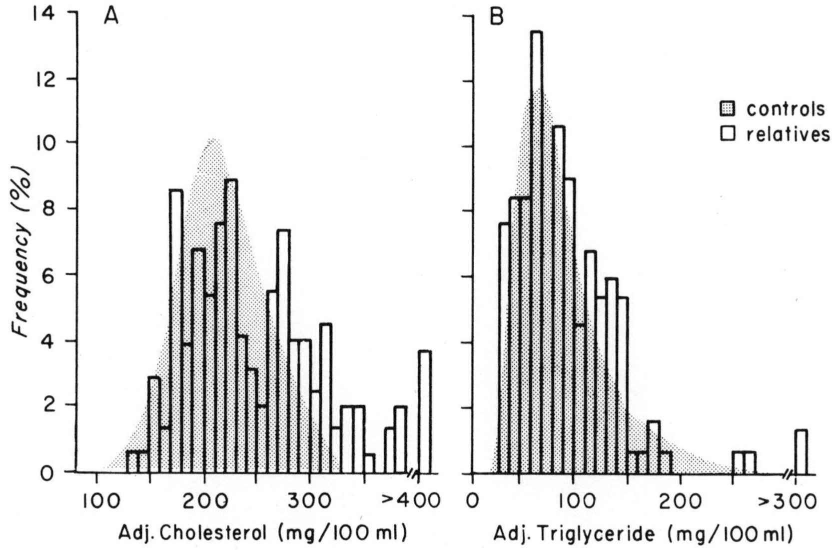

Fig. 15 Frequency distribution of adjusted lipid levels in 132 near and distant relatives of 16 survivors with familial hypercholesterolemia. Included in this analysis were 68 first-degree, 44 second-degree, 18 third-degree, and 2 fourth-degree relatives. 49 of the 132 relatives were between the ages of 6 and 20. The distribution is divided into increments of 10 mg/100 ml. The smooth, stippled curve represents a nonparametric density estimate of the control distribution. (From Goldstein <u>et al.</u>, 1973b.)

A second disorder appeared to elevate triglyceride levels alone. Termed familial hypertriglyceridemia, it was identified in the families of 23 survivors. The lipid distributions in 132 of their adult (≥ 20 years) relatives (Fig. 16) disclosed a bimodal triglyceride distribution, one mode corresponding to the normal and one distinctly elevated with a mean concentration of 180 mg percent. The cholesterol levels were distributed as one mode which corresponded to that in controls. Inspection of various pedigrees revealed many instances of vertical transmission, further evidence for the autosomal dominant mode of transmission of this disorder.

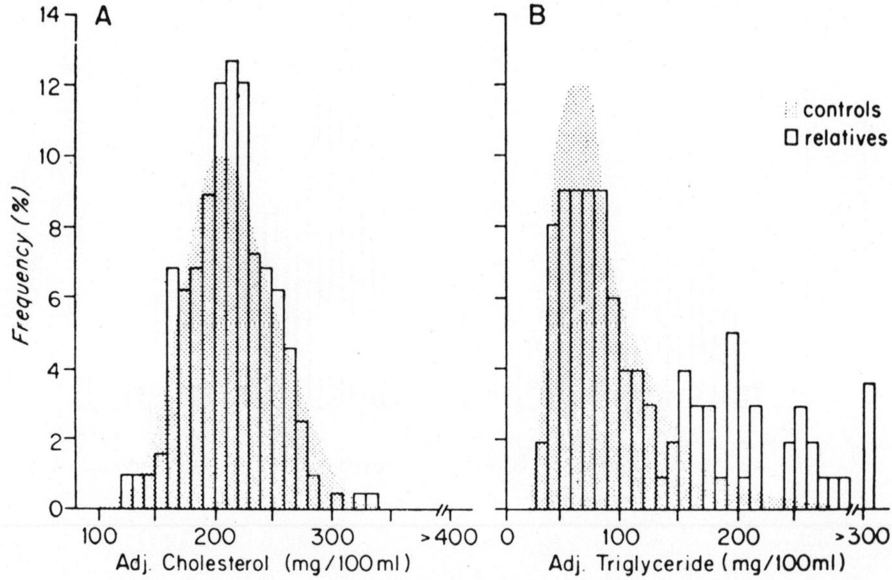

Fig. 16 Frequency distribution of adjusted lipid levels in 132 adult (≥ 20 years of age) relatives of 23 survivors with familial hypertriglyceridemia. Included in this analysis were 90 first-degree relatives, 30 second-degree relatives, and 12 third-degree relatives. The smooth, stippled curve represents a nonparametric density estimate of the control distribution.
(From Goldstein et al., 1973b.)

A third disorder, named familial combined hyperlipidemia, was discovered in the course of this study. Its presence was initially suspected in a single,large pedigree (Fig. 17) in which the propositus had elevations of both cholesterol and triglyceride. However, various hyperlipidemic relatives manifested either hypercholesterolemia or hypertriglyceridemia or both lipid elevations with no clear-cut transmission of any of the three patterns within any family subunit. Surprisingly, a total of 47 such families was identified among the hyperlipidemic survivors. Hence,it was more than twice as common as either of the two, more familiar monogenic disorders.

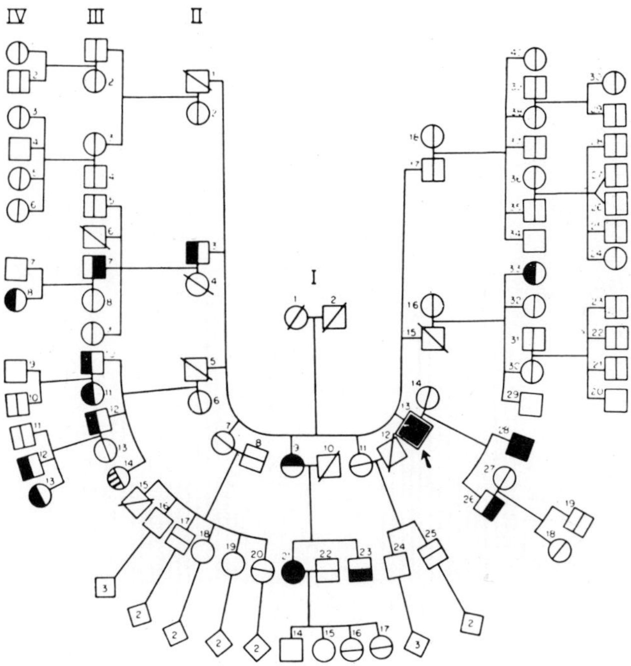

Fig. 17 Pedigree of a family with familial combined hyperlipidemia. The legend for this pedigree is: adjusted cholesterol $\geq$ 95th percentile; adjusted triglyceride $\geq$ 95th percentile; $>$90th percentile. The proband is indicated by an arrow.
(From Goldstein et al., 1973b.)

Inspection of the distribution of lipid levels in 234 first-degree adult relatives of these 47 survivors (Fig. 18) disclosed a bimodal triglyceride distribution but a unimodal cholesterol distribution, shifted to the right of the control distribution. However, further analysis of this cholesterol distribution in which the levels of those with hypertriglyceridemia were plotted separately from those without hypertriglyceridemia disclosed two subpopulations within the single curve (Fig. 19). Since a basic principle of genetics states that the closer one approaches an abnormal gene product, the more likely it is that bimodality will be seen, it was predicted that this disorder will be found to be more closely tied to triglyceride than cholesterol metabolism.

Segregation analyses of informed matings among subjects with all three disorders confirmed the predicted, approximately 50% of affected first-degree relatives and 25% of affected second-degree relatives, supporting the monogenic mode of inheritance of all three.

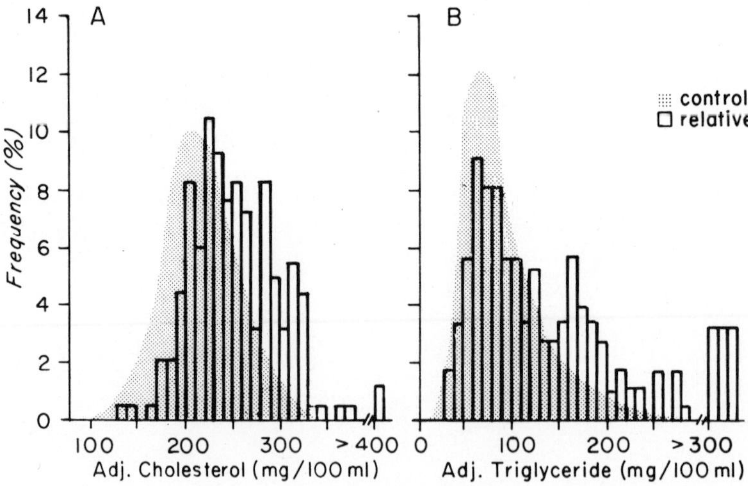

Fig. 18 Frequency distribution of adjusted lipid levels in 234 first-degree adult ($\geq$ 20 years of age) relatives of 47 survivors with familial combined hyperlipidemia. The smooth, stippled curve represents a nonparametric density estimate of the control distribution. (From Goldstein et al., 1973b.)

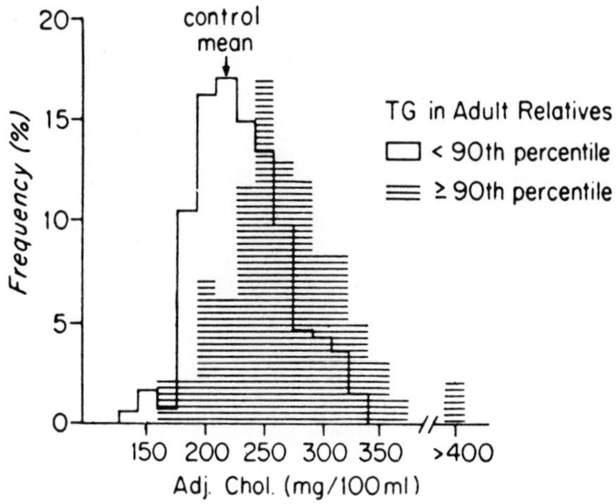

Fig. 19 Relation between the level of cholesterol and triglyceride in 234 first-degree adult (≥ 20 years of age) relatives of 47 survivors with familial combined hyperlipidemia. The 234 relatives were divided into two groups depending on whether their triglyceride level fell above (n=98) or below (n=136) the 90th percentile of controls. The mean value for adjusted cholesterol levels in controls (218 mg/100 ml) is indicated by the arrow at the top of the figure. (From Goldstein *et al.*, 1973b.)

The remainder of the hyperlipidemic survivors were felt to have either a polygenic (multifactorial) form of hypercholesterolemia or a non-genetic (*i.e.*, sporadic) form of hypertriglyceridemia (Fig. 20). Thus, among the hyperlipidemic survivors the majority had one of three monogenic forms of hyperlipidemia. These accounted for more than 20% of all survivors under age 60 but only 7.5% among those above age 60. This was in contrast with polygenic hypercholesterolemia and sporadic hypertriglyceridemia, the prevalences of which were no greater below than above age 60. Thus, the monogenic forms of hyperlipidemia appeared to account for a disproportionate share of premature coronary heart disease, clearly aggravating the age-related atherosclerotic process.

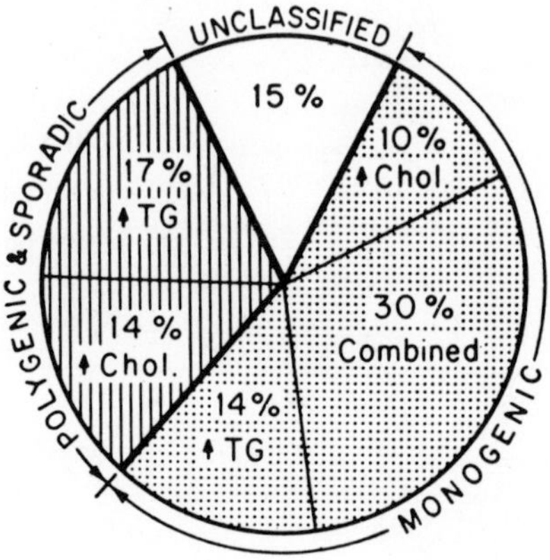

Fig. 20 Summary of genetic analysis in 157 hyperlipidemic survivors of myocardial infarction. The unclassified category represents those hyperlipidemic survivors in whom family study was not possible because of lack of availability of at least three relatives. Type III hyperlipidemia (not included here) was identified in four, or 2.4%, of these 157 hyperlipidemic survivors.
(From Goldstein et al., 1973b.)

Breaking these disorders down still further, it was evident that of the three, familial hypercholesterolemia carried the most ominous prognosis (Table III). The mean age of the 13 male survivors with this disorder was 46 years, compared to 52 years for the 36 with familial combined hyperlipidemia and 57 years for the 18 with familial hypertriglyceridemia. Despite the autosomal nature of these disorders, myocardial infarction was far less frequent among females and, when it did occur, took place at later ages: three with familial hypercholesterolemia averaged 63 years, 11 with familial combined hyperlipidemia 62 years, and 5 with familial hypertriglyceridemia 65 years of age at the time of their myocardial infarction.

The differential importance of the three disorders in the genesis of premature coronary disease was further underscored in a recent study among healthy white-collar male employees of an airplane manufacturing company in Seattle (Boman et al., 1975). Among 1,003 such individuals, familial

TABLE III

Average Age[1] of Patients With Myocardial Infarction by Lipid Characterization[2]

Category	Number of Subjects	Males Mean Age ± SD (yrs)	Age Range (yrs)	Number of Subjects	Females Mean Age ± SD (yrs)	Age Range (yrs)
Familial hyper-cholesterolemia	13	46 ± 9	30-57	3	63 ± 12	46-71
Familial hyper-triglyceridemia	18	57 ± 12	33-74	5	65 ± 14	45-77
Familial combined hyperlipidemia	36	52 ± 9	34-65	11	62 ± 9	43-72
Polygenic hyper-cholesterolemia	22	58 ± 12	35-78	6	63 ± 6	48-70
Sporadic hyper-triglyceridemia	21	59 ± 11	39-69	10	68 ± 10	49-76
Patients without hyperlipidemia	267	63 ± 11	31-87	56	67 ± 11	35-86

[1]Corrected for ascertainment by multiplying the number of patients above 60 years by 4 since only 1 of 4 above this age was sampled. All patients aged 60 and below were studied for lipid categorization.

[2](From Motulsky and Boman, 1974.)

hypercholesterolemia was detected in but one (0.1%), while both familial combined hyperlipidemia and familial hypertriglyceridemia were each present in approximately 1%. Thus, the ratio of their prevalence in coronary survivors versus a healthy middle-aged male population was increased 34-fold among those with familial hypercholesterolemia, 9.5-fold among those with familial combined hyperlipidemia, and 4.7-fold among those with familial hypertriglyceridemia (Table IV). On the other hand, the non-monogenic forms of hyperlipidemia, present in 11.4% of male myocardial infarction survivors, were detected in 8% of healthy middle-aged employees, giving rise to an enrichment in myocardial infarction of only 1.4-fold in individuals with these forms of hyperlipidemia.

TABLE IV

Genetic Characterization of Hyperlipidemia in Men[1]

	In Myocardial Infarction Survivors (n = 377)	In Healthy White-collar Employees (n = 1003)	"Risk Ratio"
Familial hyper-cholesterolemia	3.4%	0.1%	34x
Familial combined hyperlipidemia	9.5%	1%	9.5x
Familial hyper-triglyceridemia	4.7%	~ 1%	4.7x
Non-monogenic hyper-lipidemia	11.4%	8%	1.4x

[1](From Boman _et al_., 1975.)

Additional insights as to those factors affecting penetrance of these genetic disorders were gained by assessment of their prevalences in children aged 6-20. Among this group, familial hypercholesterolemia was clearly fully penetrant, familial hypertriglyceridemia only slightly increased above background (12%), and familial combined hyperlipidemia no more evident than among non-affected children. Thus, achieving maturity appears to be necessary for the expression of the two more common forms of familial hyperlipidemia associated with premature coronary disease. An additional clue as to the mechanism involved in this age-associated penetrance was the stronger relationship between relative body weight and triglyceride levels among affected relatives with familial hypertriglyceridemia versus the control population and their non-affected siblings (Brunzell et al., 1974). A similar linear relationship of triglyceride levels with relative body weight was evident among those with familial combined hyperlipidemia, but the slope of this line was not as steep as that with familial hypertriglyceridemia.

NUTRITIONAL FACTORS IN CORONARY HEART DISEASE

Thus, obesity, as one environmental influence, clearly affects the magnitude of the hyperlipidemia in one genetically so predisposed. However, despite the clustering of excess myocardial infarctions among those with genetic forms of hyperlipidemia, most persons who experience the cardiovascular sequelae of atherosclerosis do not have monogenic hyperlipidemia. Nevertheless, the close parallelism which exists between relative body weight and serum lipid levels as a function of age in both females and males in epidemiological surveys (Fig. 21) suggests that caloric balance may be a potent force in controlling lipid levels among the population at large.

The Seattle study confirmed previous observations that hypertriglyceridemia was at least as common among coronary survivors as was hypercholesterolemia. Even certain prospective studies (Carlson and Bottiger, 1972) have suggested this relationship as well. However, data from Framingham (Kannel et al., 1971) tend to interrelate the hypertriglyceridemia with other risk factors such as obesity and diabetes mellitus (also reflected in the Seattle data [Goldstein et al., 1973a]) and with hypercholesterolemia *per se* than directly with the incidence of coronary disease. Thus, whereas in Framingham there occurred a dramatic increase in cardiovascular risk with increasing cholesterol levels (Fig. 22, far more impressive among young than older males and among males than females at all ages), S_f20-400 pre-β lipoprotein concentrations (reflecting, in this instance, non-fasting triglyceride concentrations) failed to correlate with consistent increases in risk when corrected for the known interrelationship between cholesterol and S_f20-400 lipoprotein levels (Fig. 23). Thus, despite its close association with the risk of coronary heart disease, the plasma triglyceride level is seen less as a risk factor against which intervention should be directed than an index of excess body weight and secondary causes of hyperlipidemia, aggravating factors the correction of which should achieve first priority in therapeutic regimens.

Regarding dietary composition (as opposed to caloric quantity), correlations have been repeatedly drawn between cholesterol intake and death rates from coronary heart disease, presumably mediated through its hypercholesterolemic effect. Within populations consuming diets which are largely similar, as in Framingham, this effect may be lost. However, intercultural epidemiological studies have clearly demonstrated a strong correlation (Fig. 24): societies in which cholesterol intake is minimal have a low incidence of cardiovascular death; those with a high intake have the highest incidence. Notable deviations from this linear correlation do occur, such as in Finland, where the cardiovascular death rate exceeds that which would be predicted on the basis of the cholesterol intake alone, underscoring the role of other factors, presumably largely genetic, which also bear upon this rate.

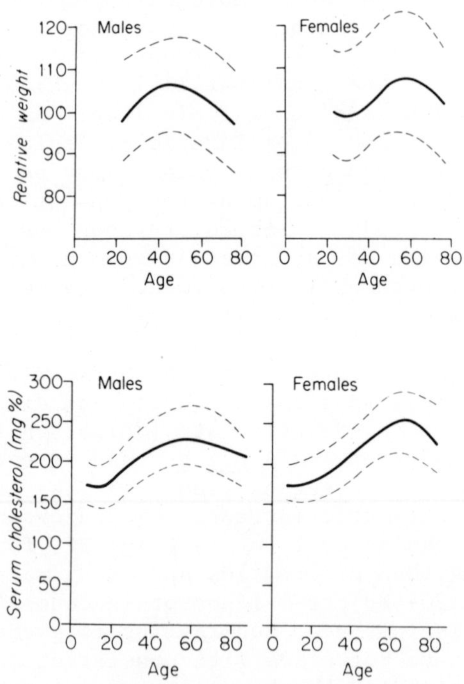

Fig. 21 Relationship between age and relative body weight (ideal=100) (upper panel) and age and serum cholesterol concentration (lower panel) in males and females in an American community, Tecumseh, Michigan. Solid lines are 50th, dashed lines 20th (lower), and 80th (upper) percentiles. (From Bierman and Hazzard, 1973, as adapted from Epstein et al., 1965.)

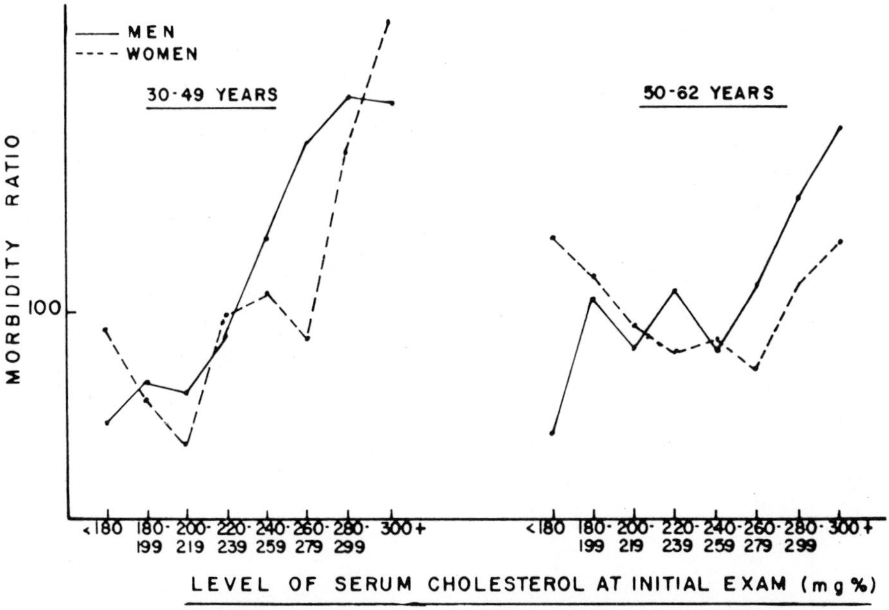

Fig. 22 Risk of coronary heart disease (14 years) according to cholesterol level: men and women age 30 to 62 at entry - Framingham study. (From Kannel et al., 1971.)

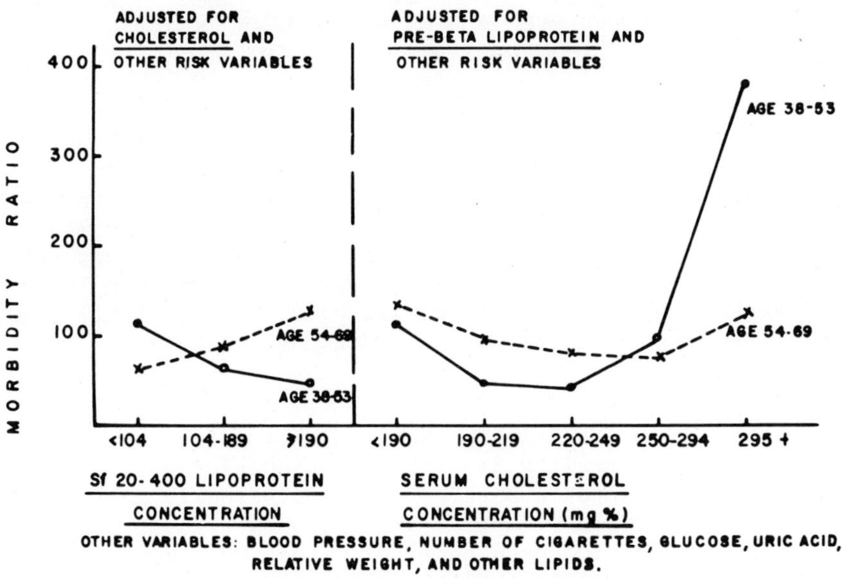

Fig. 23 Risk of coronary heart disease (in 14 years) according to serum cholesterol and S_f20-400 lipoprotein adjusted for associated variables: women, age 38 to 69 - Framingham study. (From Kannel et al., 1971.)

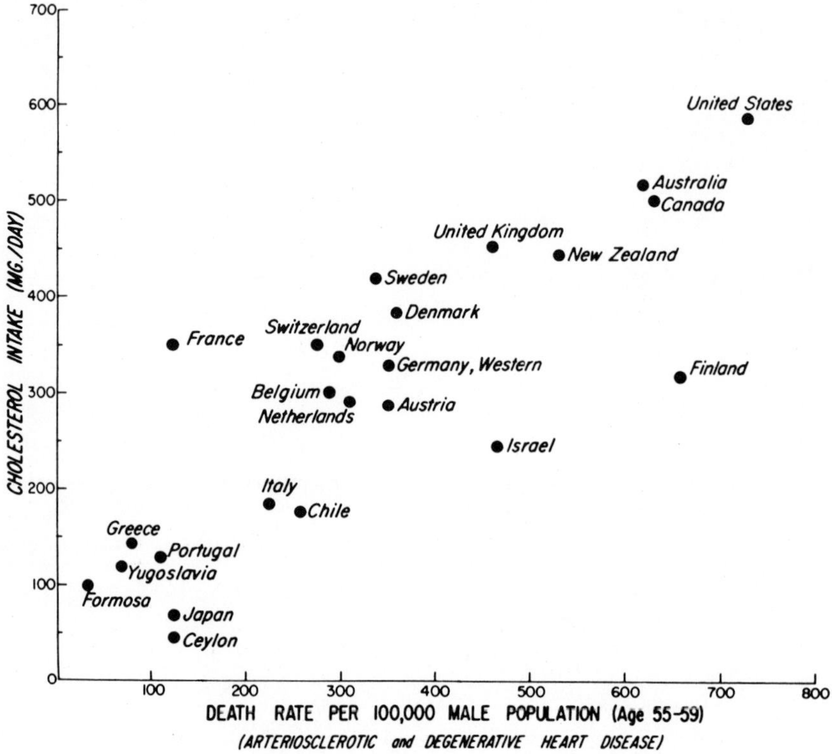

Fig. 24 The death rates from coronary heart disease (arteriosclerotic and degenerative heart disease, category B26) compared with mean daily intake of cholesterol in diet for 24 countries. The death rate is expressed in deaths per 100,000 population in men aged 55-59, 1955-1956. The mean cholesterol intake in milligrams per day per person was computed from food balance sheets for years 1952 through 1956. The correlation coefficient (r) was 0.83 and was highly significant ($p < 0.01$). (From Connor and Connor, 1972.)

Although the correlation between cholesterol intake and cardiovascular mortality is high, other characteristics of the diet of developed countries are also strongly implicated. These include (Table V) animal protein, meat, total fat, egg and sugar consumption, and total calories. Not contributing to this relationship is the intake of plant sterols, fish, vegetable fat and vegetables. Starch and vegetable protein are negatively correlated.

TABLE V

Correlations Between the Mortality Rates From Coronary Heart Disease in Men Aged 55-59 Years and the Intake of Certain Nutrients in the Diet[1]

Positive correlations ($p < 0.05$)	
Animal protein	0.782
Cholesterol	0.762
Meat	0.697
Total fat[2]	0.676
Eggs	0.666
Sugar	0.638
Total calories	0.633
Animal fat[2]	0.632
No correlations ($p > 0.05$)	
Plant sterols	0.144
Fish	0.013
Vegetable fat[2]	0.011
Vegetables	0.009
Negative correlations ($p < 0.05$)	
Starch	-0.464
Vegetable protein	-0.403

[1]Data derived from the national statistics about food consumption and deaths from thirty different countries. (From Connor and Connor, 1972, as derived from World Health Organization, 1959, and Food and Agricultural Organization of the United Nations, 1963.)

[2]Date available from only 29 countries for these nutrients.

Despite the lack of clear separation of dietary cholesterol content versus these other factors in determining cardiovascular disease incidence and the importance of endogenous cholesterol production in contributing to plasma input each day (Table VI),careful metabolic investigations have clearly established a linear increase in serum cholesterol as a function of dietary cholesterol ingestion. As demonstrated in figure 25, the slope of this linear relationship exceeds the more gentle, curvilinear relationship predicted from epidemiological data. Thus, it appears that, despite a partial suppression of endogenous cholesterol synthesis by dietary cholesterol intake, this biofeedback is imperfect, resulting in a degree of additive plasma cholesterol input from each mg of dietary cholesterol ingested.

TABLE VI

Cholesterol Balance in Man[1]

Input into the plasma-tissue pool.	
Dietary cholesterol (0-1000 mg/day)	
Synthesis by the liver and intestine (1000 mg/day)	
Output (500-1000 mg/day)	
Major pathway:	the feces
	The cholesterol and bile acids excreted in the bile and not reabsorbed.
Other pathways:	skin, urine, milk, fetus

[1](From Connor and Connor, 1972.)

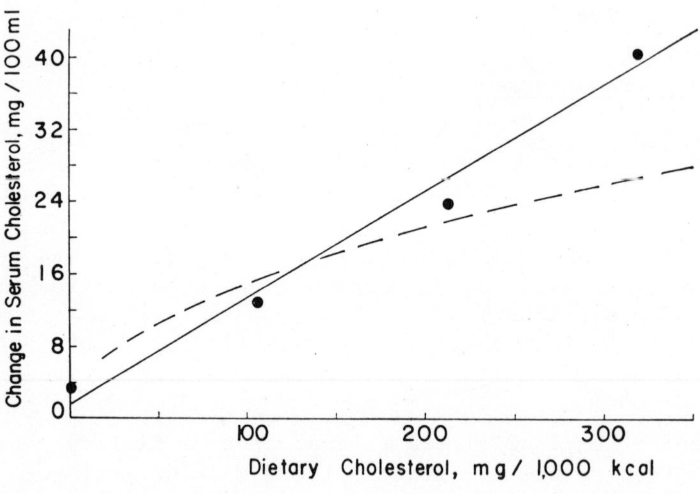

Fig. 25 Relationship between cholesterol intake and the change in serum cholesterol following 21 days on a cholesterol-free formula, ●—●. The broken line shows predicted values based on the equation of Keys et al. (1965). (From Mattson et al., 1972.)

The magnitude of the potential change in serum cholesterol from variations in cholesterol intake (the degree of polyunsaturated fat remaining constant) can be appreciated from carefully controlled metabolic studies such as that from the studies of Connor depicted in figures 26 and 27. In a group of rabbits fed a common diet high in cholesterol, a wide variation in resulting serum cholesterol levels is evident in figure 26. Thus, the degree to which a given individual responds to a given diet depends upon his genetic "set point".

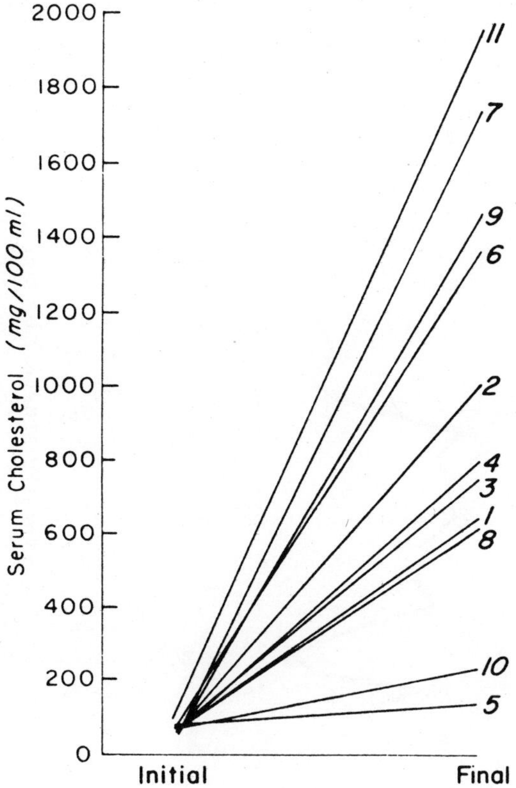

Fig. 26 The initial and final serum cholesterol concentrations for each of eleven rabbits consuming a high cholesterol diet for 24 weeks.
(From Connor and Connor, 1972.)

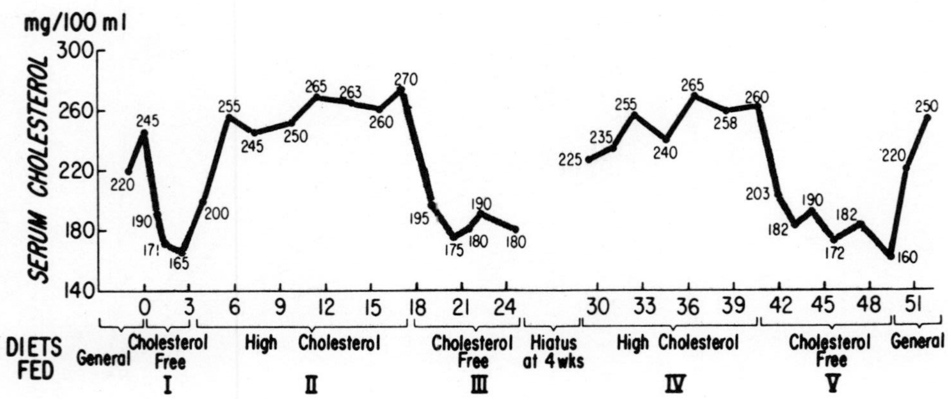

Fig. 27 The effects of dietary cholesterol upon the serum cholesterol level in a 34-year-old man over a 12 month period. The diets of mixed, general foods were either cholesterol-free or contained 2400 mg of cholesterol supplied by egg yolk. In both diets the protein was 15% of total calories, the fat 40% (14% saturated, 17% monounsaturated, and 10% polyunsaturated) and the carbohydrate 45%. The iodine number of the dietary fat in all diets was 80-85. The calories were adjusted to maintain a constant body weight. (From Connor and Connor, 1972.)

However, in the subject without hereditary hypercholesterolemia, whose study is described in figure 27, a near doubling of serum cholesterol was observed during periods of high cholesterol intake (2400 mg daily, approximately 3 to 4 times the average amount currently consumed by adult Americans). Obviously, the potential hypocholesterolemic effect of a reduction in daily cholesterol intake from 750 to 300 mg, the level currently recommended by the American Heart Association, is more modest.

The second dietary factor, the degree of polyunsaturation of the ingested triglycerides, has an equally powerful effect upon the serum cholesterol concentration. This factor may be even more amenable to practical therapeutic manipulation than the intake of cholesterol per se, which, for many middle-aged Americans, has already been reduced to low levels. The mechanism whereby polyunsaturated fats exert their hypocholesterolemic effect is still not well understood and may vary considerably among different individuals. An alarming possibility suggested by some is a displacement of cholesterol from the plasma to the tissue compartment. Other workers have disputed this claim, however, demonstrating a net increment in the fecal excretion of both cholesterol and bile acids, the primary oxidative degradation product of cholesterol catabolism, during polyunsaturated fatty acid feeding.

The magnitude of the potential change in serum lipids through a major revision in dietary habits is exemplified by the contrasting lipid levels in those consuming vegetarian diets, high in carbohydrate and plant sterols, versus those consuming the typical American diet (exemplified in Table VII). In this study among subjects age-matched with those drawn from free-living subjects in Framingham, the average serum cholesterol was reduced by 1/3 and the triglyceride only slightly increased, even when weight-matching was performed. Thus, a life-long diet low in both saturated fat and cholesterol might avoid both the age-related increase in serum lipid levels and its attendant cardiovascular consequences.

Clearly, the timing of dietary intervention might be as critical as its nature and degree in determining its effect upon cardiovascular morbidity and mortality. What is the current knowledge regarding the efficacy of dietary intervention designed to lower serum cholesterol levels and thereby reduce the incidence of cardiovascular disease?

TABLE VII

Mean Blood Lipids on Vegetarian and Conventional Diets[1]

	Age (yr)	No. of Subjects	CHOL[2] (mg/dl)	TG[2] (mg/dl)	Body Weight (kg)
VEGETARIANS[3]	16-29	(92)	123±27	58±29	-
	30-39	(15)	133±34	61±26	-
	40-62	(6)	146±43	64±34	-
	$\bar{x}$	(115)	126±30	59±29	58±9
CONVENTIONAL[4]	$\bar{x}$	(115)	184±37	86±47	73±15
	Δ	(115)	58±47	27±56	15±15
	Δ (wt. matched)	(42)	55±53	25±60	0±9

[1]Based on Sacks et al., 1975.
[2]Mean ± S.D.
[3]Staples: whole grains, beans, vegetables, seaweed, and soy products. Supplements: fruits, nuts, fish.
[4]Age-matched subjects drawn from free-living subjects in Framingham.
CHOL=Cholesterol; TG=Triglycerides

DIETARY INTERVENTION STUDIES

Four such studies might be summarized in this regard. In the National Diet-Heart Study (1968) men ages 44-55 were studied in 5 centers, each recruiting 250 subjects (Table VIII). These men were drawn from among free-living subjects selected from 18% of persons responding to a census tract mailing to middle and upper class neighborhoods. Other subjects were those confined to mental hospitals. All were free of overt cardiovascular disease at entry and had normal electrocardiograms and physical examinations. The presence of associated cardiovascular risk factors among participants was neither sought nor excluding. These subjects were instructed by a dietitian and received either "control" or "polyunsaturated fatty acid-filled" foods from a local commissary and delivered to the home. Adherence was assessed from dietary recall and measurement of the fatty acid composition in adipose tissue, red blood cells and plasma cholesterol esters. Certain notable conclusions were drawn. First, both diets were well tolerated by all participants. Thus, a

TABLE VIII

National Diet-Heart Study[1]

OBJECTIVE

To determine the feasibility of a double blind randomized trial of a cholesterol-lowering diet on preventing coronary artery disease.

DIETS		RESULTS
Diets B & C (Experimental)		Cholesterol lowering (compared to Control Diet D)
Saturated fat:	< 9%	Free-Living
Polyunsaturates (Diet B):	15% (P/S 1.7)	Diet B 10.8%
(Diet C):	18-20% (P/S 2.2)	Diet C 11.7%
Cholesterol:	350-450 mg	Confined
Diet D (Control)		Diet B 16.5%
P/S ratio of 0.4		Diet C 15.0%
cholesterol:	650-750 mg	Heart Attack Rate
		All subjects (even the controls) lost weight and decreased smoking with a reduction in coronary attack rate to about 0.5% per year (about 1/2 the expected rate).
		Projections
		To achieve a 20% reduction in coronary events would require 100,000 participants.
		Conclusion
		A full-scale national diet-heart study is not feasible.

Design:

- Men 44-55, 5 centers each recruiting 250 subjects.
- Free-living subjects selected from 18% of persons responding to a census tract mailing to middle and upper class neighborhoods. Subjects had to have good credit ratings.
- Confined subjects studied in mental hospitals.
- All subjects had normal history, EKG, and physical exams.
- Subjects with particular risk factors were not especially sought out.
- "Control" or polyunsaturate - filled foods were ordered from a local NIH commissary and delivered to the home.
- All subjects were interviewed by a dietitian.
- Adherence was assessed from dietary recall and measurements of fatty acid composition in adipose tissue, red blood cells, and cholesterol esters.
- Ten-month or five-year follow-up.

[1]National Diet-Heart Study Research Group, 1968.

reduction of cholesterol intake to 350-450 mg (roughly 56% of that among the control subjects) and ingestion of a diet enriched in polyunsaturates (with a polyunsaturated/saturated [P/S] ratio of either 1.7 or 2.2) was accepted by the study subjects. Among the free-living subjects studied for a 10-month period both experimental diets reduced cholesterol by an excess of 10%. Among the confined subjects studied for a 5-year period there occurred a 15-16.5% lowering in serum cholesterol. However, the most revealing conclusions from this study were that all subjects, even the controls, lost weight, decreased their smoking, and experienced a reduction in the coronary attack rate to about 0.5% per year, half the projected rate. Consequently, it was estimated that to achieve a 20% reduction in coronary events among free-living participants would require 100,000 volunteer subjects. Thus, from the standpoints of cost and logistical considerations, the National Diet-Heart Study failed its feasibility trial and further efforts were abandoned.

However, among those subjects confined to 7 chronic care institutions in Minnesota, important conclusions have recently been reported. Known as the Minnesota Coronary Survey, this study has had a four-year follow-up of nearly 9,000 subjects equally distributed between the two sexes (Tables IX and X). The experimental diet, enriched in polyunsaturated fatty acids without a decrease in total fat content, increased the P/S ratio from 0.23 to 2.49 and reduced the average cholesterol intake from 602 to 137 mg per day. This resulted in a dramatic fall in serum cholesterol in the treated subjects. Regarding the incidence of deaths from stroke, myocardial infarction or sudden death during the four-year follow-up period, markedly different conclusions were drawn depending on the age and sex of the groups under observation. Among men of all ages, the experimental diet had no effect upon total cardiovascular mortality; among women, a similar effect was observed. However, in the important subgroup of men below age 50, the experimental diet was associated with a decrease in cardiovascular events from 10 to 3 and total mortality from 12 to 2 (but no decrease in either cardiovascular events or total mortality among women in the same age group). Thus, it could be concluded either that this study was totally negative or that it constitutes the most powerful demonstration to date of the potential benefit of reducing cholesterol levels in younger middle-aged males. However, given the small absolute numbers of cardiovascular events in these younger men, it is unlikely that national policy decisions and dietary habits will be greatly affected.

TABLE IX

The Minnesota Coronary Survey.
Dietary Composition, Adherence and Serum Lipid Response[1]

Diet Specifications	Fat % Calories			P/S Ratio	Cholesterol mg/day
	Total	P	S		
Control	42.4	4.3	18.6	0.23	602
Experimental	44.9	19.8	8.0	2.49	137

Adherence: All meals for all participants monitored in institutional cafeterias.
Serum Lipid Response: Treatment group serum cholesterol decreased 13.8%; controls 0.6%. (Subjects on the treatment diet who missed ≤5% of their assigned meals experienced a 16% cholesterol decline.)
P = Polyunsaturated fat.
S = Saturated fat.
[1](From Brewer *et al.*, 1975.)

TABLE X

The Minnesota Coronary Survey.
Deaths From Stroke, Myocardial Infarction, or Sudden Death (Four-Year Follow-Up)[1]

	Age < 50 Years				All Ages			
	Men		Women		Men		Women	
	Exptl.	Contr.	Exptl.	Contr.	Exptl.	Contr.	Exptl.	Contr.
(n)	1192	1106	1124	1068	2505	2428	2417	2425
Events	3	10	6	6	67	78	67	51
Mortality	2	12	11	7	157	159	111	97

[1](From Frantz *et al.*, 1975.)

A third large study was that conducted in mental hospitals in Finland. This employed a cross-over design in which diets rich in polyunsaturated fatty acids were fed in two different hospitals during two different 6-year periods (Table XI). As can be seen from the table, during the six-year study period A (1959-65), patients from hospital K received the control diet and those from hospital N received the experimental diet. During study period B (1965-71), patients from hospital N received the control diet and those from hospital K received the experimental one. "Filled milk" (skim milk with butterfat replaced by soybean oil, total fat content: 3.9%) and "soft margarine" (containing 26% linoleic and 4.5% linolenic acids) were the staple dietary fats in the experimental periods. This changed the P/S ratio from 0.22-0.29 to 1.4-1.8.

TABLE XI

Finnish Mental Hospital Study[1]
on Adult Human Males

	Mean Choles-terol (mg/dl)	% Mean Adipose Tissue (18:2)	(n)	Deaths		Age-Adjusted Death Rate/1000 Persons		
				CHD	Total	CHD	Ca	Total
Control (K) Study A	268	10.2	880	24	66	15.2	3.4	40.2
Control (N) Study B	266	9.8	1023	52	151	13.0	4.5	38.8
Exptl. (N) Study A	217	26.9	1003	20	121	5.7	2.7	34.6
Exptl. (K) Study B	234	32.4	1273	14	66	7.5	7.3	35.1

CHD = Coronary Heart Disease; Ca = Cancer.
[1](From Miettinen *et al.*, 1972.)

The response was monitored by assessing the degree of polyunsaturated fat in adipose biopsies and measuring serum cholesterol. An overall reduction of 10.8% in serum cholesterol was achieved in both hospitals, although a slightly higher mean cholesterol concentration in Hospital K was ascribed to the consistently increased amounts of fat (by 8 to 30 grams) in the diet in that institution. The experimental diet was associated with a reduction in total mortality among males in both hospitals. Among females, no clear effect could be seen. Furthermore, age-adjusted *total* death rates per 1,000 person years among males were not reduced to a statistically significant degree in either hospital by the experimental diet. Thus, the statistically significant decline in coronary heart disease mortality observed during the experimental dietary period in both hospitals ($p < .06$ for Hospital K and

$p < 0.002$ for Hospital N) was negated by the continuing, presumably age-related deaths from other causes in this population. Whether or not the high general death rate might be a function of a high incidence of death from other causes unique to patients in mental hospitals could not be ascertained.

Finally, an even more impressive (and, to some, depressing) failure to influence total mortality was seen in the carefully designed study of Dayton et al. (1969, 1970) (Table XII)*. This was an 8-year, prospective study of 846 volunteer men in a Veterans Administration retirement home who were randomly assigned (regardless of cholesterol level) to a conventional diet or to one similar in all respects except for a substitution of vegetable oils for saturated fat. Prior vascular disease was not excluding, but this affected only approximately 10% of both control and experimental groups. Importantly, the mean age of participants was 65 years for both groups. Other cardiovascular risk factors were randomly and equally distributed between both groups. No subject had xanthomata suggestive of hereditary hypercholesterolemia. The mean cholesterol level was identical (234 mg percent) in both groups and both adhered to their assigned diets to roughly the same degree (approximately 50%).

Results of the 8-year follow-up revealed that fatal atherosclerotic events were more common in the control group (70 versus 48, $p < .05$). This reduction in the combined incidence of myocardial infarction, sudden death, and cerebrovascular accidents, was even more impressive when stratified for men below age 65 or among those with a high cholesterol level (Figs. 28 and 29). However, this was offset by an equivalent increase in deaths from non-atherosclerotic causes in those ingesting the experimental diet (Fig. 29), so that total mortality was similar in both groups (178 among controls versus 174 among those on the highly polyunsaturated fat diet). This was largely attributed to a borderline statistically significant ($p < .06$) increase in deaths due to carcinoma, from 17 in the control group to 31 in the experimental group (Fig. 30). The organs affected by the increased carcinoma incidence were fairly widespread, including buccal mucosa, digestive tract, lung, and genito-urinary tract (Pearce and

*DESIGN FROM TABLE XII: Male veterans in a V.A. retirement home volunteered. Subjects were randomized re diet. Diets were prepared in a single kitchen, were kept separate by color coding, and experimental and control subjects ate in separate dining rooms. Prior vascular disease was not excluding. Adherence assessed from cafeteria attendance records. Blinded follow-up.

TABLE XII

V.A. Domiciliary Study[1]

Subjects at Entry	Control	Experimental	
Number	422	424	
Mean age (yrs)	65.6	65.4	
Caucasian	383	382	
Black	29	31	
Protestant	286	289	
Catholic	115	103	
Systolic B.P.	136.0	136.5	
Weight (lbs)	156.4	153.9	
Cardiovascular Risk Factors	**Control**	**Experimental**	
LVH (left ventricular hypertrophy)	16	20	
Definite MI	30	30	
ST-T changes (on EKG)	22	24	
Angina	2	6	
Arcus senilis	210	207	
Xanthelasma	9	2	
Xanthoma	0	0	
Cigarettes (0)	86	99	
" (1/2-1 pk/day)	129	173	
Cholesterol	234	233	
Diet Adherence (%)[4]	56	49	
Results	**Control**	**Experimental**	**P**
Fatal vascular events	70	48	< 0.05
Total vascular events	96	66	< 0.01
"Soft" vascular events	70	70	N.S.
MI, sudden death, CVA (Life table 8th yr)	0.42	0.28	< 0.02
Total mortality	174	178	N.S.
Fatal cancer[2]	17	31	< 0.06
Gallstones:[3]			
# autopsied & eating 1/3 of diet	83	58	
% with stones	14	34	< 0.01
Cholecystectomy during trial	4	0	

[1](From Dayton *et al.*, 1968, 1969.) [2](From Pearce and Dayton, 1971.)
[3](From Sturdevant *et al.*, 1973.)

[4]DIET

	Control	Experimental
Fat (% of cal.)	40.1 ± 2.2	38.9 ± 1.9
Linoleic (% of f.a.)	10.0	38.4
Cholesterol (mg/day)	653	365
β-sitosterol (mg/day)	3.3	25

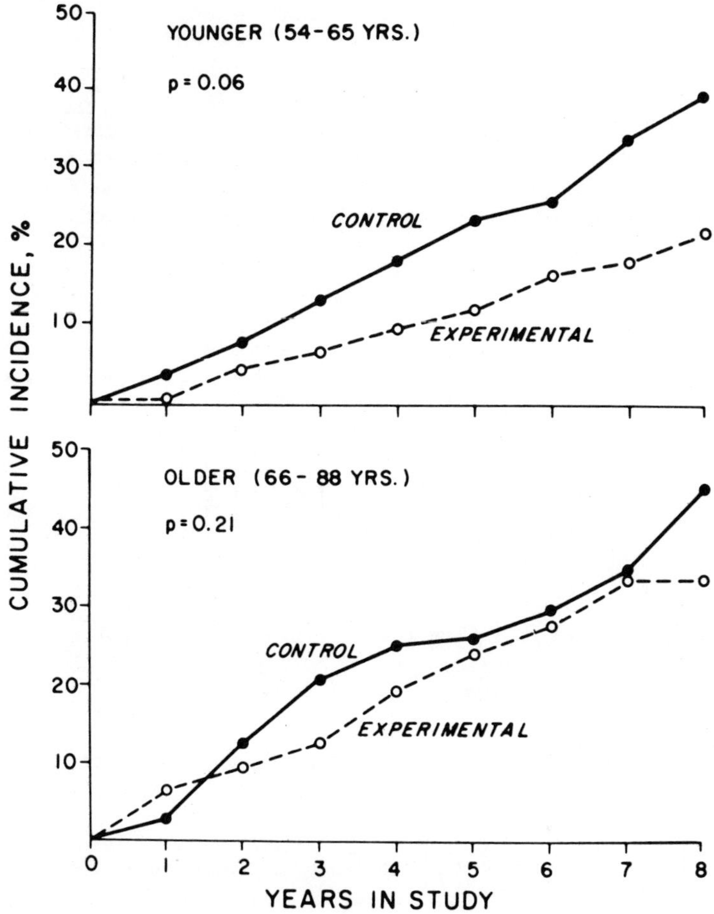

Fig. 28 VA Domiciliary Study. Combined incidence of sudden death due to coronary heart disease, definite myocardial infarction, and definite cerebral infarction, computed by the life table method and stratified by age at entry into the trial. P values apply to comparison of entire curves.
(From Dayton et al., 1970.)

Dayton, 1971). Analysis of other risk factors to neoplastic disease, such as cigarette smoking, failed to account for the increased cancer incidence in the experimental group. The significance of these findings cannot be assessed with certainty, but it has led to similar analyses of other experiences with diets enriched in polyunsaturates. This analysis has failed to confirm the experience of Dayton et al. (1968, 1969, 1970). Nevertheless, it must be viewed seriously in light of animal experiments which suggest that fat intake (especially unsaturated fat intake) can effect the incidence of certain types of neoplasm (see Pearce and Dayton, 1971).

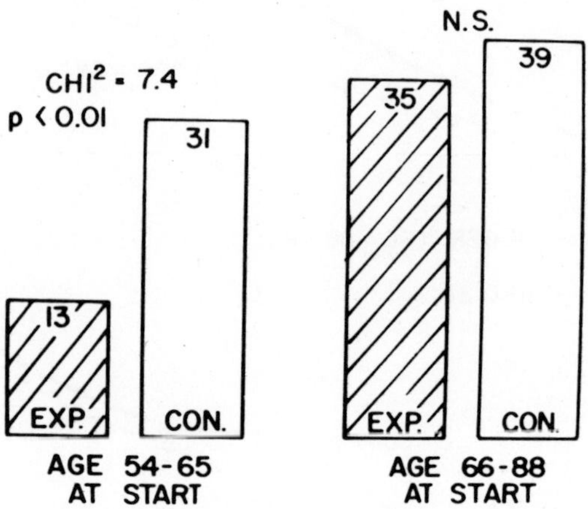

Fig. 29 VA Domiciliary Study. Number of deaths due to acute atherosclerotic events, stratified by age at entry into the trial.
(From Dayton et al., 1970.)

Another, more easily accepted and demonstrable effect of the experimental diet was an increase in the incidence of gallstones, not surprising in view of the increased lithogenicity of bile induced by polyunsaturated triglyceride ingestion.

Relevant to the question of dietary intervention in an aging population, perhaps the most logical conclusion from this study is the possibility that the experimental diet changed the cause but not the age of death. This appears likely for three reasons: (1) many of the men in this study were elderly at the outset (mean age 65 years); (2) they had a high prevalence of heavy cigarette smoking with its attendant carcinogenic potential, and (3) the prescription of the experimental diet was made independent of the serum cholesterol level of the participants. Thus, any risks of the experimental diet were not restricted to those at highest risk to atherosclerosis by virtue of an elevated cholesterol level.

Thus, despite glimmers of hope in certain young, male subgroups, dietary trials to date have suggested a degree of futility of extreme dietary manipulation among older males and among females of all ages. It should not be concluded, however, that such therapy should not be advocated but simply that it is unlikely to yield dramatic benefit. How much more appropriate would such intervention be were it of a milder degree but on a life-long basis?

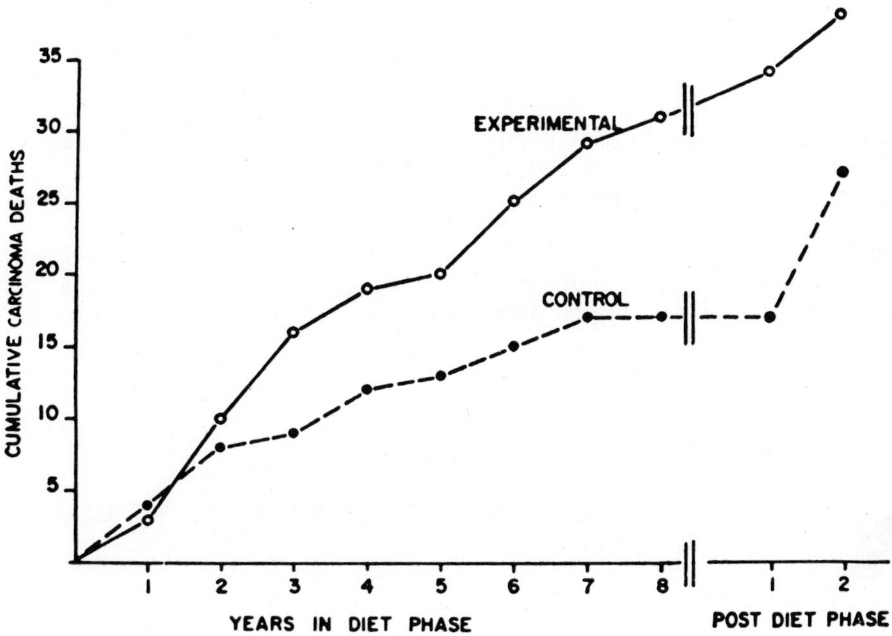

Fig. 30 VA Domiciliary Study. Cumulative carcinoma deaths in experimental and control group from time of randomization of time of death.
(From Pearce and Dayton, 1971.)

CONCLUSIONS

These data suggest the following (Fig. 31):

• First, that major risk factors to premature atherosclerosis can be readily identified and measured in population screening campaigns;

• Second, that the potential benefit of the reduction in each risk factor can be readily quantified from data derived from such prospective epidemiological surveys as the Framingham study;

• Third, that monogenic forms of hyperlipidemia account for a disproportionate share of premature atherosclerosis, whereas among the aged all forms of hyperlipidemia decline as a prominent risk factor;

• Fourth, that the typical American diet containing excessive calories and animal fat leads to a relative hypercholesterolemia in the population as a whole, while the degree to which a given individual responds to this common diet is largely genetically determined; and

• Fifth, that current evidence from several nutritional intervention trials does not justify radical alteration of that diet, particularly among the aged.

In short, in legal prose:

- Whereas all age-related diseases are (by definition) time-dependent; and
- Whereas all such processes are multifactorial in origin;
- Therefore:

  Single modality intervention late in life is unlikely to yield appreciable benefit;
  Intervention should be multifactorial and begun at an early age.

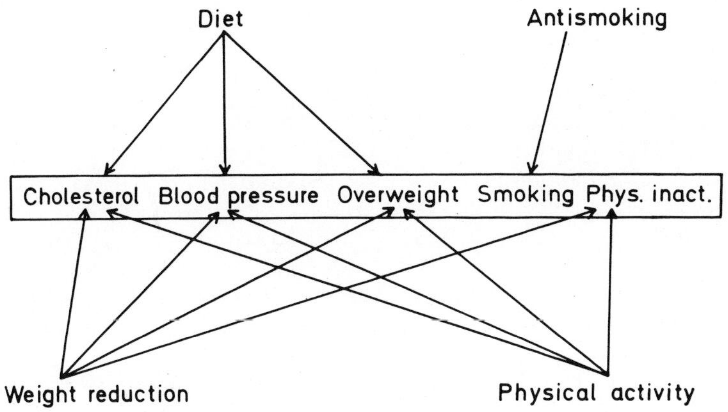

Fig. 31 Interactions of different modes of intervention against several risk factors toward coronary heart disease. (From Werkö, 1971.)

* * * * * * * * * * * * *

Reprint requests should be addressed to Dr. William R. Hazzard, Northwest Lipid Research Clinic, Harborview Medical Center, 325 Ninth Avenue, Seattle, Washington 98104.

* * * * * * * * * * * * *

REFERENCES

Armstrong, M.L., Warner, E.D., and Connor, W.E. (1970). Circ. Res. 27, 59.

Bierman, E.L. and Hazzard, W.R. (1973). In "The Biological Ages of Man: From Conception Through Old Age" (D. Smith and E.L. Bierman, eds.), pp. 154-171, W. B. Saunders, Philadelphia.

Boman, H., Hazzard, W.R., Cooper, M.M., and Motulsky, A.G. (1975). Am. J. Hum. Genet. 27, 19A.

Brewer, E.R., Ashman, P.L., and Kuba, K. (1975). Circulation 51-52, 269.

Brunzell, J.D., Hazzard, W.R., Motulsky, A.G., and Bierman, E.L. (1974). Clin. Res. 22, 462A.

Carlson, L.A. and Bottiger, L.E. (1972). Lancet 1, 865.
Connor, W.F. and Connor, S.L. (1972). Prev. Med. 1, 49.
Dayton, S., Pearce, M.L., Goldman, H., Harnish, A., Plotkin, D., Shickman, M., Winfield, M., Zager, A., and Dixon, W. (1968). Lancet 2, 1060.
Dayton, S., Pearce, M.L., Hashimoto, S., Dixon, W.J., and Tomiyasu, U. (1969). Circulation 40, 1.
Dayton, S., Chapman, J.M., Pearce, M.L., and Popjak, G.J. (1970). Ann. Intern. Med. 72, 97.
Epstein, F.H., Francis, T., Jr., Hayner, M.S., Johnson, B.C., Kjelsberg, M.O., Napier, J.A., Ostrander, L.D., Jr., Payne, M.W., and Dodge, H.J. (1965). Am. J. Epidemiol. 81, 307.
Food & Agricultural Organization of United Nations (1963). Yearbook of Food and Agricultural Statistics, Vol. 17, Rome, Italy.
Frantz, I.D., Jr., Dawson, E.A., Kuba, K., Brewer, E.R., Gatewood, L.C., and Bartsch, G.E. (1975). Circulation 51-52, 4.
Goldstein, J.L., Hazzard, W.R., Schrott, H.G., Bierman, E.L., and Motulsky, A.G. (1972). Trans. Assoc. Am. Physicians 85, 120.
Goldstein, J.L., Hazzard, W.R., Schrott, H.G., Bierman, E.L., and Motulsky, A.G. (1973a). J. Clin. Invest. 52, 1533.
Goldstein, J.L., Hazzard, W.R., Schrott, H.G., Bierman, E.L., and Motulsky, A.G. (1973b). J. Clin. Invest. 52, 1544.
Hammond, C.E. (1966). Nat. Cancer Inst. Monogr. 19, 127.
Kannel, W.B., Castelli, W.P., Gordon, T., and McNamara, P.M. (1971). Ann. Intern. Med. 74, 1.
Keys, A., Anderson, J.T., and Grande, F. (1965). Metab. Clin. Exp. 14, 759.
Mattson, F.H., Erickson, B.A., and Kligman, A.M. (1972). Am. J. Clin. Nutr. 25, 589.
Miettinen, M. (1972). Lancet 2, 835.
Motulsky, A.G. and Boman, H. (1974). In "Atherosclerosis III" (G. Schletter and A. Weizel, eds.), pp. 438-465, Springer-Verlag, Berlin, Heidelberg, New York.
National Diet-Heart Study Research Group (1968). Circulation 37, 1.
Pearce, M.L. and Dayton, S. (1971). Lancet 1, 467.
Reid, D.D. (1972). Prev. Med. 1, 84.
Ross, R. and Glomset, J. (1974). Univ. Wash. Med. 1, 3.
Sacks, F.M., Castelli, W.P., Donner, A., and Kass, E.H. (1975). N. Eng. J. Med. 292, 1148.
Seltzer, C.C. (1975). Abstr. 10th Inter. Congr. Gerontol., Jerusalen, Israel, 1975.
Stamler, J.V. and Epstein, F.H. (1972). Prev. Med. 1, 27.

Sturdevant, R., Pearce, M.L., and Dayton, S. (1973). N. Eng. J. Med. 288, 24.
Veterans Administration Cooperative Study Group on Antihypertensive Agents. (1970). J. Am. Med. Assoc. 213, 1143.
Werkö, L. (1971). Ann. Intern. Med. 74, 278.
Whyte, H.M. (1975). Lancet 1, 906.
Wilhelmsson, C., Vedin, J.A., Elmfeldt, D., Tibbin, G., and Wilhelmsson, L. (1975). Lancet 1, 415.
World Health Organization. (1959). Annual Epidemiological and Vital Statistics, 1956, Palais de Nations, Geneva, Switzerland.

NUTRITIONAL ASPECTS OF STROKE, PARTICULARLY IN THE ELDERLY

Adrian M. Ostfeld, M. D.

Department of Epidemiology and Public Health
Yale University School of Medicine
New Haven, Connecticut 06510

Nutrition and Vascular Disease of the Nervous System in an Elderly Population

Vascular diseases of the brain and nervous system represent the third leading cause of death in the United States and a major crippler of middle-aged and old people. While work on the causes of these disorders has progressed slowly, it is becoming possible to determine the relative importance of chronic disease and, alternatively, of the aging process alone in the etiology of these conditions.

The purpose of this communication is to show that normal or usual aging has relatively little etiological importance in the range of neural disorders in the elderly. Far more important etiologically are four common, related diseases: diabetes mellitus, obesity, atherosclerosis and high blood pressure. This evidence has been adduced from an extensive longitudinal inquiry conducted by this author into diseases of the nervous system in an elderly cohort.

In October 1965, a cohort study of the epidemiology and natural history of cerebrovascular attacks (CVA) was begun in Cook County, Illinois, in an elderly poor, urban population. The principal objective of that research has been to identify variables associated with the incidence of stroke. The basic hypothesis is that factors associated with risk of coronary heart disease (CHD) during middle age are also related to risk of CVA in old age (Kannel, 1967, 1971; Kurtzke, 1969). The prospective method of epidemiology was used to investigate this hypothesis in order to make possible direct assessments of the relationship between risk of stroke and the independent variables. Also, the prospective method was employed to avoid two problems which often diminish the value of data obtained by the retrospective method; namely, the possibility of bias arising from selective elimination of cases before sampling and of bias arising from systematic changes in the independent variables occurring after the clinical appearance of the disease.

What is the incidence of CVA in this population and how is this incidence related to race, sex, age, blood pressure, serum lipids, glucose tolerance, smoking habits, electrocardiogram (ECG) patterns, transient ischemic attacks, and other cardiovascular disease?

Sampling

Three probability samples were selected over a period of 14 months from the population of noninstitutionalized Negro and Caucasian persons who were 65 to 74 years of age and receiving Old Age Assistance (OAA) in Cook County, Illinois. The samples were selected in September, 1965, January, 1966, and November, 1966. At that time, eligibility for OAA required a person to be at least 65 years of age, to have been a resident of Illinois for at least 1 year, and to meet certain financial criteria which, in effect, stated that the person must be destitute and unable to obtain support from relatives. Persons residing in public institutions for the treatment of tuberculosis or mental illness and inmates of penal or correctional institutions are not eligible for OAA.

Initial Interview

Subjects were clustered geographically by postal zone and, within clusters, put into groups of 8 to 12 persons living in close proximity to one another. These groups were assigned to trained interviewers using random permutations in order to randomize effects of systematic differences among interviewers.

A letter of introduction was mailed to each subject just before assignment to an interviewer. The project was described as a study of the health of older persons with the purpose of learning how to prevent illness and promote good health during old age. Cooperation of the subjects was solicited at the initial interview. The interviewers emphasized that cooperation was entirely voluntary and in no way would affect, positively or negatively, a subject's status with the Department of Public Aid.

If the person agreed, the interviewer completed a standard questionnaire schedule which covered demographic, social, and medical topics and made an appointment for the subject to be examined at the central office.

Initial Examination

Upon arrival at the office, a subject was shown to an individual examination room where street clothes were removed and an examination gown put on. The following procedures or measurements were carried out at the initial examination:

A 12-lead electrocardiogram recorded on a Sanborn direct-writing instrument;

Response of the arterial pressure to sitting and standing after being supine while the ECG was recorded;

Oral administration of 50 gm of glucose in a lemon-lime-flavored solution to subjects denying a history of diabetes mellitus;

Height recorded to the nearest centimeter with the subject stretched to greatest height while standing against a flat surface;

Weight recorded to the nearest hectogram on balance scales;

Systolic and diastolic pressures in the left and right arms measured after 5 min. of quiet sitting;

Specimens of venous and capillary blood drawn 1 hr after administration of the glucose;

Vital capacity and 1-sec forced expiratory volume recorded on a 9-liter Collins respirometer;

A detailed history was taken and physical examination given with emphasis on the cardiovascular and central nervous systems.

The medical histories and examinations were performed by three physicians, two of whom stayed with this phase of the project from beginning to end. One physician was an ophthalmologist, the other two were internists. One internist and the ophthalmologist had received 6 weeks of special training in neurology under the supervision of a consulting neurologist. The other procedures were performed by medical technicians who had been specially trained in these techniques.

Laboratory Procedures

Hemoglobin, hematocrit, blood urea nitrogen, and plasma glucose were measured on all subjects. Protein-bound iodine, total protein, and albumin were measured on subjects in the first two samples, and protein electrophoretic patterns were measured on subjects in the first sample only.

At least two 2-ml samples of serum from each subject were placed in sealed vials and stored at -40° C. After the initial examinations were completed, these samples were used to measure total cholesterol and triglycerides on approximately three-fourths of the subjects. (Funds ran out before analyses on the remaining fourth were completed.) Except for the electrophoretic patterns, hemoglobin and hematocrit, all analyses were performed using standard AutoAnalyzer® procedures. Pooled samples, blind split samples, and commercial controls were used continuously to monitor quality of the laboratory determinations.

Diagnostic Categories

"Definite" myocardial infarction (MI) was diagnosed if there was a "definite" history of MI and/or if the ECG presented clear evidence of MI. A definite history of MI was defined as (1) the sudden -- less often gradual -- onset of chest pain or discomfort, (2) hospitalization for a period of weeks, and (3) a physician's statement that the subject had had a "heart attack". The electrocardiograms were read by one of the staff internists according to criteria used by the National Health Survey (Gordon and Garst, 1965).

"Possible" MI was diagnosed in the absence of clear ECG evidence if there was a history containing any two of the three criteria outlined above for a "definite" history.

"Definite" angina pectoris was diagnosed if there was a clear history of two or more attacks of discomfort or pain across both sides of the anterior chest wall, in the precordium or centrally under the sternum, which may have then radiated to the arms, shoulders, neck, or jaw. The discomfort or pain must have been precipitated by effort -- e.g., exercise, emotion, or exposure to cold and wind -- lasted for 30 sec to 30 min, been relieved within minutes after cessation of effort, and spontaneously described as "pressing", "tight", "heavy", "constricting", "crushing", "numbing", or "burning".

"Possible" angina pectoris was diagnosed (1) if there was only one attack meeting all criteria listed above, (2) if the pain or discomfort was described in terms other than those listed above except that lancinating, pleuritic, or throbbing pain was excluded, (3) if there was pain or discomfort as in definite angina but it began in any of the sites of radiation mentioned or in the right anterior chest or epigastrium, or (4) if the discomfort or pain subsided despite continued effort.

Angina pectoris was excluded (1) if the discomfort or pain occurred after the cessation of effort or only in relation to meals, posture, or special movements of the body, (2) if the pain was described as stabbing or lancinating in the region of the left breast, or (3) if there was localized or general chest and/or arm pain due to thoratic outlet or hyperabduction syndrome.

Congestive heart failure was diagnosed if there was dyspnea with exertion or at night, if rales were present in the lung bases, and if there was cardiac enlargement.

Peripheral arterial disease was diagnosed if any of the following were present at examination: (1) history of intermittent claudication, (2) abnormal changes in skin color with changes in position of the extremity, (3) persistent redness or cyanosis of painful ulceration or gangrene in the absence of other disease of the extremity, (4) abnormally slow return of color after blanching, (5) excessive coldness of an extremity when accompanied by atrophic changes in the skin, or (6) evidence of collateral circulation at the femoral artery.

Hypertensive heart disease was diagnosed if (1) the systolic pressure was 160 and/or the diastolic pressure was 100 mm Hg, (2) there was at least grade 1 retinopathy, and (3) there was cardiac enlargement as evidenced by the ECG or physical examination.

Stroke was diagnosed if there was a clear history of cerebral dysfunction (1) compatible with occlusive of hemorrhagic involvement of one or more neck or intracranial arteries, (2) occurring suddenly, (3) lasting for at least 24 hours, and (4) showing some improvement after the time of maximum involvement unless death occurred early.

The Follow-up

Each subject not diagnosed as having CVA at his initial examination was followed until a stroke or death occurred or through March, 1970, when the follow-up phase of the study ended. The primary purpose of the follow-up was to identify those individuals who developed new strokes or transient ischemic attacks (TIA). Several procedures were used to achieve this purpose. All subjects were visited biannually by field workers trained to observe signs of CVA and to administer a standard questionnaire about symptoms of CVA and TIA. Data from these completed evaluations were mailed daily to the central office, where they were evaluated by the research supervisor who had been trained to compare current with past results and to apply consistently certain criteria for selecting subjects for follow-up examination by a neurologist. The supervisor's decisions were regularly checked by the neurological consultant to ensure that they agreed with his own. As long as the information was negative for the possibility of CVA or TIA, the participant was reevaluated at his next biannual examination. Data suggesting the possibility of CVA or TIA led to a follow-up physician's examination. Early in the study, these examinations were done in the subject's home. Later, subjects were examined in a special follow-up clinic at the University of Illinois Hospital where, as in the home, they were examined by a board-certified neurologist or a senior resident in neurology.

Another source of information about morbidity and mortality in this cohort came from the Cook County Hospital, where the great majority of hospitalizations in this population occurred. Located directly across the street from the investigators, this hospital provided a daily list of all its admissions. Possible cases of CVA or TIA were brought to the attention of the neurologist for further workup. Diagnostic procedures such as angiography or lumbar puncture were suggested by the neurologist if they had not already been done, but no such procedures were performed on patients solely because of their participation in this study.

All diagnostic decisions were made by a neurologist according to criteria established at the beginning of the study. For living subjects, the decisions were based on examinations conducted by a neurologist or his senior resident. For deceased subjects, the diagnostic decisions were based upon the best available data -- medical and hospital records, death certificates, or coroner's examinations. Whenever sufficient data were available, differentiation was made between brain infarction and hemorrhage.

Results

The disposition of subjects initially examined is shown in figure 1. The total number of subjects examined, 3141, is 66 per cent of the target population. The reasons for non-participation are: could not be located, 9 per cent; refusal to participate, 19 per cent; and death between selection and initial contact, 6 per cent.

Information about the cohort's place of birth, years of education, marital status, and living arrangements have been published elsewhere, as have tabulations of the prevalence of major chronic illness at the initial examination (Ostfeld *et al.*, 1971).

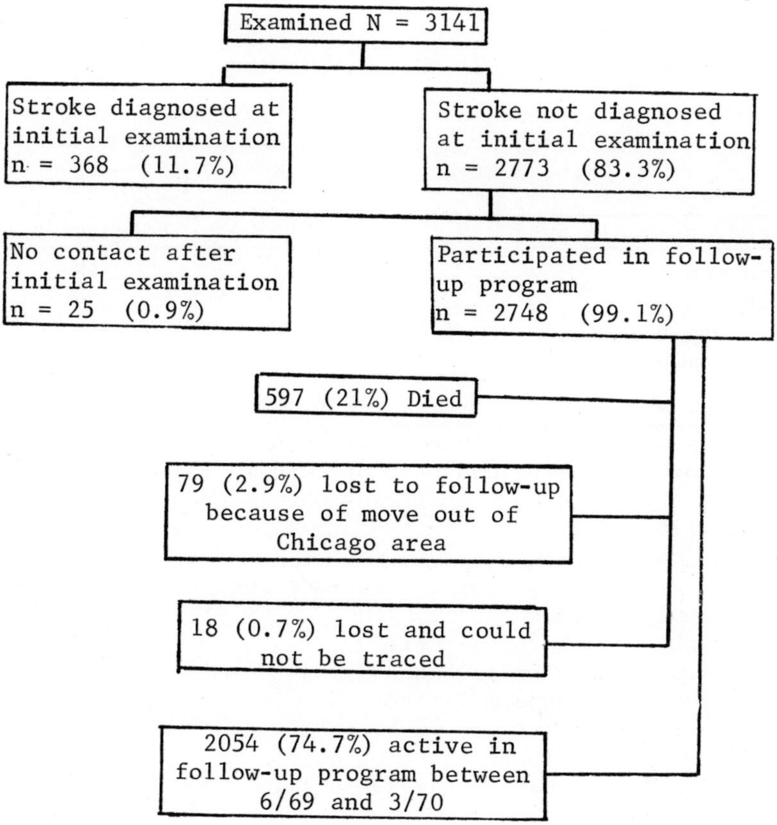

Fig. 1 Disposition of subjects initially examined - Chicago Stroke Study 9/65 - 3/70.

The distribution of subjects free of CVA at the initial examination and followed until new stroke, death, or the end of the program is shown in Table I. One of the major substantive questions of the research was whether potential risk factors for stroke, such as high blood pressure, operated to induce stroke in subjects without any evidence of cardiac or vascular disease. To evaluate this possibility, the total population at risk for stroke was divided into populations A and B. Population A consists of all persons with clinical heart disease, transient ischemic attacks, peripheral atherosclerosis, intermittent claudication, definite ECG abnormalities, histories of diabetes mellitus, blood urea nitrogen of

30 mg per dl, and health status rated as gravely ill. Population B consists of all persons without any one of these conditions.

TABLE I

Distribution of Subjects in the Follow-up Program by Sex and Race Chicago Stroke Study, 1965-67

Categories	All Subjects	Population A*	Population B*
White men	582	324	258
Black men	729	430	299
White women	619	367	252
Black women	818	526	292
Total	2748	1647	1101

*Subjects are included in Population A if any one of the following conditions was present, and in Population B if none of the following conditions were present at the initial examination:

1. Clinical heart disease
2. Clinical cerebrovascular disease, including transient ischemic attacks
3. Peripheral atherosclerosis
4. Intermittent claudication
5. Definite ECG abnormalities
6. Diabetes mellitus, by history
7. Blood urea nitrogen of 30 mg/dl
8. Health status rated as gravely ill

One hundred ninety-eight new strokes developes during the follow-up period. In 136 cases, there was a clear history with confirming signs, in 6 cases a clear history without confirming signs, in 16 a less than clear history with confirming signs at examination, in 11 cases signs only**, and in 29 cases a death certificate only. When the designation Class 1 strokes is used in this paper, it refers to those strokes with both a clear history and confirming signs at follow-up examination.

Table II shows the distribution of cases of stroke by presumed clinical category.

**Because the precise time of onset of these 11 strokes is not known, they have not been included in determinations of incidence.

TABLE II

Distribution of Cases by
Presumed Clinical Diagnosis
Chicago Stroke Study, 9/65 - 3/70

Diagnostic Category	Frequency	Per Cent
	All Strokes	
Nonembolic infarction	158	79.8
Hemorrhage	23	11.6
Embolus	2	1.0
Unknown	15	7.6
Total	198	100.0
	Class 1 Strokes Only	
Nonembolic infarction	114	83.8
Hemorrhage	15	11.0
Embolus	2	1.5
Unknown	5	3.7
Total	136	100.0

Table III shows the three-year incidence of stroke by sex, race, and age. Incidence rates and their standard errors have been computed by life table procedures. When indicated, these estimates have been adjusted for sex, race, and age to the 1960 U.S. population. The substantially higher incidence of strokes in blacks in each group is noteworthy. Stroke incidence was also higher at ages 70 to 74, for each race and sex category, than at 65 to 69; for all categories, it rose from 41 per 1000 to 83 per 1000.

Table IV indicates the three-year incidence of stroke by history of diabetes and reported mode of treatment. The incidence of stroke is significantly higher ($p < 0.05$) among those with a positive history of diabetes than those without a history of diabetes both for all strokes and Class 1 strokes only.

TABLE III

Three-Year Incidence of Stroke,
by Sex, Race, and Age
Chicago Stroke Study, 9/65 - 3/70

Category	Number of subjects	Number of strokes	3-year rate/1000	Standard error
	Age 65-69			
White men	269	7	30	11
Black men	374	25	78	15
White women	218	8	44	15
Black women	309	21	75	16
All (adjusted)	1170	61	41	9
	Age 70-74			
White men	313	19	76	17
Black men	355	26	89	17
White women	401	29	85	15
Black women	509	52	122	16
All (adjusted)	1578	126	83	10
	Age 65-74 (adjusted)			
White men	582	26	50	10
Black men	729	51	82	11
White women	619	37	62	11
Black women	818	73	94	12
All (adjusted)	2748	187	59	7

Incidence rates and their standard errors have been computed by life table procedure. Where indicated, these estimates have been adjusted for sex, race, and age to the 1960 U.S. population.

TABLE IV

Three-Year Incidence of Stroke, by History of Diabetes Mellitus and Reported Mode of Treatment Chicago Stroke Study, 9/65 - 3/70

		All Strokes			Class 1 Strokes Only		
Categories	Subjects	Strokes	Rate/ 1000	S.E.	Strokes	Rate/ 1000	S.E.
History +, no Rx	278	32	119	20	19	73	16
History +, diet only	65	7	69	25	5	44	20
History +, oral med.	128	12	70	22	10	63	21
History +, insulin	53	5	123	50	4	98	47
All history +	524	56	111	15	38	75	13
All history -	2223	131	67	6	88	47	5
All	2747	187	75	6	126	52	5

One subject (no stroke) omitted because of missing data.

In Table V, the three-year incidence of stroke by diagnostic category of heart disease at initial examination is shown. Subjects with hypertensive heart disease (HHD), but not CHD or other heart disease, were at substantially and significantly higher risk of developing stroke ($p < 0.05$) than those free of heart disease. Table VI depicts the three-year stroke incidence by diagnosis of peripheral vascular disease. For both all strokes and Class 1 strokes, there was a significantly higher incidence ($p < 0.05$) among persons with peripheral atherosclerosis (PA).

Continuously distributed variables were divided into quintiles to evaluate the relationship between their levels and stroke incidence. The relationship between stroke incidence and systolic blood pressure quintiles is shown in Table VII; between stroke incidence and diastolic pressure in Table VIII; between stroke incidence and plasma glucose in Table IX and between stroke incidence and ponderal index in Table X. Table XI depicts the results of testing for linear trends in incidence rates of stroke within the quintiles based on distributions of systolic and diastolic blood pressure, serum cholesterol, plasma glucose, cigarette smoking, and ponderal index. The procedure is described in Snedecor and Cochran's

(1967) statistical methods. Table XI indicates that the slopes of the relationship between stroke incidence on the one hand and systolic pressure, diastolic pressure, and ponderal index on the other hand differ significantly from 0, both for all subjects and for population A (the ill group). No such relationship exists between stroke incidence and serum cholesterol, plasma glucose, and cigarette smoking for population A. No significant relationship of any kind was found to exist for stroke incidence and all of these factors among population B.

TABLE V

Three-Year Incidence of Stroke, by Diagnostic Categories of Clinical Heart Disease at Initial Examination
Chicago Stroke Study, 9/65 - 3/70

		All Strokes			Class 1 Strokes Only		
Categories	Subjects	Strokes	Rate/ 1000	S.E.	Strokes	Rate/ 1000	S.E.
AP+, HHD-	175	4	33	17	1	11	11
MI+, HHD-	112	6	82	33	3	45	25
HHD+	600	77	147	20	54	115	19
Other HD	217	10	53	18	8	39	15
HD absent	1644	90	62	6	60	42	5
All	2748	187	75	6	126	52	5

AP = Angina pectoris; HHD = Hypertensive heart disease;
MI = Myocardial infarction; HD = Heart disease

TABLE VI

Three-Year Incidence of Stroke, by Diagnosis of Peripheral Atherosclerosis at Initial Examination
Chicago Stroke Study, 9/65 - 3/70

		All Strokes			Class 1 Strokes Only		
Categories	Subjects	Strokes	Rate/ 1000	S.E.	Strokes	Rate/ 1000	S.E.
PA present	245	24	125	25	18	94	22
PA absent	2503	163	72	6	108	49	5
All	2748	187	75	6	126	52	5

PA = Peripheral atherosclerosis

TABLE VII

Three-Year Incidence of Stroke, by Level of Systolic Blood Pressure at Initial Examination Chicago Stroke Study, 9/65 - 3/70

		All Strokes			Class 1 Strokes Only		
Quintiles	Subjects	Strokes	Rate/ 1000	S.E.	Strokes	Rate/ 1000	S.E.
		All Subjects					
1	482	26	58	12	16	30	7
2	599	27	51	10	15	30	8
3	564	34	68	12	24	49	10
4	514	31	67	13	24	56	13
5	557	66	134	16	45	94	14
All*	2716	184	75	6	124	52	5
		Population A Only					
1	245	15	63	16	10	38	12
2	326	16	56	14	8	29	11
3	327	22	74	16	14	51	14
4	320	23	86	21	18	73	20
5	407	58	158	20	39	110	18
All*	1625	134	90	8	89	61	7
		Population B Only					
1	237	11	51	17	6	20	8
2	273	11	47	14	7	32	12
3	237	12	53	15	10	42	13
4	194	8	50	18	6	42	17
5	150	8	56	19	6	45	18
All*	1091	50	54	8	35	39	7

*34 subjects (3 strokes) omitted because of missing data.

TABLE VIII

Three-Year Incidence of Stroke, by Level of Diastolic Blood Pressure at Initial Examination*
Chicago Stroke Study, 9/65 - 3/70

		All Strokes			Class 1 Strokes Only		
Quintiles	Subjects	Strokes	Rate/ 1000	S.E.	Strokes	Rate/ 1000	S.E.
All Subjects							
1	534	28	57	11	12	28	8
2	529	32	65	13	22	45	11
3	646	43	75	11	31	57	10
4	444	30	91	17	21	67	16
5	563	51	95	14	38	73	12
All	2716	184	75	6	124	52	5
Population A Only							
1	311	20	65	15	8	32	12
2	306	21	76	19	16	59	18
3	365	28	88	16	19	65	15
4	262	22	109	24	14	73	21
5	381	43	115	18	32	88	16
All	1625	134	90	8	89	61	7
Population B Only							
1	223	8	49	19	4	20	10
2	223	11	67	22	6	39	17
3	281	15	60	15	12	50	14
4	182	8	66	24	7	61	23
5	182	8	44	15	6	34	14
All	1091	50	54	8	35	39	7

*Rates of incidence and their standard errors were computed by life table methods, and have been adjusted by giving equal weight to each of the 8 sex-race-age specific estimates. 34 subjects (3 strokes) omitted because of missing data.

TABLE IX

Three-Year Incidence of Stroke, by Level of Plasma Glucose at First Examination in Persons Denying History of Diabetes Mellitus*
Chicago Stroke Study, 9/65 - 3/70

		All Strokes			Class 1 Strokes Only		
Quintiles	Subjects	Strokes	Rate/ 1000	S.E.	Strokes	Rate/ 1000	S.E.
		All Subjects					
1	432	22	59	13	15	41	11
2	415	27	72	14	15	41	11
3	431	27	73	14	18	52	13
4	435	29	71	13	23	57	12
5	445	22	59	13	14	39	11
All	2158	127	67	6	85	47	5
		Population A Only					
1	199	11	61	18	6	35	15
2	205	17	81	19	11	54	16
3	216	16	94	25	11	72	23
4	240	16	64	16	13	54	15
5	231	17	85	22	9	52	19
All	1091	77	79	9	50	55	8
		Population B Only					
1	233	11	55	17	9	47	16
2	210	10	58	18	4	25	12
3	215	11	55	16	7	36	13
4	195	13	78	21	10	59	18
5	214	5	29	13	5	29	13
All	1067	50	56	8	35	40	7

*590 subjects (60 strokes) omitted; 524 (50 strokes) because they had a history of diabetes mellitus at initial examination, and 66 (4 strokes) because of missing data.

TABLE X

Three-Year Incidence of Stroke, by Level of Ponderal Index at Initial Examination*
Chicago Stroke Study, 9/65 - 3/70

		All Strokes			Class 1 Strokes Only		
Quintiles	Subjects	Strokes	Rate/ 1000	S.E.	Strokes	Rate/ 1000	S.E.
		All Subjects					
1	508	35	72	12	25	53	11
2	502	39	95	15	30	74	14
3	493	35	74	12	23	51	11
4	498	32	69	12	22	47	10
5	508	23	45	10	16	33	10
All	2509	164	72	6	116	52	5
		Population A Only					
1	318	29	90	17	20	63	14
2	301	25	103	21	20	86	20
3	290	23	81	17	18	67	16
4	308	25	81	16	16	52	13
5	286	15	52	14	10	34	12
All	1503	117	83	8	84	61	7
		Population B Only					
1	190	6	40	17	5	35	16
2	201	14	85	22	10	61	19
3	203	12	73	21	5	33	16
4	190	7	45	16	6	36	14
5	222	8	39	14	6	32	13
All	1006	47	55	8	32	39	7

*239 subjects (23 strokes) omitted because of missing data.

TABLE XI

Tests of Linear Trends in Incidence Rates of Stroke*
Chicago Stroke Study, 9/65 - 3/70

Statistic	All Subjects		Population A Only		Population B Only	
	All Strokes	Class 1 Only	All Strokes	Class 1 Only	All Strokes	Class 1 Only
			Pondera1 Index			
Slope	-8.0	-6.7	-9.6	-8.9	-4.6	-3.2
Standard deviation	2.21	2.15	1.92	2.06	0.90	0.75
			Plasma Glucose			
Slope	-0.1	1.1	2.8	3.1	-3.3	-0.5
Standard deviation	0.03	0.36	0.49	0.69	0.68	0.13
			Serum Cholesterol			
Slope	-0.5	0.9	3.0	3.0	-5.7	-1.3
Standard deviation	0.14	0.28	0.58	0.68	1.09	0.30
			Diastolic Blood Pressure			
Slope	10.1	11.1	13.1	12.6	-0.8	5.4
Standard deviation	2.78	3.61	2.64	2.99	0.16	1.23
			Systolic Blood Pressure			
Slope	17.5	15.8	24.3	20.2	1.2	6.3
Standard deviation	4.81	5.17	4.87	4.80	0.24	1.49
			Cigarette Smoking*			
Slope	-1.0	-1.3	-5.9	-6.3	4.2	3.4
Standard deviation	-0.23	0.37	0.96	1.27	0.71	0.66

*Smoking category "2+ pk/day" omitted from analysis because of small numbers of subjects.
Standard deviation ≥ 1.645 are associated with $P \leq 0.05$.

Discussion

These data make tenable several inferences about stroke incidence in this population. Stroke incidence was higher among blacks than whites and higher at ages 70 to 74 than at ages 65 to 69. Strokes occurred significantly more often in those with transient ischemic attacks (Ostfeld et al., 1973), peripheral vascular disease, and hypertensive heart disease than in those without these diagnoses. The risk of stroke increases significantly with increasing levels of systolic and diastolic pressure and decreases significantly with increasing ponderal increase. These relationships hold both for the entire population and for the ill group only. It is essential, in this connection, to recall that ponderal index is inversely related to body ponderosity. No association between stroke incidence and serum cholesterol or cigarette smoking was demonstrated.

The absence of any statistically significant relations between levels of potential risk factors and stroke incidence in the initially well population is striking. The data suggest that by the time hypertensive people have reached age 65, those with some target organ damage are susceptible to more target organ damage, i.e., stroke, and those without it are less susceptible to stroke.

In one sense, such abnormalities as TIA and peripheral vascular disease are not risk factors for stroke. They are more properly evidence of atherosclerosis occurring concomitantly with CVA and implying that when fatty plaques are present in the legs they are also likely to be in the neck and head.

What implications do these data have for progress of stroke prevention in this age group? Clearly, little is to be gained by lowering serum cholesterol or reducing cigarette smoking, two procedures which are likely to reduce CHD incidence in younger persons. Would it do any good to reduce blood pressure and rigorously control diabetes? The data are not conclusive but suggest certain inferences. It may be desirable to lower blood pressure among those with higher pressures and other evidence of cardiovascular disease, but not in those without the latter. In this cohort, untreated diabetes and those receiving insulin had a higher stroke incidence than the diabetics receiving diet or oral agents. An obvious inference is that mild diabetics have fewer strokes than more severe ones, and that the underlying character of the disease, rather than success of treatment, influences stroke incidence. The evidence that ponderal index is inversely related to stroke incidence suggests that weight reduction may be helpful but provides no assurance that such action would be beneficial.

Even though no risk factors for stroke were discernible in population B, strokes still occurred in that group. The operation of unidentified risk factors comes to mind.

These findings suggest that hypertension in those with target organ damage is a risk factor for stroke and in those without such damage is not a risk factor. These observations may have implications for primary prevention of atherosclerotic disease and indicate the need for more knowledge about the natural history of hypertension.

Summary

The data signify that even in the elderly, the stroke-prone persons can be identified. In this cohort, risk of stroke is higher among blacks, older persons, and those with preexisting cardiovascular disease manifested as TIA, peripheral vascular disease, diabetes, and hypertensive heart disease. Among those with preexisting cardiac and vascular disease, systolic and diastolic pressures and ponderal index were significantly related to risk of stroke. Among the group free of preexisting disease, no gradient of risk could be demonstrated with any variable measured.

After these data analyses and interpretations were completed, we returned to the data to examine the relationship between stroke incidence and level of hemoglobin. Because hemoglobin is positively correlated with blood viscosity and therefore with propensity to clot, we expected that higher hemoglobin levels would be associated with a higher stroke incidence. We observed that the actual relationship between hemoglobin level and stroke incidence was more complex than that. The relationship was U-shaped (Table XII). Both extremes of hemoglobin levels were associated with higher stroke incidence than intermediate levels. The lower hemoglobin levels in this population were clearly related to an iron deficiency anemia. The results suggest, but do not prove, that iron supplementation of the diet will prevent some strokes in the aged.

TABLE XII

Hemoglobin Concentration and Risk of Stroke in Elderly

Study group Hemoglobin (g/dl)	≤12.2	12.3-12.9	13.0-13.8	13.9-14.4	≥14.5	All
3-year incidence rates/1000 for all strokes						
All persons	101	71	49	88	87	73
H-, CS-[a]	79	37	31	34	82	52
3-year incidence rates/1000 for definite stroke, probably nonembolic brain infarction						
All persons	63	37	21	61	62	44
H-, CS-[a]	65	9	22	22	40	30
Number of participants						
All persons	621	483	542	535	567	2748
H-, CS-[a]	272	187	208	187	150	1004

[a]Neither hypertensive (H) nor cigarette smokers (CS)

The Aging Peripheral Nervous System

Although stroke is the most devastating common disease of the nervous system in old age, other milder dysfunction is much more frequently encountered. The findings of leg weakness, loss of deep tendon reflexes, and absent sense of vibration and position occur so commonly in the aged that they have been usually assumed to be a part of the aging process. To evaluate the relative importance of normal aging and of atherosclerosis-related disease to these changes in the aging neural system, we employed data from the same longitudinal study.

Only scant information is available about the function of the normal nervous system in the aged. Following the early work of Critchley (1931), it has been recognized that the objective findings on detailed neurologic examination of aged persons without known neurologic disease may differ in some respects from the findings in a similar population at a younger age. These differences occur so frequently that they are discounted as evidence of any disease process (Critchley, 1939, 1956; Howell, 1949). It has been proposed that these alterations in neurologic function occur as part of the normal aging process and not as a reflection of any superimposed pathologic involvement of the nervous system of the aging individual (Critchley, 1956). A number of generalized or at least bilaterally symmetrical changes are included in this category and believed not to be of pathologic significance. These include such phenomena as loss of tendon reflexes, alterations of pupillary responses and diminution of vibratory sensibility.

There are at least three possible explanations for these alterations. They could be a reflection of functional and structural changes in the nervous system itself, occurring as part of the normal process of aging. These changes would not be due to alterations of the vasculature of the brain or other non-neuronal influences, but a part of the normal life cycle of the nervous system. Secondly, the clinically detectable changes could be due to neuronal functions which have been altered as a result of diseases which are common in an aged population, e.g., diabetes mellitus or hypertension. The third mechanism which has been suggested is that the changes in neurologic findings could be the result of degenerative changes in the non-nervous tissues which are carrying out part of the response. In this way the loss of tendon reflexes has been attributed to changes in the tendons themselves (Critchley, 1956).

At the present time, the exact incidence of the various changes attributed to normal aging and the interrelationships among these changes are unknown. Furthermore, no systematic study has as yet investigated whether these alterations are related to disease processes such as hypertension, peripheral atherosclerosis, and diabetes mellitus.

The purpose of this analysis is to investigate certain aspects of the neurologic examination performed on a randomly selected elderly population.

Methods

The persons included in this study were members of the cohort which was selected in order to study the epidemiology of stroke in an elderly poor urban population (Ostfeld *et al.*, 1971).

Results and Discussion

The prevalence per 1000 of bilaterally absent reflexes is shown in Table XIII. The Achilles reflexes were unobtainable bilaterally more frequently than either the patellar or biceps reflexes. The prevalence of bilaterally absent

Achilles reflexes was 703 per 1000 while the prevalence of bilaterally absent patellar reflexes was 108 and the prevalence of bilaterally absent biceps reflexes was 42 per 1000. These observations are consistent with Critchley's (1931, 1956) findings that the Achilles reflex is bilaterally absent more frequently than any other tendon reflex in elderly persons. The finding that the patellar reflexes were bilaterally absent more frequently than the biceps reflexes differs from the impression of Critchley (1956), who reported that arm reflexes were more frequently absent than patellar reflexes. Critchley, however, did not remark whether or not he used reinforcement in attempting to elicit patellar reflexes; in this study reinforcement was not performed.

TABLE XIII

Prevalence Per 1000 of Reflex Findings, by Age in Persons 65 to 74, Without Known Neurologic Disease Chicago Stroke Study, 9/65 - 8/67

Type of Finding	65-69 N=385	70-74 N=542	Total N=927
Achilles reflex bilaterally absent	665	731	703
Patellar reflex bilaterally absent	104	111	108
Biceps reflex bilaterally absent	34	48	42
Snout reflex present	161	173	168
Jaw jerk present	55	50	52
Ankle clonus present	0	0	0
Babinski reflex bilaterally present	3	2	2
Chaddock reflex bilaterally present	3	0	1
Hoffman reflex bilaterally present	0	0	0

The prevalence with which these reflexes -- Achilles, patellar, and biceps -- were bilaterally absent increased with age, but the differences are quite small. If these neurologic findings were due to increasing age and had no pathologic significance, larger differences between age groups might be expected. This observation suggests that increasing age may not be the sole factor in the occurrence of bilaterally absent reflexes.

Table XIII also lists the prevalence of several other reflexes in individuals without known neurologic disease. Bilateral extensor responses were rarely elicited by either the method of Babinski or Chaddock. This confirms Critchley's (1956) findings that bilateral extensor responses are unusual in this type of population. Finger flexion elicited as a Hoffman reflex and sustained ankle clonus are also rare in this population. An increased jaw jerk was more common, having a prevalence of 52 per 1000. A snout reflex was even more common at 168 cases per 1000. The appearance of the snout reflex and other primitive reflexes in the aged has been attributed to diffuse bilateral and irreversible central nervous system disease (Paulson and Gottlieb, 1968). The frequency of the snout response in this population casts doubt on the concept that the appearance of this reflex is always associated with clinically apparent cerebral dysfunction.

The relationships between pairs of reflexes are shown in Table XIV. It is unusual for an individual to have unobtainable patellar or biceps reflexes if the Achilles reflexes are not also bilaterally absent. In individuals with one or both Achilles reflexes present, the prevalence of absent biceps reflexes is 11 per 1000 and of bilaterally absent patellar reflexes is 14 per 1000. In individuals with bilaterally absent Achilles reflexes, on the other hand, the prevalence of bilaterally absent biceps reflexes is fivefold greater (55 per 1000) while that of bilaterally absent patellar reflexes is tenfold greater (147 per 1000). This observation suggests that individuals with bilaterally absent biceps and patellar reflexes come from the population with bilaterally absent Achilles reflexes.

TABLE XIV

Prevalence Per 1000 of Bilaterally Absent Deep Tendon Reflexes, by Status of Other Deep Tendon Reflexes in Persons 65 to 74 Without Known Neurological Disease Chicago Stroke Study, 9/65 - 8/67

Status of other deep tendon reflexes	Prevalence per 1000 of bilaterally absent deep tendon reflexes		
	Biceps	Patella	Achilles
Biceps reflex:			
Bilaterally absent, n = 39	-	641	923
Not bilaterally absent, n = 888	-	84	694
Patellar reflex:			
Bilaterally absent, n = 100	250	-	960
Not bilaterally absent, n = 827	17	-	672
Achilles reflex:			
Bilaterally absent, n = 652	55	147	-
Not bilaterally absent, n = 275	11	14	-

The relationship among bilaterally absent tendon reflexes can be seen in other ways. In individuals with one or both of the biceps reflexes present, the prevalence per 1000 of bilaterally absent patellar reflexes was 84 and of bilaterally absent Achilles reflexes was 694. Among individuals with bilaterally absent biceps reflexes, however, the prevalence of bilaterally absent patellar and Achilles reflexes increased to 641 and 923 per 1000, respectively. This same trend is true for bilaterally absent biceps and Achilles reflexes in relationship to the status of patellar reflexes. The fourfold point correlations between status of biceps and patellar reflexes, biceps and Achilles reflexes, and between patellar and Achilles reflexes are 0.36, 0.10, and 0.20, respectively. These correlations are significantly greater than zero ($p < .005$). These findings all demonstrate the close relationship between absent pairs of tendon reflexes and are consistent with the hypothesis that a single mechanism could be related to the absence of all three pairs of tendon reflexes. These data by themselves cannot give any information as to whether this mechanism is neuronal or extraneuronal since generalized structural changes of all tendons could perhaps yield these results.

The relationship of bilateral lower extremity weakness to status of deep tendon reflexes is shown in Table XV. The overall prevalence of bilateral lower extremity weakness -- including proximal weakness only, distal weakness only, and both proximal and distal weakness combined -- was 134 per 1000. The prevalence was similar in males and females and in both sexes the prevalence increased slightly with increasing age. The prevalence per 1000 of lower extremity weakness is 115 among individuals in whom neither the Achilles nor patellar reflexes are bilaterally absent, 129 among those in whom only one of these reflexes is bilaterally absent, and 221 among those in whom both the Achilles and patellar reflexes are bilaterally absent. This association between prevalence of bilateral lower extremity weakness and status of Achilles and patellar reflexes is significantly different from zero ($p < .05$) when testing for a linear trend in proportions. This relationship between bilaterally absent reflexes and clinically detectable weakness in the lower extremities suggests that the loss of tendon reflexes is related to neuromuscular function and may not be just a function of factors related to the tendons themselves.

Since it is rare for individuals to have bilaterally absent patellar reflexes without also having bilaterally absent Achilles reflexes, almost all individuals listed in Table XV as "only one reflex bilaterally absent" had absent Achilles reflexes, while those listed as "both reflexes bilaterally absent" had lost both Achilles and patellar reflexes. It is the loss of the second reflex which is associated with a marked increase in the prevalence of weakness. This suggests that the status of the patellar reflex is more significant in relation to strength than the status of the Achilles reflex.

TABLE XV

Prevalence of Bilateral Lower Extremity Weakness, by Status of Achilles and Patellar Reflexes,* in Persons 65 to 74 Without Known Neurological Disease Chicago Stroke Study, 9/65 - 8/67

Status of Achilles & patellar reflexes	Total Subjects	Bilateral lower extremity weakness	
		Frequency	Prevalence/1000
Both reflexes not bilaterally absent	270	31	115
Only one reflex bilaterally absent	558	72	129
Both reflexes bilaterally absent	95	21	221
Total	923	124	134

*The association between prevalence of bilateral lower extremity weakness and status of Achilles and patellar reflexes is significantly different from zero ($p < .05$) when testing for a linear trend in proportions. Four subjects have been omitted from this table (1 from the upper row, 2 from the middle row, and 1 from the lower row) because data on lower extremity weakness were missing. The age-adjusted rates, giving the younger and older groups equal weight, are 114, 128 and 210 cases per 1000 for rows 1 to 3, respectively.

Bilateral upper extremity weakness (71 cases per 1000) is less common than bilateral lower extremity weakness (134 per 1000). Bilateral upper extremity weakness was unrelated to the status of the biceps reflex, which was the only arm reflex tested.

The prevalence per 1000 of bilateral loss of vibratory and position senses are shown in Table XVI. Loss of these forms of sensation are relatively common in this population but are quite similar in both age groups. Loss of vibration limited to both lower extremities only is the commonest anomaly, with an overall prevalence of 515 per 1000. Bilateral loss of vibratory sensibility in both upper and lower extremities occurs with a prevalence of 310 per 1000, while bilateral loss in the upper extremities only is quite unusual (17 per 1000). The relative distribution of bilateral alteration of position sense is quite similar to the distribution of alterations of vibratory sensation, even though the overall prevalence is much lower. Bilateral loss of position sense is most commonly limited to the lower extremities only (112 per 1000). Bilateral position sense loss in both upper and lower extremities is next in frequency (48 per 1000), while loss in only the upper extremities is rare (3 per 1000).

TABLE XVI

Prevalence per 1000 of Bilateral loss in Vibratory and Position Sense, by Site of Loss and Age in Persons 65 to 74 Without Known Neurological Disease Chicago Stroke Study, 9/65 - 8/67

Type & Site of Sensory Loss	65-69 N=385	70-74 N=540	Total N=925
Vibration sense:			
Upper extremities only	10	22	17
Lower extremities only	538	459	515
Both upper & lower extremities	291	323	310
Total	839	844	842
Position sense:			
Upper extremities only	3	4	3
Lower extremities only	109	115	112
Both upper & lower extremities	34	58	48
Total	146	177	163
Vibration and/or position sense:			
Upper extremities only	10	22	17
Lower extremities only	530	487	505
Both upper & lower extremities	312	359	339
Total	852	868	861

Two subjects have been omitted from this table because data on vibratory and position sense were missing.

The overall prevalence of alterations in either position or vibratory sensation (861 per 1000) is only slightly higher than the overall prevalence of alterations in vibratory sensation (842 per 1000). This observation suggests that individuals with loss of position sense come from the population with loss of vibratory sensation and is consistent with the hypothesis that a single neuronal mechanism may be the basis for alterations in both position and vibratory sensation.

The relationship between bilateral loss of vibratory and position sense and absent tendon reflexes is shown in Table XVII. The prevalence of bilateral loss of either position or vibratory sensibility in both upper and lower extremities is 292 per 1000 among individuals in whom neither the Achilles nor patellar reflexes are bilaterally absent. If either of these reflexes is bilaterally absent, the prevalence of sensory alteration is 347 per 1000, while, if both pairs of reflexes are bilaterally absent, the prevalence increases to 417 per 1000. This finding demonstrates a definite correlation between loss of position and vibratory sensibility and loss of tendon reflexes, and is consistent with the hypothesis that a single neuronal mechanism is related to alterations of tendon reflexes in elderly persons as well as position and vibratory sensibility.

TABLE XVII

Prevalence of Bilateral Loss of Vibratory or Position Sense in Both Upper and Lower Extremities, by Status of Achilles and Patellar Reflexes in Persons 65-74 Without Known Neurological Disease. Chicago Stroke Study, 9/65 - 8/67

Status of Achilles bilaterally absent	Total	Bilateral loss of vibratory or position sense in both upper and lower extremities	
		Frequency	Prevalence/1000
Both reflexes not bilaterally absent	270	79	292
Only one reflex bilaterally absent	559	194	347
Both reflexes bilaterally absent	96	40	417
Total	925	313	338

The association between loss of sensibility and status of reflexes is statistically significant ($P < .05$) when tested for a linear trend in proportions. Two subjects were omitted from this table because data on vibratory and position senses were missing. The age-adjusted rates, giving equal weight to both the younger and older groups, are 294, 340 and 414 cases per 1000 for rows 1 to 3, respectively.

The data presented above support the concept that certain alterations seen in the neurologic examination in an elderly population are related to a single neuronal mechanism. It does not suggest any particular mechanism.

The relationship between bilateral loss of deep tendon reflexes and hypertension, diabetes mellitus or hyperglycemia, and peripheral atherosclerosis is shown in Table XVIII. For this study, hypertension has been defined as a systolic pressure of 160 or greater and/or a diastolic pressure of 95 or greater. Hyperglycemia has been defined as a positive history of diabetes mellitus or a plasma glucose level of 205 mg/dl or greater one hour after an oral 50 gram glucose load. The diagnosis of peripheral atherosclerosis was based on a history of intermittent claudication or alterations on physical examination described previously (Ostfeld et al., 1971).

The relationship between bilateral loss of pairs of reflexes and hyperglycemia or a history of diabetes mellitus is statistically significant ($X^2 = 7.84$, $p < .01$), as is the relationship to peripheral atherosclerosis ($X^2 = 5.09$, $p < .05$). The relationship to hypertension is not statistically significant ($p < .20$). The relationship between the loss of both the Achilles and patellar reflexes and these three factors is shown in another way. If none of these factors is present, the prevalence per 1000 of bilateral loss of both reflexes is only 56. If one factor only is present, the prevalence per 1000 is 110, and if two or all three factors are present, the prevalence per 1000 is 139. This trend is also statistically significant ($p < .01$).

The relationship between loss of deep tendon reflexes and these conditions is not due to age alone since the age-adjusted rates, giving equal weight in the adjustments to persons 65-69 and to those 70-74, are 54, 108 and 135 per 1000, respectively, for individuals with none, one only, and two or all three of the conditions. This finding suggests that normal aging is not the sole factor in the alterations seen in neurologic examination in the elderly. It suggests that these alterations are frequently related to disease states which are common in this population (Critchley, 1931).

Summary and Conclusion

The results of neurologic examination in an elderly poor urban population without known neurologic disease have been presented. Bilateral loss of deep tendon reflexes and bilateral loss of positions and vibratory sensation were the most frequent alterations noted. Bilateral loss of lower extremity tendon reflexes was related to clinically detectable lower extremity weakness. Bilateral loss of tendon reflexes

TABLE XVIII

Prevalence of Bilaterally Absent Achilles and Patellar Reflexes, by Blood Pressure, Plasma Glucose Level, and Signs of Peripheral Atherosclerosis in Persons 65 to 74 Without Known Neurologic Disease Chicago Stroke Study, 9/65 - 8/67

Categories		Number of subjects	Achilles and patellar reflexes bilaterally absent		Statistical significance
			Frequency	Prevalence/1000	
Hypertension SBP $\geq$ 160 and/or DBP $\geq$ 95	P	386	46	119	X^2 = 1.99
	A	521	46	88	P < .20
Hyperglycemia and/or history of diabetes mellitus	P	471	61	130	X^2 = 7.84
	A	436	31	71	P < .01
Peripheral Atherosclerosis	P	131	21	160	X^2 = 5.09
	A	776	71	91	P < .05
Number of above conditions present	None	251	14	56	Z = 2.80
	One	362	40	110	P < .01
	2 or 3	294	38	129	

Twenty subjects have been omitted from this table because of missing data. The age-adjusted rates for persons with none, one, and 2 or 3 of the above conditions are, respectively, 54, 108 and 135 cases per 1000, giving equal weight in the adjustment to both the younger and older groups.
P = Present; A = Absent; SBP = Systolic Blood Pressure; DBP = Diastolic Blood Pressure.

was also related to loss of position or vibratory sensation. These observations suggest that a common neuronal mechanism is the basis of loss of tendon reflexes and loss of position and vibratory sensation in this population. The loss of tendon reflexes was related to hyperglycemia and peripheral atherosclerosis. This observation suggests that the loss of deep tendon reflexes may be a concomitant of these disease states and not just of normal aging of the nervous system.

Senile Dementia

Finally, we employed all the data available to us to determine the incidence of senile dementia or chronic brain syndrome. Among the 3141 persons we followed for 3 years, only 12 cases of chronic brain syndrome occurred, an incidence of about 1.3 cases per 1000 per year. In another group of 401 persons aged 61-84 followed for 2 years, only 4 cases occurred. Those who developed chronic brain syndrome had a mean blood pressure of 159/88 and the mean pressure of those who remained free of this disorder was 149/81. These results, admittedly meager, suggest the need for further study of high blood pressure as a precurser of chronic brain syndrome.

Our results have led, overall, to the conclusion that specific diseases, diabetes, high blood pressure, atherosclerosis and obesity have far more to do with nervous system disease in the elderly than the presumed nervous system changes of aging.

Nutrition and Neural Disease

Each of the four diseases enumerated above is closely related to problems of nutrition. The evidence that a diet high in saturated fats leads to atherosclerosis is now very substantial (Epstein, 1965; Simberg, 1970). There is no longer any question that obesity leads to hypertension and that weight loss lowers blood pressure (Fletcher, 1959; Kagan et al., 1959; Florey and Cuadrado, 1968); and the relationship between adiposity and adult-onset diabetes is so well known that it does not require documentation here.

A lifelong diet excessive in calories, in saturated fat, and in refined sugars has far more to do with disease of the nervous system of elderly man than any changes with age that have yet been identified.

REFERENCES

Critchley, M. (1931). Lancet 1, 1119.
Critchley, M. (1939). In "Problems of Ageing" (E. V. Cowdry, ed.), pp. 483-500, Williams and Wilkins, Baltimore.
Critchley, M. (1956). J. Chronic Dis. 3, 459.
Epstein, F. H. (1965). J. Chronic Dis. 18, 735.
Fletcher, A. P. (1959). Q. J. Med. 23, 331.
Florey, C. duV. and Cuadrado, R. R. (1968). Human Biol. 40, 189.
Gordon, T. and Garst, C. C. (1965). "Coronary Heart Disease in Adults, United States, 1960-1962". PHS Publication No. 1000, Ser. 11, No. 10. U. S. Government Printing Office, Washington, D. C.
Howell, T. (1949). Brit. Med. J. 56, 121.
Kagan, A., Gordon, T., Kannel, W. B., and Dawber, T. R.(1959). In "Framingham Study Council High Blood Pressure Res." Vol. 7, pg. 53.
Kannel, W. B. (1967). "Epidemiology of Stroke". PHS Publication No. 1607, U. S. Government Printing Office, Washington, D. C.
Kannel, W. B. (1971). Stroke 2, 295.
Kurtzke, J. F. (1969). "Epidemiology of Cerebrovascular Disease". Springer-Verlag, New York.
Ostfeld, A. M., Shekelle, R. B., Tufo, H. M., Wieland, A. M., Kilbridge, J. A., Drori, J., and Klawans, H. (1971). Am. J. Public Health 61, 19.
Ostfeld, A. M., Shekelle, R. B., and Klawans, H. (1973). Stroke 4, 980.
Paulson, G. and Gottlieb, G. (1968). Brain 91, 37.
Simberg, D. W. (1970). J. Chronic Dis. 22, 515.
Snedecor, G. and Cochran, W. (1967). "Statistical Methods", Ed. 6. Iowa State University Press, Ames, Iowa.

THE ROLE OF NUTRITION TO DIABETES IN RELATION TO AGE

George C. Gerritsen

The Upjohn Company
Kalamazoo, Michigan 49001

Although the clinical symptoms of diabetes were reported 3,500 years ago in the Egyptian Ebers Papyrus, diabetes mellitus and its manifestations are still poorly understood. In general terms, diabetes can be characterized by hyperglycemia, glycosuria and relative or absolute insulin deficiency. It is the insulin deficiency which is probably responsible for abnormalities in carbohydrate, lipid and protein metabolism.

In very broad terms, there are two general forms of the disease. One is referred to as juvenile-type diabetes. Individuals having this form require insulin and are prone to ketoacidosis which is indicative of severe metabolic disorders. The second and more common form of diabetes is referred to as insulin-independent diabetes or diabetes not requiring insulin administration. With full cooperation of the patient, this less severe form can generally be managed by appropriate diet and exercise (Krall and Joslin, 1971). If diet and exercise fail, addition of oral antidiabetic agents frequently can be used successfully in this type (Krall, 1971). This second type of diabetic generally develops diabetes after middle age; therefore, this form of the disease has been referred to as maturity-onset diabetes. The common terms, juvenile-onset and maturity-onset diabetes found in the literature can be misleading since there are insulin-requiring diabetics who became symptomatic after middle age and there are noninsulin-requiring diabetics which developed the disease prior to age 20.

Although there is general agreement that diabetes is inherited in man, there is considerable disagreement as to the mode of inheritance. The first to recognize that diabetes was a familial trait was Rondelet (1628). Pincus and White (1933) were the first to do quantitative genetic studies and postulated an autosomal recessive mechanism of inheritance. However, numerous other mechanisms for inheritance of diabetes have been postulated such as autosomal dominant, juvenile-onset type as homozygous, adult-onset type as heterozygous, sex-linked and multifactorial (Rimoin, 1970). Much of the confusion appears to be due to different methodology for collection of data, such as death certificates, questionnaires, interviews or blood and urine sampling under a variety of experimental conditions as well as differing definitions of diabetes. Another complication correctly pointed out by Neel _et al_. (1965) is that blood and urine sugar are far removed from the genetic defect(s) and therefore are poor endpoints for genetic analysis.

Recent data suggest that diabetes may be a series of syndromes since there is considerable variation in diabetic phenotypes between various ethnic groups such as Amish and Navajo (Rimoin, 1968) and the Pima indians (Genuth _et al_., 1967). Furthermore, Tattersall and Fajans (1975) have presented evidence for genetic heterogeneity of diabetes in young people. In one type, diabetes is of the classical insulin-dependent type, but in the other group diabetes is very mild and does not require insulin despite early onset.

The classic studies in monozygotic twins by Pyke _et al_. (1970), Tattersall and Pyke (1972) and others show 60% concordance for diabetes. This suggests that environmental factors such as infectious disease, stress (or lack of it), nutrition, etc., may interact with their genotype to either cause or prevent onset of diabetes.

There appears to be little doubt that obesity is a risk factor for adult-onset diabetes (West and Kalbfleisch, 1970). Seventy-five percent of there patients are obese at the time of diagnosis of diabetes (West, 1975). Furthermore, Genuth (1966) and Grodsky and Benoit (1969) have shown marked improvement in plasma insulin levels after weight reduction. Obesity implies nutritional excess of one type or another, thus dietary components have long been suspected as risk factors for development of diabetes if the proper genotype was present. Recent epidemiological studies in aboriginal societies have revealed a 10-fold increase in the rate of diabetes as dietary habits have changed from a primitive to a more refined, westernized-type diet (West, 1974).

Strong arguments have been made for increased dietary sucrose and/or refined starch intake as a contributor to the increased incidence of diabetes (Cohen _et al_., 1972; Cleave, 1974; West and Kalbfleisch, 1970; West, 1974). However, others feel that sucrose does not correlate with increased risk for diabetes. For example, Keen (1974) felt that the present evidence is inconclusive since he observed populations with high rates of obesity which had low sugar consumption. Himsworth and Marshall (1935) reviewed data which suggested that dietary carbohydrate protects against diabetes and that high dietary fat intake is a risk factor for diabetes.

Recently Trowel (1974, 1975) has suggested that the very low crude fiber content of the western-style diet contributes to the etiology of diabetes. Hunt et al. (1975) have hypothesized that caloric density of the diet is related to obesity and thus to possibly diabetes as well. It should be pointed out that risk factors for diabetes such as obesity, excessive caloric intake or qualitative dietary changes are difficult to evaluate since two or more variables frequently change simultaneously. The data cited on increased incidences of diabetes in developing countries are complicated by changing life styles; such as shifts from rural to urban societies, decreased exercise, different occupations, crowding, infectious disease, and increased pollution. However, West (1975) stated that "high rates of diabetes have not been reported in any society in which obesity is rare".

There is little doubt that diabetes mellitus is a major health problem in most developed countries. The data suggest that the incidence of diabetes has increased steadily during this century. At the turn of the century, diabetes was ranked 27th as a cause of death by disease but, in 1972, ranked fifth as an underlying cause of death by disease in the United States (Tokuhata et al., 1975). In 1973, diabetes ranked fourth as the underlying cause of death following cardiovascular-renal diseases, cancer and pulmonary diseases (Metropolitan Life Statistical Bulletin, 1974).

The lack of recognition of diabetes as a major cause of death for some time may, in part, be attributed to the system employed in reporting mortality data, since only one disease is counted as the underlying cause of death even though other related diseases may be present in the same patient. As an example, Tokuhata et al. (1975) reviewed 200,000 death certificates filed with the Pennsylvania State Health Department; of these 10,170 certificates indicated diabetes as a cause of death. "Of this total, 2,639 recorded diabetes as the underlying cause, whereas the remaining 7,531 listed diabetes as a contributary cause". Therefore, if only the underlying cause is considered, Tokuhata calculated a death rate of 22.4/100,000 in the population. The contributary cause calculated out as 63.9 per 100,000. Thus, if both categories are combined, the figure would then be 86.3 deaths per 100,000 in the population related to diabetes. Tokuhata has extrapolated from his sample and estimates that there could be as many as 300,000 deaths annually related to diabetes in the United States. This would make diabetes third as a cause of disease-related deaths in the United States.

There is little doubt that life expectancy of the diabetic is less than that of the nondiabetic, primarily due to premature vascular disease (Marks, 1965). During the past twenty years, 76 percent of the 27,966 diabetics seen at the Joslin Clinic died of cardiovascular-renal disease (Marks, 1971). Furthermore, Marks' data suggest that the earlier the onset of diabetes and dependence on insulin, the greater the effect on vascular disease and survival. In other words, there appears to be some correlation between decreased survival and the severity of diabetes. Perhaps the clearest demonstration of the effect of diabetes on cardiovascular mortality has come from the Framingham study (Garcia et al., 1974). During the 16 years of very careful study, 42 of 55 diabetics died of cardiovascular disease. Figure 1 shows the ratio of observed deaths (diabetics) to expected deaths (nondiabetics) due to cardiovascular disease. In diabetics, three times as many deaths occurred from cardiovascular disease than in the nondiabetic cohort. Most of the deaths were due to nonsudden coronary heart disease (CHD) whereas deaths due to sudden CHD, cerebral vascular accidents (CVA) and other cardiovascular problems were about evenly distributed. Cardiovascular mortality according to type of diabetes management is shown in figure 2. It is of interest that the ratio of diabetic to nondiabetic deaths was significantly elevated regardless of treatment, suggesting that current therapy does not normalize the excessive cardiovascular disease risk in diabetics.

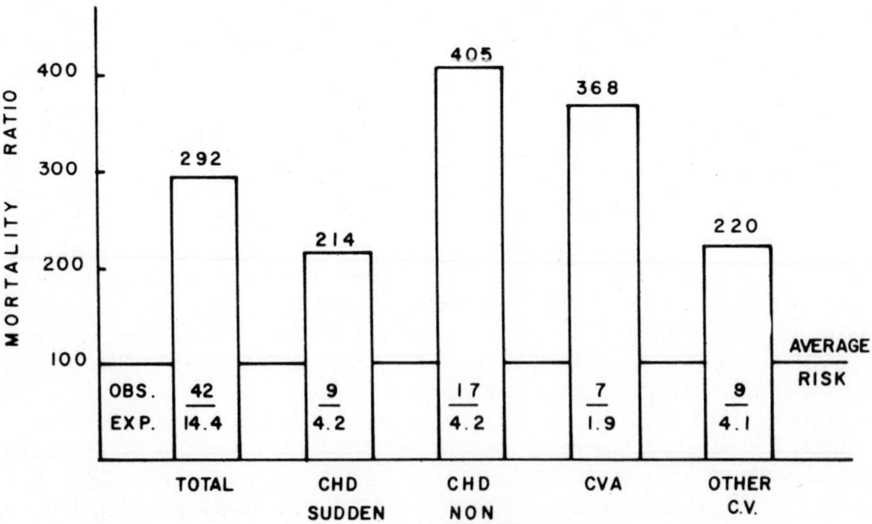

Fig. 1 Risk of cardiovascular death in diabetics (16 years) men and women: Framingham study. CHD=coronary heart disease. CVA=cerebral vascular accidents. CV=other cardiovascular problems. (From Garcia et al., 1974.)

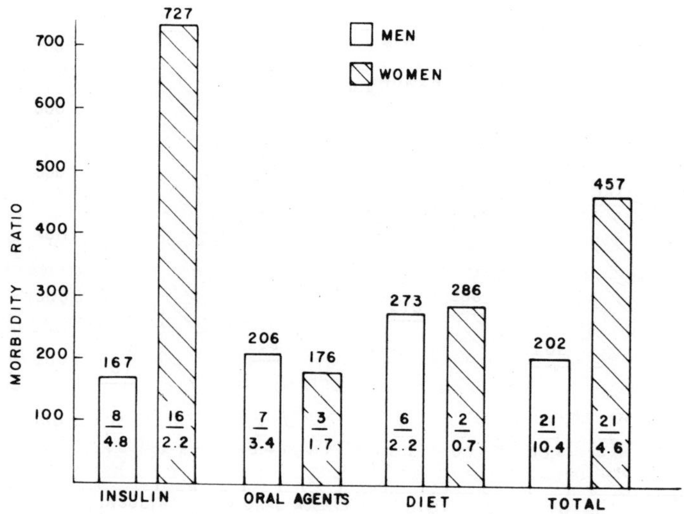

Fig. 2 Cardiovascular mortality according to type of diabetes management men and women 30-62 years of age, at entry: Framingham study. (From Garcia et al., 1974.)

It is of considerable interest that insulin-treated women have such an incredibly high cardiovascular mortality ratio of 7 to 1 compared with insulin-treated men (ratio = 1.7 to 1). Unfortunately, Garcia et al. (1974) don't have an explanation for this finding. However, the data suggest that premature death due to cardiovascular disease may in some way be linked to the severity of diabetes. However, mild diabetics who were managed by diet had a cardiovascular mortality ratio similar to the diabetics requiring oral agents. The mortality ratio for diabetic men managed by diet was higher than that of men treated with insulin. Earlier studies done in Bedford, England (Keen et al., 1962) and Tecumseh, Michigan (Ostrander et al., 1965) support the conclusions of the Framingham study (Garcia et al., 1974).

It is reasonable to assume that diabetes causes premature cardiovascular disease but the mechanism is obscure. The earliest detectable changes are in the microcirculatory system and have been referred to as diabetic microangiopathy or the English equivalent, "diabetic small blood vessel disease" (Ditzel and Sagild, 1954). Blood vessel changes in the diabetic retina were described by Jager (1855), 34 years prior to the classic experiments of von Mering and Minkowski (1889) which demonstrated that diabetes follows pancreatectomy. McMillan (1975), in an excellent review on the deterioration of the microcirculation in diabetics, points out that the succession of events leading to premature cardiovascular disease appear to be: "1. altered local blood flow, 2. progressive reversible dilatation of small veins, 3. periodic arteriolar vasoconstriction, 4. sclerosis of the walls of arterioles, small veins, and capillaries, and 5. slowly progressive microcirculatory decompensation".

There is no doubt that muscle capillary basement membrane thickness is increased in diabetics compared with nondiabetics of the same age and sex (Kilo _et al._, 1972). Furthermore, Kilo _et al_. (1972) demonstrated that nondiabetic capillary basement membranes also thicken with age. It is of some interest to note that blood sugar levels and, in particular, glucose intolerance increase with age (O'Sullivan, 1974), but it is not clear if this glucose intolerance correlates with basement membrane thickening. However, the diabetic's capillary basement membrane thickens at a faster rate. In other words, the basement membrane of a 20-year old diabetic of 4 years duration is similar in thickness to that of a 40- to 50-year old nondiabetic. In some ways this rapid basement membrane thickening can be thought of as premature aging of the diabetic microcirculatory system which may lead to the documented premature cardiovascular mortality in diabetics.

The increased mortality of diabetics appears related to severity or management of the disease (Krall and Joslin, 1971). Stone (1961), West (1973) and many others have shown that careful regulation of caloric intake (generally 1,500-2,000 kcal/day) and composition of the diet (25-35% calories fat, 20% protein and the remainder primarily from complex carbohydrates) will tend to normalize the metabolism of the diabetic. However, West (1973) has pointed out that it is extremely difficult to motivate people to adhere to their prescribed diets. Therefore, there are no data from human studies which show that normalization of metabolism by diet will prevent complications of diabetes or extend longevity.

Due to the extreme difficulty in demonstrating a direct beneficial effect of treatment on the longevity of diabetic humans, an experimental animal model has been adopted. The Chinese hamster spontaneously develops a type of diabetes which is remarkably similar to that observed in man. The diabetic animals have elevated blood sugar, abnormal glucose tolerance and some display ketonemia and ketonuria (Gerritsen and Dulin, 1967). Like man, mildly diabetic animals respond to sulfonylureas but severe cases do not (Gerritsen and Dulin, 1966). Time of onset when normalized for the life span of the hamster is also similar to that of man (Schmidt _et al._,

1970). In the diabetic hamster, plasma and pancreatic insulin levels (Dulin et al., 1970), β-cell granulation (Carpenter et al., 1967; Luse et al., 1967) and insulin synthesis in vitro (Chang, 1970) are generally decreased. Pancreatic insulin and glucagon responses in vitro in response to stimuli are also impaired (Frankel et al., 1974; Grodsky et al., 1974). Hepatic gluconeogenic enzymes are increased while glycolytic enzymes are decreased, as was glucose production from pyruvate increased in diabetic hamsters (Chang and Schneider, 1970). Glucose utilization by muscle and fat in diabetic hamsters is normal (Gerritsen and Dulin, 1967) and the animals are not obese (Gerritsen and Blanks, 1974). The diabetic animals have retinal lesions (Federman and Gerritsen, 1970; Soret et al., 1973, 1974), kidney lesions (Shirai et al., 1967; Conforti, 1972; Soret et al., 1974), and neurological changes (Luse et al., 1970; Schlaepfer et al., 1974). The changes observed in the various hamster tissues mentioned are similar (remarkably so for the nervous system) in most respects to those observed in diabetic humans. Vascular changes have been observed in the Chinese hamster (Chobanian et al., 1974a, b; McCombs et al., 1974). It should be pointed out that although the biochemical changes in blood vessels are highly significant, the morphological changes (as in most rodents) are minimal. The mode of inheritance of diabetes in this animal appears to be polygenic (Butler, 1967; Butler and Gerritsen, 1970). As in man, both sexes are affected by the disease (Gerritsen et al., 1974b).

The Chinese hamster colony has been developed over the last 14 years and sublines have been inbred and selected for and against diabetes. Therefore, control or nondiabetic animals come from a genetic background in which no diabetics have been observed for over 10 generations of continuous brother to sister mating. All animals are tested biweekly for urine glucose and if glycosuric they are also tested for urine ketones.

Animals used in the studies to be described were defined as follows: nondiabetics are defined as described above; aglycosurics have a diabetic genotype but have never tested positive for glycosuria; diabetics continuously test 4+ for urine sugar or maximum by Lilly Testape®; ketonurics continuously rate "large" for urine ketones by Ames Ketostix®.

An epidemiological study of the Chinese hamster was done to determine whether diabetes in this animal reduces life span as it does in man. Details of this study have been published (Gerritsen et al., 1974a). The populations of Chinese hamsters studied had fixed, reproducible genetic backgrounds. This was possible since all breeders used to produce the populations were selected from sublines that had been inbred by continuous brother-sister mating for a minimum of 8 generations so that at least 85-90% of their genetic material was fixed in the homozygous state. Four sublines that produce diabetics and four nondiabetic-producing sublines were used to provide breeders. A male and female pair were always from different inbred sublines so that the populations studied were hybrid to avoid the possibility of an inbreeding influence on longevity. Data analyzed by life table analysis technique (Cutter and Ederer, 1958) demonstrate a significant inverse correlation between severity of diabetes and survival in the Chinese hamster (Fig. 3). Fifty percent of the ketonuric diabetics survived approximately 1.5 years, but 50% of nonketonuric diabetics survived over 2 years. In contrast, 50% of aglycosurics survived over 3 years. It should be pointed out that all animals represented in figure 3 have a similar diabetic genotype since the three phenotypes represented are siblings from inbred diabetic parents. The data suggest that abnormal metabolism, and not genotype, reduced survival in the Chinese hamster. This point is supported by the data presented in figure 4 in which survival curves of aglycosurics with diabetic genotype and diabetic parents are compared with nondiabetics. It was obvious that there was no significant difference in the survival rate of the two populations. This, again, suggested that it was abnormal metabolism and not genotype which reduced longevity.

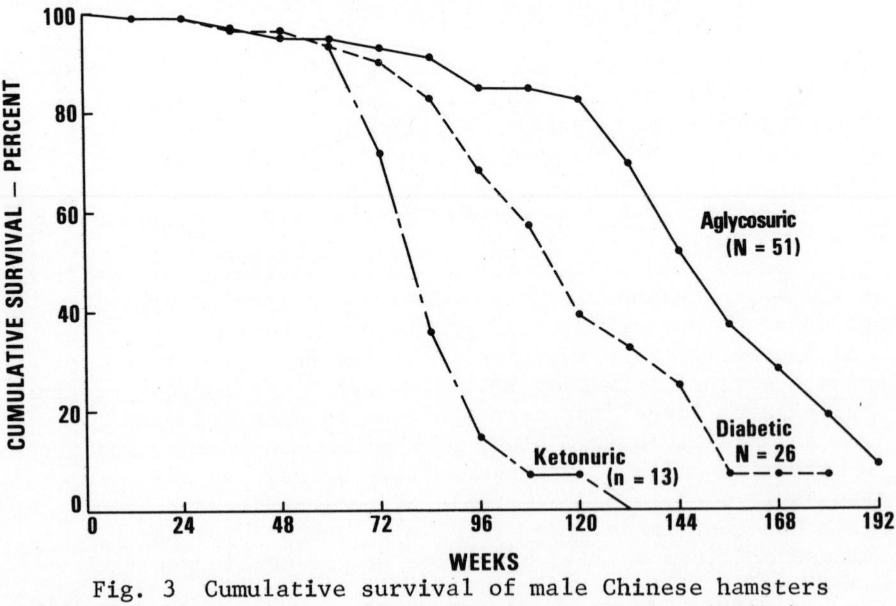

Fig. 3 Cumulative survival of male Chinese hamsters with diabetic parents. (From Gerritsen et al., 1974b.)

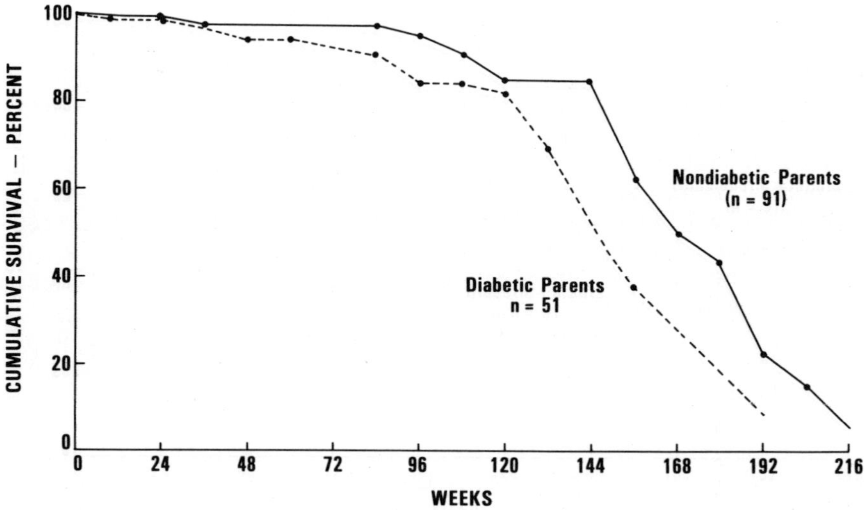

Fig. 4 Cumulative survival curves of aglycosuric male Chinese hamsters (diabetic genotype and diabetic parents) compared with male nondiabetic Chinese hamsters (nondiabetic genotype and nondiabetic parents). (From Gerritsen _et al._, 1974b.)

Mating of two ketotic Chinese hamsters resulted in 100% incidence of diabetes in their offspring (Gerritsen _et al._, 1970) and, therefore, hamsters from that genetic background could be identified as prediabetic at birth. During the asymptomatic period from birth until development of glycosuria, they were defined as prediabetic. Prediabetic Chinese hamster pups had similar blood sugar levels, and plasma and pancreatic insulin levels compared with nondiabetics but consumed 40% more food than the nondiabetic controls (Gerritsen and Blanks, 1970).

To determine if the apparent hyperphagia of prediabetic Chinese hamsters had an effect on subsequent development of diabetes in these animals; so, food intake was normalized. The methodology of these experiments has been detailed previously (Gerritsen _et al._, 1974a). The effect of hyperphagia on the change from the prediabetic to the diabetic state was studied by limiting the diet of prediabetics from: a) birth to 150 days, b) birth to weaning, and c) weaning to 30 months of age. Food intake was limited during the preweaning period by fostering one-half of each prediabetic litter into nondiabetic ones to make large heterogeneous litters (consisting of 2 prediabetic plus 5 nondiabetic pups). The prediabetic litters averaged 4 pups while the nondiabetic litters were adjusted to 5. Thus, 2 prediabetics were fostered into the nondiabetic litters and forced to compete with the 5 nondiabetic pups, while their 2 prediabetic siblings were left with their natural mother and did not have to compete for available nutrition. After weaning, diet limitation to within normal range was accomplished by feeding prediabetic animals 2.5 g/day of Purina Mouse Breeder Chow®; nonlimited prediabetic siblings were allowed food ad libitum.

In the initial studies, prediabetic hamsters were switched from 2.5 g/day to nonrestricted feeding at 150 days of age. This was done to prove that these animals were actually prediabetic. In two subsequent studies, effect of preweaning diet limitation by the fostering technique alone and the effect on the development of diabetes of postweaning diet limitation (2.5 g/day) for 30 months were evaluated (Gerritsen et al., 1974a). Fostering prediabetics into large litters was an effective procedure for limitation of dietary intake since body weight of the fostered prediabetics was significantly less than their nonfostered siblings at 15 days (Fig. 5). The significant difference in body weights of the fostered and nonfostered prediabetics was maintained during the last 9 days of suckling but growth rates during this period appear to be similar since the slopes of the curves are similar. Despite the fact that the 2 fostered prediabetics had significantly lower body weights than their own natural nonfostered siblings at 15 days, they still gained significantly more weight than the 5 nonprediabetic offspring of their foster mothers.

The significant difference in weaning body weights was maintained by limiting diet of fostered pups to an intake of 2.5 g/day (Fig. 6). The fostered prediabetics were maintained at a significantly lower body weight than their nonfostered and ad libitum-fed siblings for the entire 150 days of diet limitation. The only exception was at 94 days, the time of sexual maturity in the Chinese hamster. The diet-limited animals had a rapid growth spurt after the switch to nonrestricted feeding, so that after 14 days they no longer were significantly lighter than their ad libitum-fed siblings. The growth rate of the prediabetics limited to 2.5 g/day was normalized as shown in figure 7. Growth curves of nondiabetic weanlings fed ad libitum were similar to those of the prediabetics limited to 2.5 g/day that were of similar initial weights. The mean daily food consumption for the nondiabetics was 2.45 g/day.

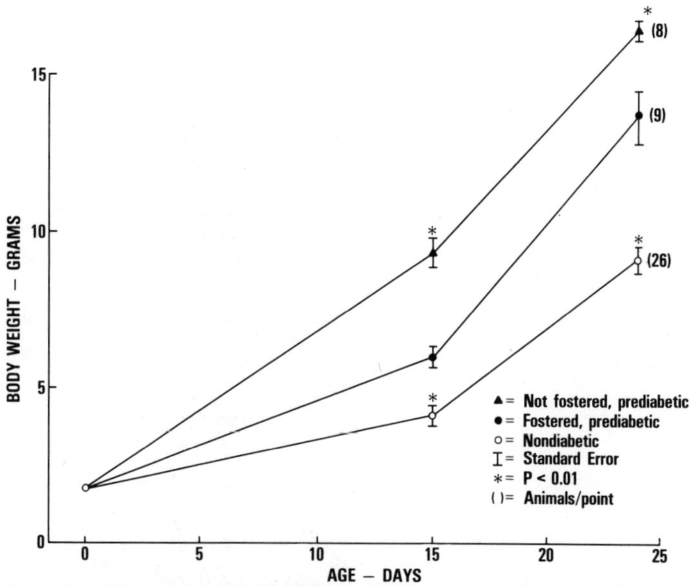

Fig. 5 Preweaning Chinese hamster body weights of nonfostered prediabetics of litter size 2 and fostered prediabetics with nonprediabetics of total litter size 7. (From Gerritsen _et al_., 1974a.)

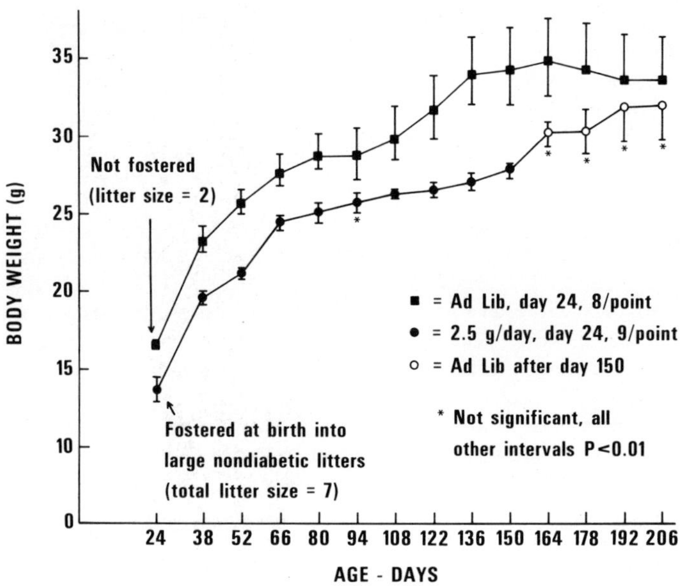

Fig. 6 Effect of food restriction on body weights of prediabetic Chinese hamsters. (From Gerritsen _et al_., 1974a.)

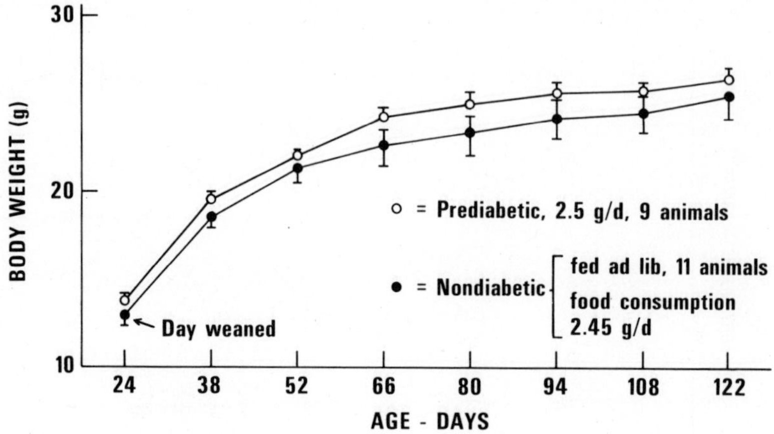

Fig. 7 Comparison of growth rates of nondiabetic Chinese hamsters fed ad libitum with growth rates of prediabetics limited to 2.5 g of food per day. (From Gerritsen et al., 1974a.)

Diabetes developed very rapidly in the prediabetic hamster pups that were not limited to a normal food intake (Fig. 8). At 40 days of age, 7 of 8 prediabetics on nonrestricted food intake had developed glycosuria (4+ Testape® value). In contrast, only 3 of the 9 prediabetics that were limited to a normal quantity of food developed mild glycosuria (2+ Testape®) by 50 days of age and remained at 2+. When switched to nonrestricted feeding, glycosuria increased to 4+ within a few days. The other 6 prediabetics that were fostered and subsequently limited to 2.5 g/day did not develop glycosuria as long as they were limited to this quantity of food intake. However, within 50 days after placing these animals on nonrestricted diet they all showed mild glycosuria (2+ to 3+). Furthermore, these animals remained very mildly diabetic for their entire life span. Seven out of the eight hamsters fed ad libitum also developed ketonuria, but this never developed in their siblings that were diet-limited for the first 150 days.

It was also observed that 5 of 8 of the hamsters fed ad libitum died prior to 300 days of age (Fig. 9). The 3 that survived beyond 300 days died prior to 18 months of age. In contrast, all the siblings that were diet-limited for the first 150 days survived beyond two years.

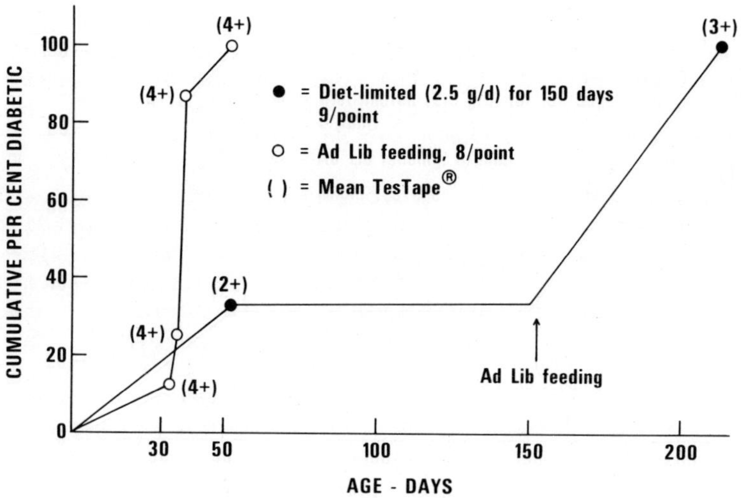

Fig. 8 Comparison of age of onset and severity of diabetes of diet-limited with _ad libitum_-fed prediabetic Chinese hamsters. (From Gerritsen _et al._, 1974a.)

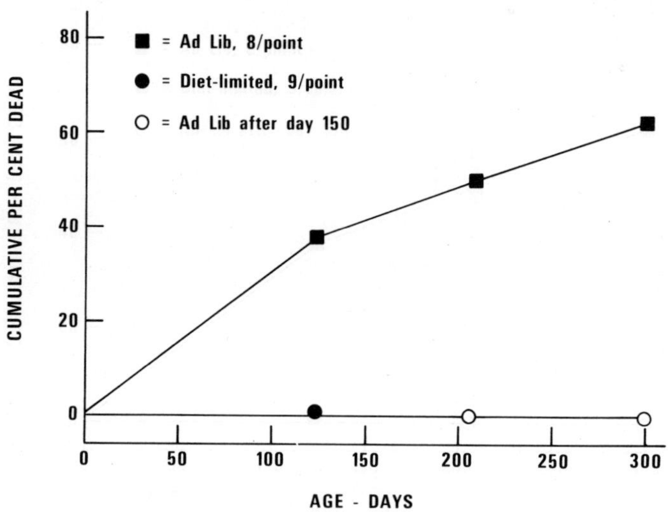

Fig. 9 Mortality of _ad libitum_-fed versus diet-limited Chinese hamsters. (From Gerritsen _et al._, 1974a.)

The significant effect on body weight of prediabetics due to fostering into large litters was overcome during the first 14 days of nonrestricted feeding after weaning. Preweaning diet-limitation alone had no significant effect on onset of severity of diabetes, development of ketonuria or survival in these prediabetic Chinese hamsters. The results were similar to data shown for *ad libitum*-fed animals in figures 8 and 9.

Limitation of diet to 2.5 g/day after weaning resulted in a reduced growth rate, but these diet-limited prediabetics slowly caught up to their *ad libitum*-fed siblings (Fig. 10). At 200 days of age, body weights were no longer significantly different. However, development of glycosuria was markedly different in these prediabetic hamsters (Fig. 11). The *ad libitum*-fed siblings developed diabetes very rapidly; in some, diabetes progressed to ketonuria and premature death. Again, only 3 of the 12 animals which were kept on 2.5 g/day for 30 months showed a trace of glycosuria, which was intermittent. They have never progressed to consistent mild glycosuria and the other nine have never shown any glycosuria. These prediabetics with diet limited to 2.5 g/day were killed after the 30 month diet limitation. Postmortem examinations revealed no pathology that could be linked to diabetes. Their pancreata, kidneys and vascular systems appeared similar to age- and sex-matched nondiabetic Chinese hamsters.

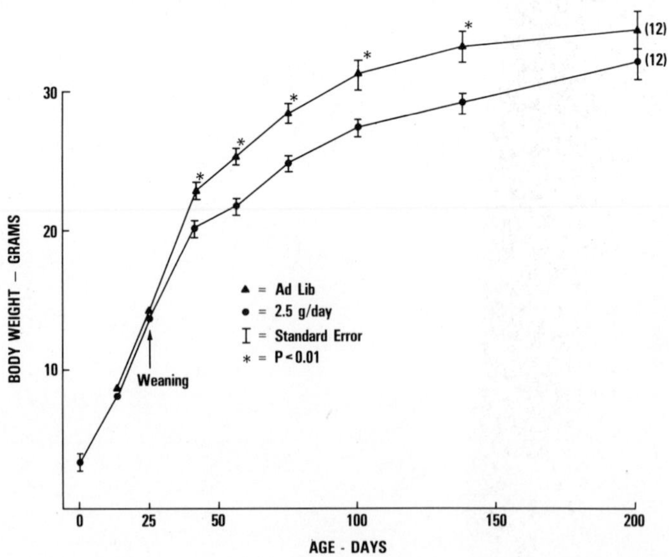

Fig. 10 Effect of diet restriction after weaning on body weight of prediabetics. (From Gerritsen *et al.*, 1974a.)

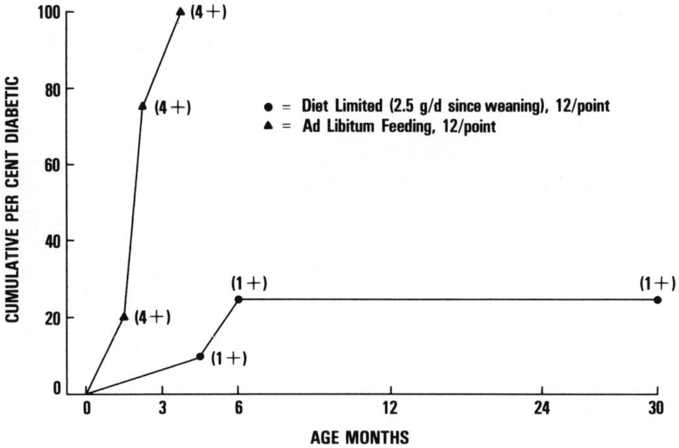

Fig. 11 Comparison of incidence and age of onset of diabetes of *ad libitum*-fed with postweaning diet-limited prediabetics. (From Gerritsen *et al.*, 1974a.)

Whether the hyperphagia of these prediabetic Chinese hamsters is of genetic etiology, related to environmental factors such as uterine environment or maternal hyperglycemia and/or ketonemia or to a combination of these factors is unclear. Considerable research will have to be conducted to gain insight into this complex problem.

However, it is quite evident that excessive caloric intake interacts with the diabetic genotype. This interaction results in onset of diabetes, severe metabolic derangement and premature death. It is also clear that if caloric intake is normalized in this animal with a diabetic genotype, onset of diabetes is markedly delayed or prevented. Furthermore, premature death related to severe metabolic derangement such as glycosuria and ketonuria was prevented and pathological lesions in pancreata, retina, kidney and nerves described previously were not apparent. It should be pointed out that these animals were not starved but were simply limited to a normal caloric intake. This suggests that the excessive caloric intake interacted with the diabetic genotype and caused onset of diabetes in prediabetic hamsters fed *ad libitum*.

Limitation of diet by fostering only for the weaning period did not alter the development of diabetes or its sequelae. However, starting diet limitation to 2.5 g/day at weaning essentially prevented the disease for the 30 months during which caloric intake was maintained within normal limits.

It may be concluded from these studies that normalizing food intake of the hyperphagic, prediabetic Chinese hamster has a marked influence on onset and severity of the disease. The increase in longevity suggests the benefits of delaying the development and/or reducing the severity of the disease. It appears that continued diet limitation will essentially keep the prediabetic free of clinical symptoms of diabetes and normalize life span.

Although prediabetic hamsters are not obese, whether the early increase in eviscerated carcass lipid prior to hyperglycemia contributes to early development of diabetes is not known (Gerritsen et al., 1974a). This, however, is possible since obesity has been implicated in the development of spontaneous diabetes in other laboratory animals (Coleman and Hummel, 1967; Nakamura and Yamada, 1967) and also of maturity-onset diabetes.

Unfortunately, there has been no report in the literature as to the effects of diet limitation on human prediabetics. There is, however, a suggestion that emotional problems and stress during the prediabetic years may lead to poor nutritional habits which may have an effect on development of diabetes (Stein and Charles, 1971). Other circumstantial evidence suggests that severe caloric restriction during wars can decrease the prevalence of diabetes (Bouchardat, 1883; Pyke, 1968).

It is important to recognize that the data suggest that, if environmental factors can be understood and manipulated properly, the clinical symptoms and, perhaps, the consequences of abnormal metabolism such as premature death may be prevented in the diabetic.

Recently, evidence has been obtained which suggests that decreased fat and/or increased protein content of the diet improved the metabolic state of the ketonuric Chinese hamster. Grodsky et al. (1974) observed that ketonuria disappeared when ketonuric diabetic animals were inadvertently placed on a 4% fat diet (Feedstuffs Processing Co. of San Francisco) rather than the standard 11% fat Purina Mouse Chow®.

Longitudinal studies have been done in our laboratories on the San Francisco diet (SFD) compared with Purina Mouse Chow® (PMC). The SFD contains 4% fat, 23% protein and 54% carbohydrate (available kcal/g = 3.4), whereas Purina Mouse

Chow® contains 11% fat, 17% protein and 53% carbohydrate. (available kcal/g = 3.8).

The data in figure 12 show that diet has a significant effect on glycosuria. Although caloric intake was the same on both diets, fed ad libitum, glycosuria was significantly reduced on the low-fat high protein SFD. Furthermore, when both diets were restricted to 3.0 g/day, glycosuria was again significantly lower on the SFD. In addition, glycosuria was similar when the low-fat SFD fed ad libitum was compared with 3 g/day of 11% fat diet despite the fact that total caloric intake was twice as high while on the SFD ad libitum regimen.

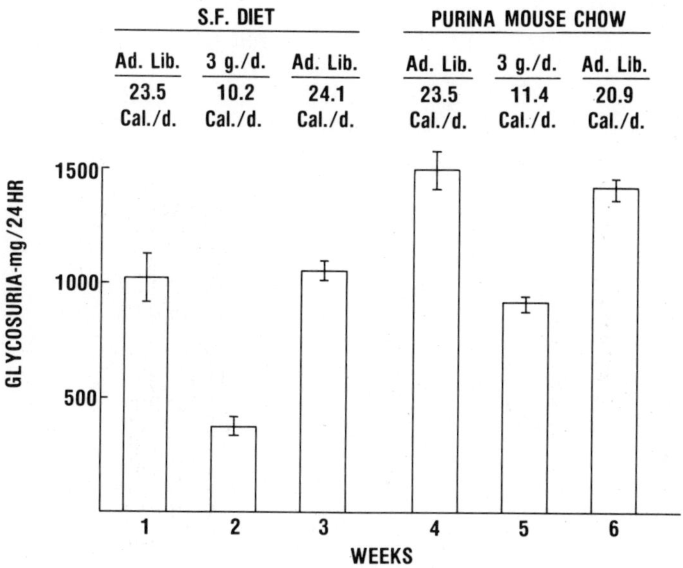

Fig. 12 Effect of high and low fat content diets on glycosuria of ketonuric diabetic Chinese hamsters.

The effects of these diets are even more striking when β-hydroxybutyrate excretion was measured (Fig. 13). The low-fat SFD reduced β-hydroxybutyrate levels to normal limits, but even restriction of high-fat diet to 50% of normal intake did not reduce β-hydroxybutyrate excretion. It is important to note that total dietary fat intake was similar on SFD ad libitum compared with PMC restricted to 3 g/day. This suggests that the effects observed in the Chinese hamster are more complex than simple quantitative fat intake but may be related to the relative amounts of individual nutrients in the diet.

Ketonemia was also reduced to normal levels on the SFD but remained elevated even on restricted PMC. Plasma insulin levels were not altered, but after 3 weeks on SFD granulation of the beta cells appeared to be greater and there was a suggestion that hydropic degeneration of the islets of Langerhans was less. It is not clear if the SFD per se or the reduced ketonemia had a beneficial effect on the beta cells. It will be of considerable interest and importance to determine if a low-fat diet fed chronically to ketonuric Chinese hamsters will normalize or lengthen their survival time and/or retard or reverse pathological lesions.

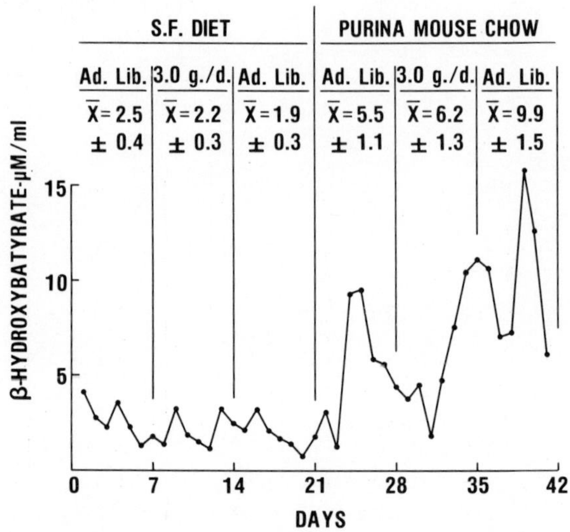

Fig. 13 Effect of high and low fat content diets on ketonuria of Chinese hamsters.

Although it is dangerous to extrapolate observations in animals to humans, the effect of high-fat diets on Chinese hamsters are in line with the old observations of Himsworth (1935) that dietary fat may be diabetogenic. These Chinese hamster data are also supported by the observations of Miki and Maruyama (1970) who reported an increasing incidence of dietary fat consumption and juvenile-type diabetes in Japan.

It has been known for some time that in vivo age is inversely correlated with in vitro life span of mass cultures of human fibroblasts (Hayflick, 1965). Seven years ago work by Goldstein et al. (1969) suggested that plating efficiency of human fibroblast cultures from individuals with two diabetic parents was decreased. Goldstein referred to these subjects as "prediabetics" but due to the previously mentioned heterogeniety of diabetes and the well known fact that all individuals with 2 diabetic parents do not necessarily develop diabetes make Goldstein's data difficult to interpret. During the past seven years, several papers appeared that cited or reproduced Goldstein's original data (Martin et al., 1970; Goldstein et al., 1975; Vracko and Benditt, 1975). However, only Vracko and Benditt (1974) show reduced cell doublings of fibroblasts from 3 diabetics to substantiate Goldstein's original observation.

Recently in our laboratories, preliminary data on tissue cultures derived from nondiabetic, prediabetic and diabetic neonatal pancreas of Chinese hamsters have been obtained (Kupiecki and Adams, personal communication). The hamsters used were as previously defined. Kupiecki and Adams have shown that β-cell monolayer cultures form readily from nondiabetic hamsters, produce insulin and survive for approximately 40 days. Under similar conditions, explants from prediabetic and diabetic pancreata attach to the culture dish but do not spread out into β-cell monolayers. After initial attachment they tend to "ball up", become granular and die, but cultures derived from nondiabetics continue in healthy functional monolayer form.

Vracko has presented strong arguments that cells of diabetic individuals are more susceptible to injury and premature death. This may be related to premature development of microangiopathy since his data indicate that accelerated rates of cell death and cell replenishment may be related to accumulation of multiple layers of basal lamina in the small vessels of the diabetic (Vracko, 1974a, b; Vracko and Benditt, 1970; Vracko and Benditt, 1974). Vracko's hypothesis becomes quite attractive since Garcia et al. (1974) pointed out emphatically that the tremendous increase in mortality of the diabetic due to cardiovascular disease cannot be explained simply on the basis of combined risk factors for cardiovascular disease, but that there must be some unknown factor which predisposes the diabetic to premature aging of the cardiovascular system. Vracko's concept of the diabetic's cells susceptibility to injury and premature death and the unexplained high incidence of cardiovascular mortality of diabetics is supported by the fact that individuals with premature aging syndromes (metageria, pangeria, progeria and total lipodystrophy) also have cardiovascular diseases and diabetes (Gilkes et al., 1974). (The only exception appears to be acrogeria.)

In the limited space available, it was not possible to discuss in detail the incredible amount of information on the inordinately complex interrelationships between diabetes, nutrition and aging. An attempt has been made to summarize what appear to be some of the more important aspects of this very complex problem. It is very clear that the longevity of the diabetic is reduced and this reduction appears to be related to premature microangiopathy. In many cases, nutrition and obesity are in some way related to the etiology of diabetes. There is also substantial evidence to indicate that diabetes is a heterogenic disease and therefore suggests that all diabetics should not be treated by the same diet or other therapeutic measures.

Human (Marble, 1971) and animal data clearly show that nutrition affects the metabolic state of the diabetic. When caloric intake of diabetic hamsters was controlled so that excessive caloric intake did not interact with genotype, their metabolic state and longevity was markedly improved. Unfortunately, at the present time chronic caloric control has not been evaluated or proved practical for the human diabetic.

Preliminary tissue culture studies in both man and Chinese hamster suggest a genetic defect which affects cell longevity. It is tempting to speculate that there is a genetic defect in the β-cell wall of the Chinese hamster since diabetic and prediabetic β-cells did not attach to the petri dish and form monolayers. Much remains to be done in order to understand the complex interrelationships of genetics, nutrition and premature aging of the diabetic.

ACKNOWLEDGEMENT

The author gratefully acknowledges the invaluable assistance of Donald Galow and Naomi Walker of the Upjohn technical library. Special thanks are due Cindy Shattuck for preparation of the manuscript.

REFERENCES

Bouchardat, H. (1883). De la Glucosurie du Diabète Sucré. Paris.

Butler, L. (1967). Diabetologia 3, 124.

Butler, L. and Gerritsen, G. C. (1970). Diabetologia 6, 163.

Carpenter, A-M., Gerritsen, G. C., Dulin, W. E., and Lazarow, A. (1967). Diabetologia 3, 92.

Chang, A. Y. (1970). In "The Structure and Metabolism of the Pancreatic Islets. Wenner-Gren Symposium No. 16" (S. Falkner, B. Hellman, and I. B. Tähjedal, eds.), pp. 515-526, Pergamon Press, Oxford and New York.

Chang, A. Y. and Schneider, D. I. (1970). Diabetologia 6, 180.
Chobanian, A. V., Gerritsen, G. C., Brecher, P. I., and McCombs, L. (1974a). Diabetologia 10, 589.
Chobanian, A. V., Gerritsen, G. C., Brecher, P. I., and Kessler, M. (1974b). Diabetologia 10, 595.
Cleave, T. L. (1974). "The Saccharine Disease". John Wright and Sons, Ltd., Bristol.
Cohen, A. M., Teitelbaum, A., and Saliternik, R. (1972). Metabolism 21, 235.
Coleman, D. L. and Hummel, K. P. (1967). Diabetologia 3, 238.
Conforti, A. (1972). Acta Diabetol. Lat. 9, 655.
Cutter, S. J. and Ederer, F. (1958). J. Chronic Dis. 8, 699.
Ditzel, J. and Sagild, U. (1954). New Engl. J. Med. 250, 587.
Dulin, W. E., Chang, A. Y., and Gerritsen, G. C. (1970). In "Les Mutants Pathologiques chez l 'Animal, Leur Intérêt dans la Recherche bio-medicale" (M. Sabourdy, ed.), pp. 131-155, Centre National de la Recherche Scientifique, Paris.
Federman, J. L. and Gerritsen, G. C. (1970). Diabetologia 6, 186.
Frankel, B. J., Gerich, J. E., Hagura, R., Fanska, R. E., Gerritsen, G. C., and Grodsky, G. M. (1974). J. Clin. Invest. 53, 1637.
Garcia, M. J., McNamara, P. M., Gordon, T., and Kannell, W. B. (1974). Diabetes 23, 105.
Genuth, S. M. (1966). Diabetes 15, 798.
Genuth, S. M., Bennett, P. H., Miller, M., and Burch, T. A. (1967). Metabolism 16, 1010.
Gerritsen, G. C. and Blanks, M. C. (1970). Diabetologia 6, 177.
Gerritsen, G. C. and Blanks, M. C. (1974). Diabetologia 10, 493.
Gerritsen, G. C. and Dulin, W. E. (1966). Diabetes 15, 331.
Gerritsen, G. C. and Dulin, W. E. (1967). Diabetologia 3, 74.
Gerritsen, G. C., Needham, L. B., Schmidt, F. L., and Dulin, W. E. (1970). Diabetologia 6, 158.
Gerritsen, G. C., Blanks, M. C., Miller, R. L., and Dulin, W. E. (1974a). Diabetologia 10, 559.
Gerritsen, G. C., Johnson, M. A., Soret, M. G., and Schultz, J. R. (1974b). Diabetologia 10, 581.
Gilkes, J. J. H., Sharvill, D. E., and Wells, R. S. (1974). Br. J. Dermatol. 91, 243.
Goldstein, S., Littlefield, J. W., and Soeldner, J. S. (1969). Proc. Natl. Acad. Sci. 64, 155.
Goldstein, S., Niewarowski, S., and Singal, D. P. (1975). Fed. Proc. 35, 56.
Grodsky, G. M. and Benoit, F. L. (1969). In "Proceedings, VI Congress of the International Diabetes Federation,

Stockholm, 1967" (J. Östman, ed.), p. 540, Excerpta Medica, Amsterdam.

Grodsky, G. M., Frankel, B. J., Gerich, J. E., and Gerritsen, G. C. (1974). Diabetologia 10, 521.

Hayflick, L. (1965). Exp. Cell Res. 37, 614.

Himsworth, H. P. and Marshall, E. M. (1935). Clin. Sci. 2, 117.

Hunt, J. N., Cash, R., and Newland, P. (1975). Lancet II, 905.

Jager, E. (1855). Beiträge zür Pathologie des Auges. Vienna.

Keen, H. (1974). In "Is the Risk of Becoming Diabetic Affected by Sugar Consumption?" (S. S. Hillebrand, ed.), pp. 14-27, International Sugar Research Foundation, Bethesda.

Keen, H., Rose, G., Pyke, D. A.,Boyns, D., Chlouverakis, C., and Mistry, S. (1962). Lancet 2, 1188.

Kilo, C., Vogler, N., and Williamson, J. R. (1972). Diabetes 21, 881.

Krall, L. P. (1971). In "Joslin's Diabetes Mellitus" (A. Marble, P. White, R. F. Bradley, and L. P. Krall, eds.), pp. 304-315, Lea & Febiger, Philadelphia.

Krall, L. P. and Joslin, A. P. (1971). In "Joslin's Diabetes Mellitus" (A. Marble, P. White, R. F. Bradley, and L. P. Krall, eds.), pp. 262-272, Lea & Febiger, Philadelphia.

Kupiecki, F. P. and Adams, L. D. (1976). Personal communication.

Luse, S. A., Caramia, F., Gerritsen, G. C., and Dulin, W. E. (1967). Diabetologia 3, 97.

Luse, S. A., Gerritsen, G. C., and Dulin, W. E. (1970). Diabetologia 6, 192.

Marble, A. (1971). In "Joslin's Diabetes Mellitus" (A. Marble, P. White, R. F. Bradley, and L. P. Krall, eds.), pp. 287-301, Lea & Febiger, Philadelphia.

Marks, H. H. (1965). Am. J. Public Health 55, 417.

Marks, H. H. (1971). In "Joslin's Diabetes Mellitus" (A. Marble, P. White, R. F. Bradley, and L. P. Krall, eds.), p. 227, Lea & Febiger, Philadelphia.

Martin, G. M., Sprague, C. A., and Epstein, C. J. (1970). Lab. Invest. 23, 86.

McCombs, L., Gerritsen, G. C., Dulin, W. E., and Chobanian, A. V. (1974). Diabetologia 10, 601.

McMillan, D. E. (1975). Diabetes 24, 944.

Metropolitan Life Statistical Bulletin (Feb. 1974). 10.

Miki, E. and Maruyama, H. (1970). In "Diabetes Mellitus in Asia" (S. Tsuji and M. Wada, eds.), Excerpta Medica, Amsterdam.

Nakamura, M. and Yamada, K. (1967). Diabetologia 3, 212.

Neel, J. V., Fajans, S. S., Conn, J. W., and Davidson, R. T. (1965). In "Genetics and the Epidemiology of Chronic Diseases" (J. V. Neel, M. Shaw, and W. Schull, eds.), p. 105, U. S. Public Health Service Publication 1163.
Ostrander, L. D., Francis, T., Hayner, N. S., Kjelsberg, M. O., and Epstein, F. H. (1965). Ann. Intern. Med. 62, 1188.
O'Sullivan, J. B. (1974). Diabetes 23, 713.
Pincus, G. and White, P. (1933). Am. J. Med. Sci. 186, 1.
Pyke, D. A. (1968). In "Clinical Diabetes and its Biochemical Basis" (W. G. Oakley, D. A. Pyke, and K. W. Taylor, eds.), p. 245, Blackwell, London.
Pyke, D. A., Cassar, J., Todd, J., and Taylor, K. W. (1970). Br. Med. J. 4, 649.
Rimoin, D. L. (1968). Arch. Intern. Med. 124, 695.
Rimoin, D. L. (1970). In "Diabetes Mellitus: Theory and Practice" (M. Ellenberg and H. Rifkin, eds.), pp. 566-569, McGraw-Hill, New York.
Rondelet, G. (1628). In "Operaomina Medica", CopXLII, p. 525, Chouet, Geneva.
Schlaepfer, W. W., Gerritsen, G. C., and Dulin, W. E. (1974). Diabetologia 10, 541.
Schmidt, F. L., Leslie, L. G., Schultz, J. R., Gerritsen, G. C. (1970). Diabetologia 6, 154.
Shirai, T., Welsh, G. W., 3rd, and Sims, E. A. H. (1967). Diabetologia 3, 266.
Soret, M. G., Dulin, W. E., and Gerritsen, G. C. (1973). In "Early Diabetes, Advances in Metabolic Disorders", Supplement 2 (R. Camerini-Davalos and H. S. Cole, eds.), p. 291, Academic Press, New York.
Soret, M. G., Dulin, W. E., Mathews, J., and Gerritsen, G. C. (1974). Diabetologia 10, 567.
Stein, S. P. and Charles, E. (1971). Am. J. Psychiat. 128, 700.
Stone, D. B. (1961). Am. J. Med. Sci. 241, 64.
Tattersall, R. B. and Fajans, S. S. (1975). Diabetes 24, 44.
Tattersall, R. B. and Pyke, D. A. (1972). Lancet 2, 1120.
Tokuhata, G. K., Miller, W., Digon, E., and Hartman, T. (1975). J. Chronic Dis. 28, 23.
Trowell, H. (1974). Lancet 2, 998.
Trowell, H. (1975). Diabetes 24, 762.
von Mering, J. and Minkowski, O. (1889). Arch. Exp. Pathol. Pharmakol. 26, 371.
Vracko, R. (1974a). Diabetes 23, 94.
Vracko, R. (1974b). Am. J. Pathol. 77, 314.
Vracko, R. and Benditt, E. P. (1970). J. Cell Biol. 47, 281.
Vracko, R. and Benditt, E. P. (1974). Am. J. Pathol. 75, 204.
Vracko, R. and Benditt, E. P. (1975). Fed. Proc. 34, 68.

West, K. M. (1973). Ann. Intern. Med. 79, 425.
West, K. M. (1974). Diabetes 23, 841.
West, K. M. (1975). Nutr. Rev. 33, 193.
West, K. M. and Kalbfleisch, J. M. (1970). Diabetes 19, 656.

NUTRITION, AGING AND OBESITY[1]

Albert J. Stunkard

Department of Psychiatry and Behavioral Sciences
Stanford University School of Medicine
Stanford, California 94305

This paper is a review of the relationship between obesity and aging. Since the evidence directly relating aging to obesity is so scant, much of what follows will deal with the critical factor with which they are both associated -- nutrition.

This review considers first the influence of nutrition upon obesity and aging in laboratory animals. It assesses the effect upon obesity and life span of four kinds of dietary interventions:

1. Retardation of growth produced by restriction of food intake beginning early in life.

2. Restriction of food intake beginning after the attainment of maturity.

3. Changes of dietary constituents.

4. Dietary self-selection.

The second part of the review consists of a highly selective look at four topics:

1. Effects upon blood pressure of change in weight status from childhood to adult life.

2. Relationship of obesity and weight reduction to coronary risk factors.

3. Results of efforts at weight reduction.

---

[1]Supported in part by National Institute of Mental Health Grant # 28124-01.

4. Effects of dietary changes upon the health of persons in an old age home.

ANIMAL STUDIES: RETARDATION OF GROWTH PRODUCED BY RESTRICTION OF FOOD INTAKE BEGINNING EARLY IN LIFE

The first dramatic evidence that the life span of organisms was not immutably fixed by their constitution first became apparent to the scientific world less than 50 years ago. The idea that life could be prolonged beyond the time span seemingly allotted to each species had bemused thinkers and dreamers since the beginnings of recorded history. However, the more we learned about biology, the less likely the possibility seemed. The discovery of Clive McCay that life span could be significantly extended by dietary means were thus more than just another scientific finding. At a time when it seemed that scientific progress was bought at the price of our most cherished illusions, the work of McCay gave substance to an age-old dream of mankind.

McCay's basic finding was that dietary restriction, sufficiently stringent to retard growth, could extend the life span. His first study, reported during the boom year of 1929, was carried out on trout (McCay *et al.*, 1929), and demonstrated that retardation of growth by the feeding of a low protein diet beginning early in life resulted in a longer life span. Shortly thereafter, there ensued the Great Depression and McCay and his colleagues turned their attention from trout to rats. In a series of three studies, these pioneers clearly demonstrated the impact of retardation of growth upon life span (McCay *et al.*, 1935, 1939, 1941). These studies were undertaken at a time when the conventional wisdom held that diets which promoted growth and development also increased life span. McCay's findings were almost directly contradictory: restriction of caloric intake sufficient to retard growth of rats resulted in significant increases in life span. A measure of the impact of McCay's findings is conveyed by figure 1. On the left is the "aged" last survivor of a group of rats fed a standard laboratory diet *ad libitum* for 900 days (McCay, 1953). The young-looking rat on the right is the same age -- its life span had been extended by dietary restriction. Clearly, dietary restriction sufficient to retard growth could postpone aging. What are the limits of this effect?

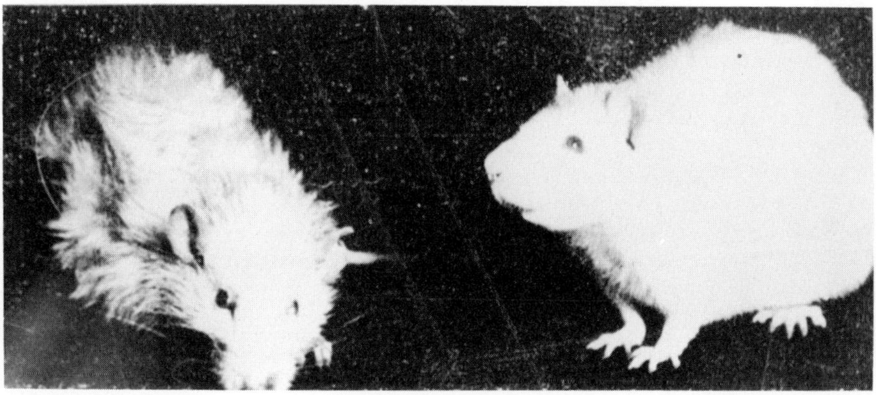

Fig. 1 Photographs of two rats, aged 100 days. The effects of early dietary restriction are clearly evidenced in the rat on the right, as compared with the "aged" rat on the left which had been fed standard laboratory chow throughout its life. (From McCay, 1953.)

The experimental design of McCay's most ambitious study is shown in the quaint outline in figure 2 (McCay, 1953). Time is displayed on the horizontal axis, weight on the vertical. We see the very low body weight of rats whose diets have been restricted and the remarkable increase in body weight of different groups when they were allowed to feed _ad libitum_. This photograph was taken when the rats were 1,000 days of age. All of those who had grown normally passed through their life cycle and died, so that the position under the curve at the extreme left is empty. Rats allowed to mature after 300, 500, and 1000 days of retardation are shown under the vertical lines representing the time at which they received access to _ad libitum_ feeding. The rat under the 300-day curve was one of only three survivors of 10 rats which began to feed _ad libitum_ at 300 days. The "young" rat on the extreme right had just been given free access to food and was just beginning to grow after 1,000 days of retardation.

The growth of rats fed restricted diets was permanently stunted and none reached the weight of those which had been fed _ad libitum_. Pathological examinations added a dimension to the picture illustrated by the survival data. The most striking finding was that growth retardation produced a significant delay in the development of diseases of the lungs, kidney and middle ear and of tumors of all kinds (McCay et al., 1935). Furthermore, McCay reported what appears to be the first experimental evidence of the deleterious effects of obesity. Rats which became obese suffered an increased incidence of all age-associated disease.

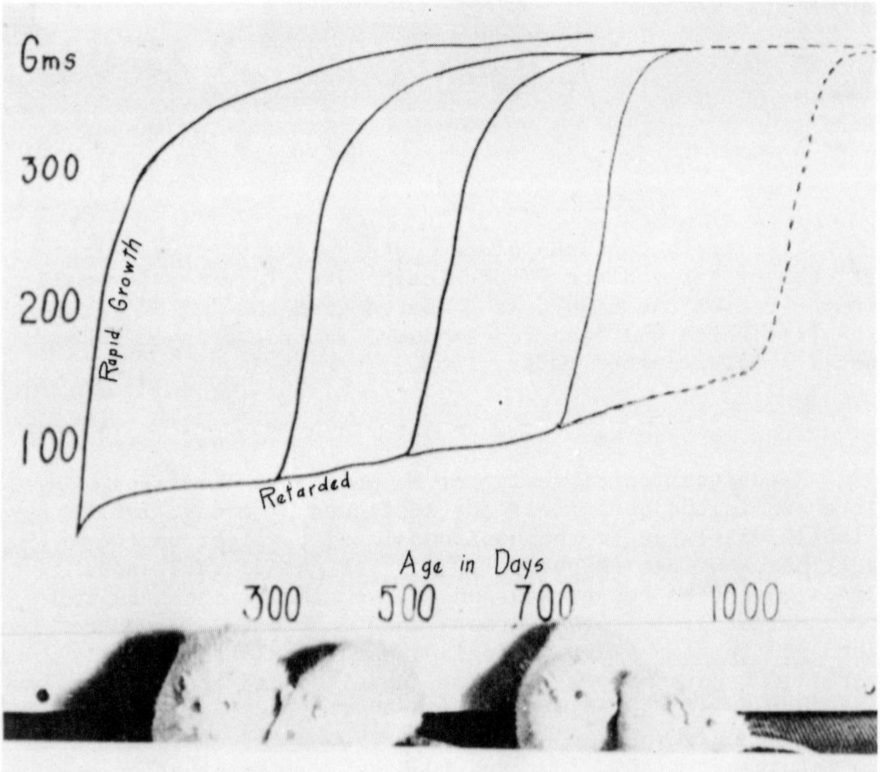

Fig. 2 Experimental design of McCay's largest study. Time in days is indicated on the horizontal axis, body weight in grams on the vertical one. Survivors of the different regimens are shown beneath the figure which represents the age at which they were accorded free access to food intake. At 1000 days there are no survivors of the group which had no limitation on food intake, and only three survivors of the ten rats with free access at 300 days. (From McCay, 1953.)

McCay's findings have been confirmed by investigation conducted in at least three different laboratories. The most ambitious of these was carried out by Ross, who provided overwhelming additional evidence for the effects of dietary restriction early in life on increasing life span in a study of over 1,000 male Charles River rats (Ross, 1961). In the course of this research, Ross observed two trends, the full significance of which was not appreciated until much later. The first was the suggestion that the effects upon the life span and incidence of disease exerted by different dietary constituents depended in part upon the time in life when the constituents were fed. The data suggest that an increase in protein early in life and a decrease later in life were associated with a prolongation in life span. The second finding was that animals could voluntarily alter their selection of diets in such a manner as to extend their life span. Thus, Ross fed his rats four diets with differing proportions of protein and carbohydrate: high protein, high carbohydrate; high protein, low carbohydrate; low protein, high carbohydrate; and low protein, low carbohydrate. The group of rats fed a diet low in protein and high in carbohydrate voluntarily restricted its intake and thereby extended its life span.

Further confirmation of the influence of dietary restriction upon life span in rats was obtained by Berg and Simms (1962). A decrease in intake of a standard laboratory diet, begun early and continued throughout life, increased life span by 25%. Furthermore, rats on an unrestricted diet, with a life span which averaged 800 days, showed a 40% incidence of kidney disease by 500 days of life. By contrast, it was 1,000 days before the rats fed a restricted diet reached a comparable incidence of kidney disease.

Quite recently Barrows (1972) has shown that the life span of C57 black mice can be extended by diets severely restricted in protein. Thus, a diet restricted to 4% protein, a level which significantly decreased the life span in rats, produced the greatest increase in life span of these mice.

All of these demonstrations that dietary restriction could increase life span were achieved by restriction of diet early in life with associated retardation in growth. Does this effect upon life span depend upon retardation in growth? If so, these findings have limited clinical applicability, since far less severe dietary restriction in human infants and children have serious deleterious effects upon higher nervous activity and upon susceptibility to disease.

If, however, dietary restriction after the attainment of maturity extended life span, clinical application might be feasible. Indeed, anything that can be learned about the impact of variations in diet upon health indices of animals following the attainment of maturity is important. That is because, in contrast to our knowledge of nutritional requirements for growth and development of the rat, we know very little about these requirements for optimal health in the mature animal. Despite the vast potential clinical significance of nutrition in adult life, it was more than 20 years after McCay's original findings before it was investigated.

ANIMAL STUDIES: RESTRICTION OF FOOD INTAKE BEGINNING AFTER THE ATTAINMENT OF MATURITY

Systematic study of the influence of dietary restriction and weight loss in adult life has been carried out only during the past five years. It is, therefore, striking that near unanimity has been achieved in the results of these investigations. There is general agreement that restriction of food intake in adult life increases the life span of animals over that of those permitted unlimited access to food throughout their lives. It also appears that the level of dietary restriction necessary to produce these results is limited to a rather narrow range and that diets outside this range have deleterious effects. Thus, dietary restriction and weight loss in adult life can increase life span but our present limitations in knowledge make this undertaking a dangerous one.

The most extensive investigations are those of Ross (1972) carried out with more than 1,300 male Charles River rats. Some of these findings are summarized in Table I. We see that the earlier the dietary restriction, the greater its effect upon life span. Thus, restriction at an early age -- 70 days -- and to the low level of 6 grams per day was sufficient to produce a marked reduction in body weight and a reduction in the mortality ratio to 35 percent.*

When dietary restriction is begun at a later age, it can still produce a decrease in the mortality ratio, but this

*Mortality ratio values were computed by dividing the number of deaths occurring at each age period in an experimental group by the number of deaths that would have occurred had that group experienced the same risk as a standard or controlled population. The age-specific mortality rates of the group of rats within each experimental series that had been maintained on ad libitum rations throughout post-weaning life were used as the standard rate. Ratio values of less than 100 are indicative of the life-prolonging influence of the experimental dietary regimen; values more than 100, the life-shortening influence.

exercise is fraught with far greater danger than is produced by dietary restriction at an earlier age. Thus, we see that restriction of food intake to 6 grams a day actually produces a significant rise in the mortality ratio of rats restricted at 300 days and an even more pronounced rise in the mortality ratio of those restricted at 365 days of life. An increase in food intake of no more than 2 grams a day reverses this effect and lowers the mortality ratio to 49% and 79%, respectively, and an even greater dietary allotment is necessary for optimal life span of the rats which were restricted at 365 days. This level of dietary restriction -- 10 grams per day -- resulted in a life expectancy of these latter rats which was almost equivalent to that of the rats restricted to 6 grams a day at 70 days of age.

TABLE I

Effects of Dietary Restriction at Different Ages on Mortality Ratio in Rats

Unrestricted Feeding	Size of Diet (Grams)	Body Weight at Change	Maintenance	Mortality Ratio (%)
Throughout life	--	--	915	100
To 70 days	6	364	200	35
To 300 days	6	733	215	241
	8	722	285	49
To 365 days	6	748	220	320
	8	784	280	79
	10	800	350	44

(After Ross, 1972.)

Ross concludes that the level of restriction most conducive to an increase in length of life changes with age. The rats that were severely restricted in their intake of food throughout post-weaning life lived the longest. When the same level of restriction was imposed at later ages, life expectancy progressively decreased; in older rats, the duration of life was drastically curtailed. The length of life of older and heavier rats, however, could be extended by a restriction which was less severe (Ross, 1972). An alternative view of these findings is suggested by the body weight as well as the food intake of the rats. Ross did not relate his findings to weight at the time of dietary restriction, maintenance weight or percent of weight reduction. Table I, however, suggests that one or more of these parameters may predict life span and mortality ratio as adequately as the level of dietary intake. Studies of Ross described later have shown that body weight early in life and maximum body weight are powerful predictors of such age-associated diseases as tumors (Ross and Bras, 1965).

Ross's findings have already been confirmed and extended in no less than four different laboratories. The results of Stuchlíková et al. (1975) are particularly impressive, for they have been carried out with no less than three different species of rodents. The effects of four different dietary regimens were tested: restriction throughout life; ad libitum feeding throughout life; restriction for the first year followed by ad libitum feeding for the second year; and, finally, ad libitum feeding for the first year followed by restriction during the second year. The effects of these four different dietary regimens upon two species of rodents are illustrated in the life tables in figure 3. Rodents fed ad libitum throughout both years of the study showed the lowest survival rate, followed by those who were restricted for two years of the program. These results are fully in accord with the earlier studies of the life-extending effects of dietary restriction early in life. The rodents which were fed ad libitum for the first year and then restricted had the next longest survival. Finally, the longest survival rate was achieved by rodents which were restricted during the first year of life and ate ad libitum during the second.

Stuchlíková's study is noteworthy in being the only one to find that rodents restricted throughout life had lower survival rates than those that were fed ad libitum either early or late in their lives. This finding is particularly significant in its suggestion that dietary restriction in adult life may, under certain circumstances, be even more efficacious than dietary restriction throughout life.

Another highly significant finding involved those animals whose food intake was restricted for the first year and which were then permitted to feed ad libitum. Stuchlíková notes that when these rodents were given unlimited access to food, they overate and became obese. Despite this obesity, they had the longest life span of any of the groups! This finding runs counter to almost everything we know about obesity and its effects on, or associations with, health and disease. If it could be confirmed, it would provide invaluable evidence that at least some forms of obesity do not automatically confer health disadvantages.

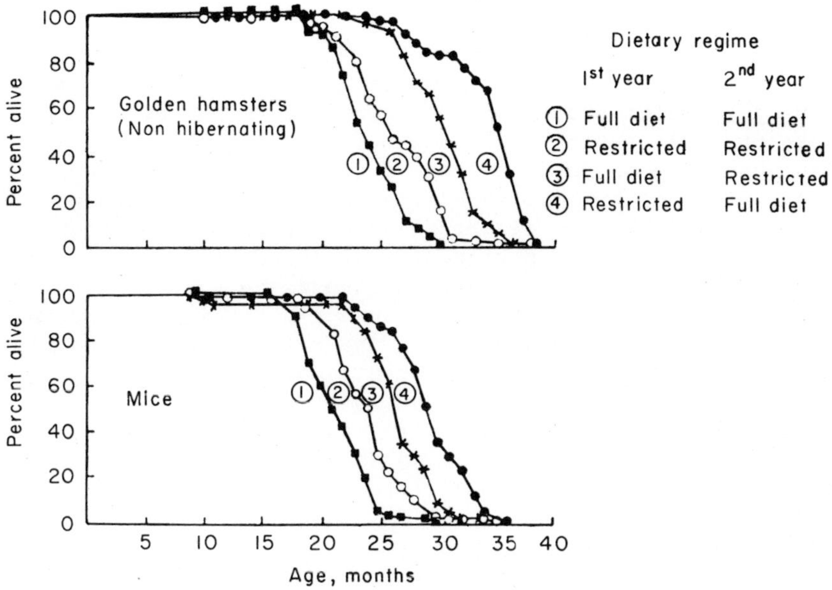

Fig. 3 Life tables illustrating survival of golden hamsters and mice under four different dietary regimens. In each species there is an orderly increase in survival rate from the first to the fourth regimen. (From Stuchlíková *et al*., 1975.)

In an ambitious study of 700 Simonsen rats of both sexes, Nolen (1972) also reported that dietary restriction in adult life resulted in life span greater than that of animals permitted *ad libitum* feeding throughout life. He found, as had Stuchlíková, that animals restricted early in life and then permitted *ad libitum* feeding developed obesity. In contrast to Stuchlíková's rodents, this obesity was not only not associated with increased life span but instead with a life span no greater than that of rats fed *ad libitum* throughout life. It was further associated with "disturbed biological characteristics such as smaller vital organs", fatty livers, and a marked increase in liver cholesterol.

A third study utilizing the same experimental design as Stuchlíková and Nolen, obtained results similar to Stuchlíková (Beauchene, 1976). Rats which were restricted in intake initially and then switched to *ad libitum* feeding developed obesity. Beauchene found, as Stuchlíková did and as Nolen did not, that this early restriction and later obesity was associated with greater longevity. He also found that rats with restriction in food intake either early or later in life had a significantly lower incidence of age-associated changes in kidney function.

Thus, three different studies have two different implications for health and for life expectancy among animals made obese by early restricted and later ad libitum feeding. This discrepancy seems important and a question deserving resolution. At least one difference in experimental design which could account for the discrepancy is apparent from the published work. Nolen's period of restricted food intake lasted only 12 weeks, Stuchlíková's and Beauchene's 12 months. Other critical differences of perhaps even greater importance, however, cannot be ascertained from the rather limited description of methods published in these reports.

Quite recently, an increase in life span produced by dietary restriction in adult life has been reported by another group. Barrows (1976) has shown that the institution of a diet containing 12% casein as late as 16 months produced an increase in life expectancy of 25% in rats.

ANIMAL STUDIES: CHANGES IN DIETARY CONSTITUENTS

Research in nutrition has not been confined to efforts at investigating the effects of alterations in the caloric content of food intake. Alterations in the constituents of food intake have been studied as intensively. These studies have revealed that alterations in the constituents comprising the diet can also alter the life span and such alterations are even more effective in producing obesity.

It has been more than 20 years since Mickelsen first produced obesity in rats by feeding them a high fat diet (Mickelsen et al., 1955; Schemmel et al., 1969). Since then, several investigators have repeated and extended this work until the use of a high fat diet has become one of the standard methods of producing experimental obesity in animals. French, for example, showed that rats fed a high fat diet became obese and had a shorter life span than rats raised on a high carbohydrate diet, even when the high fat diet was lower in calories (French et al., 1953). Similarly, the Silberbergs showed a decrease in the life span of the males of two strains of mice fed a high fat diet (Silberberg and Silberberg, 1954). Finally, Lane and Dickie (1958) produced dramatic evidence that constitution was not destiny in the case of genetically-obese (ob/ob) mice, for reducing their food intake significantly increased their life span. In fact, if the food intake of these mice was so restricted as to maintain their body weight at the same level as that of their non-obese siblings, their mean life span increased from 457 days to 795 days. These normally short-lived mice thus lived even longer than their non-obese siblings, whose life span was 747 days. One factor may help to explain this remarkable extension of life, even beyond that of the non-obese siblings. Even on the restricted diet the body carcass of the ob/ob mice contained a larger percent of body fat than did the body carcass of their non-obese siblings. Thus, in terms of lean body mass, the dietary restriction of the ob/ob mice was even greater than that of their non-obese siblings.

A significant advance in our understanding of the influence of different dietary constituents was made by Miller and Payne (1968). These authors started their investigations from the premise that the nutritional requirements of animals must vary at different stages in their development, and that in free-living animals these changing metabolic needs must find expression in the consumption of diets of differing nutritional constituents. They thus explored the effects of varying the protein content of diets according to their estimates of protein requirements early and late in life. Rats fed a stock diet consisting of 12 percent protein until the age of 120 days and then shifted to a diet containing 4 percent protein (B) showed a life expectancy greater than that of rats fed a variety of other diets. Figure 4 shows the very low survival rate of rats fed a 4 percent protein diet throughout life (D) and the only slightly greater survival rate of rats fed either a stock diet (A) or a 6 percent protein diet throughout their lives (C). The rats of Group B, fed the constituents of Diet A early in life and of Diet D later in life, demonstrate survival rates considerably greater than those of the rats that subsisted on either diet alone.

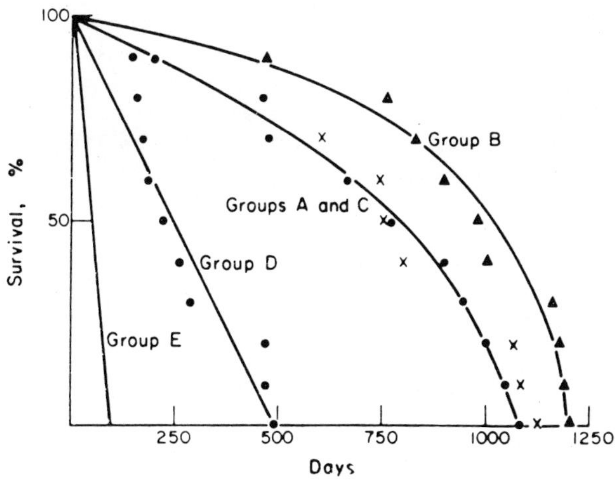

Fig. 4 Influence of diets of differing composition upon survival rates of five groups of ten hooded female rats. (From Miller and Payne, 1968.)

TUMORS: A SPECIAL CASE

A particularly interesting aspect of the influence of nutrition upon life span is that exerted upon the development of tumors. Ross has found a 40 percent incidence of tumors in rats raised on a variety of nutritional regimens (Ross and Bras, 1965). Tumors thus rank only behind kidney disease (with an incidence of 75 percent), and together with cardiovascular disease (with an incidence of 40 percent) as one of the three major forms of disease afflicting rats under varying experimental circumstances. Approximately half of these tumors were malignant. Clearly, tumors are major determinants of the life span of rats under laboratory circumstances, and are determined to an unusual degree by the state of nutrition of the animal. In fact, age and caloric intake (or the resultant body weight) are the two major determinants of the incidence of tumors.

Figure 5 shows the remarkably strong relationship between maximum body weight, which reflects the preceding level of caloric intake, and the incidence of tumors. The "Tumor Incidence Ratio" (TIR) shown in figure 5 is computed by dividing the actual number of tumors observed at each age period in an experimental group by the expected number of tumors, had the group experienced the same risks as a standard population. Clearly, over-nutrition promotes the development of tumors, under-nutrition impedes it. Indeed, the influence of food intake and consequent body weight upon the incidence of tumors is so strong that weight at 70 days predicts tumor incidence as long as a year later with an accuracy comparable to that shown for maximum body weight in figure 5.

If tumors are so dependent upon nutrition and upon the rate of growth, the question arises as to the influence of nutritional factors upon the master gland which regulates growth -- the pituitary. Ross has found that nutrition exerts a tumorigenic influence upon the organ regulating growth and development as potent as that upon the body organs which it regulates (Ross *et al.*, 1965). Food intake and consequent body weight are directly related to the incidence of chromophobe adenomas (Ross, 1969). Figure 6 shows that increases in maximum body weight are directly related to increases in the number of chromophobe adenomas.

Similar interesting relationships are found between nutrition and other forms of tumors. Increase in growth of the organ is associated with increase in the incidence of

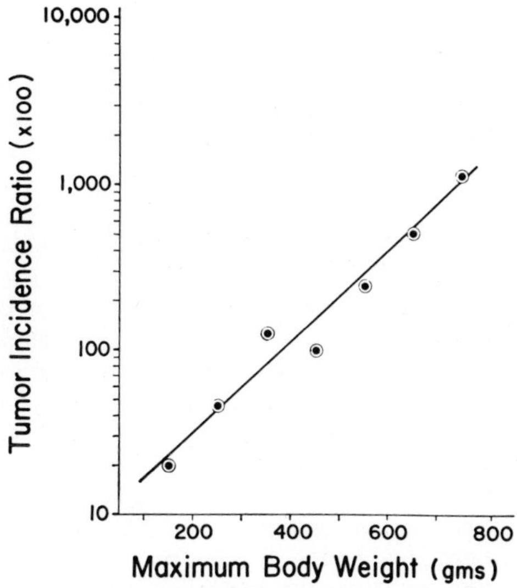

Fig. 5 Correlation between maximal body weight and tumor incidence ratio (TIR). (Rats with maximal body weights of from 400 to 500 grams were used as the standard population for computation of TIR values.) Compared with the standard population, TIR values lower than 100 indicate the degree of beneficial effect and more than 100 the degree of deleterious effect. (From Ross and Bras, 1965.)

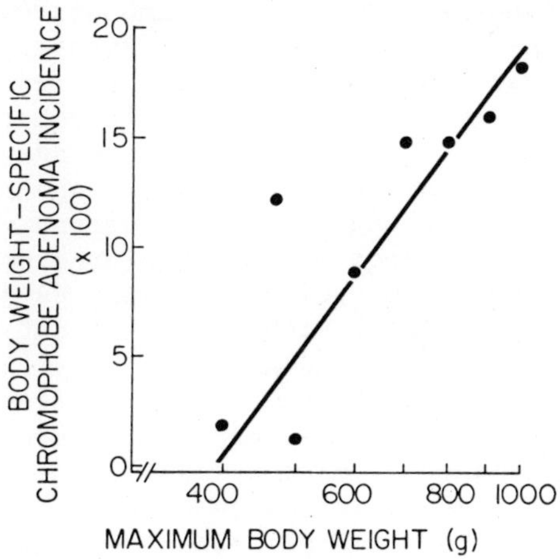

Fig. 6 Correlation between maximum body weight and risk of tumors of the anterior pituitary gland among ad libitum-fed rats. Body weight-specific incidence was computed as the ratio of the number of rats with chromophobe adenomas within a weight class to the number of rats without such tumors in that weight class. (From Ross, 1969.)

tumors of that organ and vice versa. For example, a diet low in cystine retards the occurrence of mammary tumors in mammary tumor-prone mice (White, 1961). Agents which increase the growth of the mammary gland, such as estrogen implantations or a high fat diet early in life, increase the incidence of mammary tumors (Tannenbaum, 1942; White, 1961).

ANIMAL STUDIES: DIETARY SELF-SELECTION

The studies which we have reviewed up to this point investigated the influence of diets of fixed composition under two types of experimental conditions. A prime example of the first type of condition is exemplified by those which either restricted food intake or permitted _ad libitum_ feeding, an experimental manipulation going back to the original studies of McCay. In the second kind of condition, the composition of the diet was varied, as exemplified by studies which altered the fat content of the diet to produce or restrain obesity. Both kinds of investigation have been fruitful, but they provide, at best, a limited number of experimental conditions; conditions which are indeed very far from those encountered by animals in the free-living state.

Many years ago, the pioneering work of Curt Richter introduced the idea of dietary self-selection into the repertoire of the animal experimentalist. Over a long career, Richter established that rats in a free-feeding situation are able to select essential nutrients in amounts sufficient to sustain life, to grow and to reproduce (Richter _et al_., 1938). These studies showed that rats deprived of vitamins developed highly sensitive "specific hungers" for foodstuffs containing even minute amounts of these vitamins (Barelare _et al_., 1938). Similarly, rats subjected to adrenalectomy and parathyroidectomy developed specific hungers for sodium and calcium salts which enabled them to select foods containing no more than traces of these elements out of a wide variety of possible alternatives (Richter, 1936; Richter and Echert, 1937). Nowhere has Walter Cannon's "wisdon of the body" been more elegantly expressed than in this remarkable ability of animals to respond to specific metabolic needs with these highly selective specific hungers (Cannon, 1939).

Ross was the first to introduce dietary self-selection into the study of aging. He has noted the particular advantages of this experimental approach: "The diet selected is of physiologic significance to the individual, at least during the growth period of life; it more closely approximates the natural condition; and the arbitrary decisions made by the investigator as to the quality of the diet without considering the needs of the individual are avoided. In addition, by permitting the animals to display their preferences, it may be possible to assess on an individual basis the long-term consequences of dietary habits at different stages of life." (Ross and Bras, 1975). What has this approach taught us about the effects of dietary self-selection upon longevity? How successful are experimental animals at selection of diets that will increase their life span?

The first such study was carried out in 1951 by Mayer and his coworkers (Mayer _et al._, 1951). They studied the preference in a free-choice situation of the genetically-obese (ob/ob) mouse for three diets containing, respectively, 90 percent of the calories as protein, fat or carbohydrate. The obese mice differed from their non-obese siblings in two fundamental ways. First, they ate significantly more -- a total of 25.5 ± 5 calories per day -- compared to 20 ± 4.4 calories a day. Second, there was a striking difference in the character of the diet which they chose. The obese mice selected a diet composed of 52 percent fat, compared to the 29 percent fat diet chosen by their non-obese siblings. Mayer did not assess the effects of these self-selected diets upon longevity. But everything that we have learned about the influence of high fat diets in the last 25 years leads us to expect that the diet chosen by the obese mice not only facilitated the development of their obesity but also had a deleterious effect upon their life span.

This first study of dietary self-selected, thus showed little "wisdom of the body" on the part of the genetically-obese mice. In fact, in terms of what we know about the effect of high fat diets on life span, it showed the direct opposite. However, we must keep in mind the fact that these mice were genetically selected for their ability to become obese and presumably also for behavior which might facilitate the development of their obesity. What about animals with no such predisposition? Does their dietary self-selection manifest a wisdom of their bodies?

Only one study has as yet addressed this problem, but its results are equivocal. Ross studied the influence upon life span of diets with protein contents of 10 percent, 22 percent, and 51 percent given either singly or all together in a free-choice situation (Ross and Bras, 1974). No two rats on the self-selection regimen exhibited the same dietary preferences. Within the first five weeks of feeding, however, most had established the level of protein and carbohydrate that they would continue to select for a prolonged period. Despite variation in relative preference for the three diets or in the amount of food consumed, the protein-carbohydrate ratio of the resulting diet was maintained for as long as 700 days. Rats which selected their own diets in the free-choice situation grew more rapidly and attained a greater body weight than rats fed the diet separately. After an initial rapid increase in the amount of food consumed, the daily intake of each rat remained relatively constant for as long as one year of age. By this time 90 percent of the rats had showed a marked and progressive increase in food intake. Self-selection thus apparently helps rats to optimum growth and development. What effect does it have upon life span?

The influence of a self-selected dietary regimen upon the prevalence of age-related diseases is illustrated in Table II.

TABLE II

Effects of Dietary Regimens on Incidence of Disease in Rats

	Single-Fixed Protein			Self-Selected Protein
	10%	22%	51%	10%, 22%, 51%
Tumors	26	29	28	62**
Kidney disease	38	56	73**	90*
Myocardial fibrosis	11	42	48**	67*
Prostatitis	5	10	12	62**

* p <.003
**p <.001
(After Ross and Bras, 1974.)

The three columns on the left of the table show the increasing prevalence of diseases of the kidney, heart and prostate as the percentage of protein in the single fixed diet is increased. The effects of self-selection are illustrated in the right hand column. Here we see that self-selection results in far greater prevalence of disease. It will be noted that the prevalence of disease is considerably higher than 100 percent, a fact explained by the presence of multiple afflictions of the same animal. Thus, 66 percent of the animals on the self-selected diet had at least three of the four diseases.

The first study of dietary self-selection dealt with its influence upon the prevalence of disease. A year later Ross reported upon the effects of dietary self-selection upon life expectancy (Ross and Bras, 1975). The results were consistent with earlier findings on fixed dietary regimens: rats that ate more died sooner. Rats permitted to select their own diets ate more and had a life expectancy from weaning of only 630 days. Overall, a 10 percent increase or decrease in food intake resulted in a corresponding 8 percent change in mortality.

The composition of the diet as well as its caloric content influenced life span. Furthermore, the different elements of the diet had different effects at different times in life. Thus, before 50 days, life span correlated most highly with the protein content of the diet, high protein being associated with longer life expectancy. From 50 to 300 days, the strongest correlations were with caloric content, lower caloric content being associated with longer life expectancy. After 300 days, a combination of low protein content and fewer calories had the highest correlation with life span.

The greatest influence of dietary components upon life span occurred during the adolescence of the rat -- between 100 and 200 days. Table III shows the remarkably strong effects of differences in caloric content at that time upon subsequent life span. Thus, during this period, a difference of no more than one gram per day resulted in changes in life span of 26 days.

TABLE III

Life Span of Rats Permitted Freedom of Dietary Choice: Relationship to Food Intake

Food Intake (g/day) Mean ± S.E.	Food Intake (g/day) Range	N	Life Span	Age for 50% Survival	Mortality Ratio
			(days, mean ± S.E.)	(days)	
18.3 ± 0.8	16.2 - 19.2	20	733 ± 117	690	62
19.8 ± 0.3	19.4 - 20.2	20	653 ± 126	650	97
20.7 ± 0.3	20.3 - 21.1	20	630 ± 111	630	103
21.6 ± 0.2	21.2 - 21.9	20	612 ± 115	610	108
22.4 ± 0.4	22.0 - 22.9	20	600 ± 113	580	121
24.1 ± 1.0	23.0 - 26.6	21	556 ± 106	540	162

Rats are classified according to the mean daily food intake during age period 100-199 days. The age for 50% survival was estimated from survival curves. The mortality ratio reflects the relative death risk at all ages. It is computed as 100 times the actual number of deaths divided by the expected number of deaths. Values less than 100 indicate the extent of reduction in risk relative to ... (continued on page 270)

Table III (continued) ... "standard" population; those greater than 100 indicate the extent of increase in relative risk. Age-specific mortality rates for all rats (n=121) were used as standard rates in deriving the expected number of deaths at consecutive age periods for each of the subclasses.

Finally, Ross conducted an ingenious analysis of the influence of diet on life expectancy, comparing life-time dietary records of the 30 longest-lived rats with those of the 30 shortest-lived rats. The mean life span of the first group was 787 days and that of the second 473 days. Figure 7 shows the dietary patterns of these two groups. The longer-lived rats selected diets early in life which provided about equal parts of protein and carbohydrate and they maintained this selection throughout their lives. The short-lived rats, on the other hand, self-selected diets which provided precisely the wrong constituents for extending life span. Thus, early in life, when a high protein diet has beneficial influences upon life span, they selected a low protein diet. Later in life, when low protein diets increase life span, they selected high protein diets. This particular dietary combination was associated with far shorter life spans than those of rats eating any one of the diets.

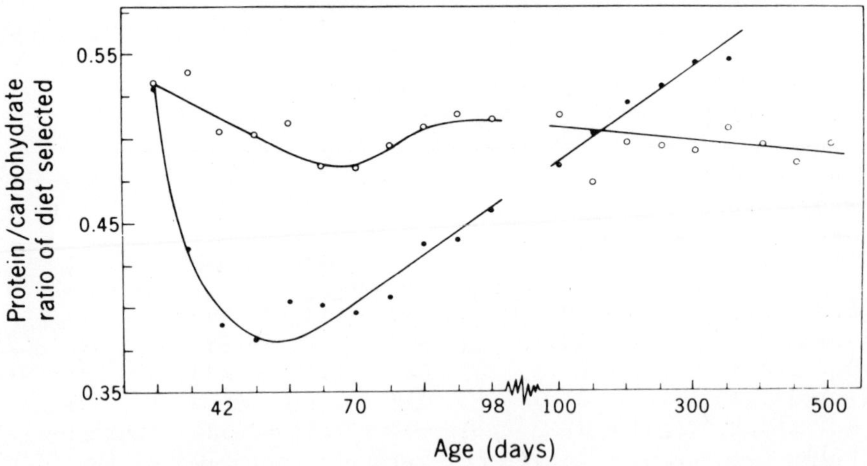

Fig. 7 Protein/carbohydrate ratio of diet selected by 30 of the shortest-lived rats (solid circles) and 30 of the longest-lived rats (open circles). Each class represents 25% of the total population. The protein/carbohydrate ratio of the diet selected by the short-lived rats was significantly different from that selected by long-lived rats ($p < .05$ for weeks 7 to 13). (From Ross and Bras, 1975.)

It is tempting to ascribe the lowered life expectancy of the short-lived rats to the diet which they chose. In fact, this seems the most logical explanation of these events. We cannot, however, rule out the possibility that some factor underlies both the dietary selection and the shorter life span. It may be that rats destined to die young also prefer certain protein:carbohydrate ratios, which they eat when they are able to choose their food. However, they might die just as young if they had eaten a completely different diet. Only further research can give the answer.

In the meantime, the weight of evidence rests on the proposition that some rats, when allowed free access to different diets, select those with the worst possible effect upon their life expectancy. These events have led Ross to modify the old adage "one man's meat is another man's poison" to "one rat's food is that same rat's poison" (Ross, 1976). What is the biological significance of this curious and apparently perverse phenomenon?

These deleterious effects of dietary self-selection can be viewed from two standpoints - the welfare of the individual and the welfare of the species. From the standpoint of the individual the results appear perverse. When we consider the welfare of the species they make uncommonly good sense, for food choices during dietary self-selection seem to optimize conditions for the maintenance of the species. Thus, rats self-select diets which are optimal for growth and development, which bring the individual to sexual maturity as soon and in as healthy a state as possible. Once these individuals have fulfilled their procreative function, their service to the species is at an end. From the standpoint of view of the species, therefore, it is best that they die and leave the food supply - and the future - to their progeny.

This "wisdom of the body" is thus primarily a wisdom in the service of the species. Cannon's classic investigations of such phenonema as the automatic physiological responses to danger which prepare the organism for fight or flight are instances when this wisdom is in the service of the individual (Cannon, 1939). In such circumstances, the welfare of the individual and the welfare of the species coincide; survival of the individual is necessary for the survival of the species. The new research on aging, however, has uncovered a situation which may be unprecedented in biological research. Here the welfare of the individual and the welfare of the species may not only not coincide - they may be in direct conflict. Under these circumstances, when the welfare of the individual conflicts with the welfare of the species, the welfare of the species takes precedence. This biological imperative is, perhaps, the outstanding lesson to be learned from the so-far limited research on self-selection of dietary regimens.

HUMAN STUDIES: EFFECTS UPON BLOOD PRESSURE OF CHANGE IN WEIGHT STATUS FROM CHILDHOOD TO ADULT LIFE

When we turn from animal studies to those involving humans, we find even less information about the influence of nutrition upon aging, and surprisingly little even about its influence on obesity. One notable exception is a study conducted in Hagerstown, Maryland on a population which has been followed by the Public Health Service since the 1920's. In 1971 Abraham and his coworkers (Abraham et al., 1971) reported the results of a follow-up study of 717 white males who had first been examined between 1923 and 1928, when they were between nine and thirteen years old. At the time of the reexamination their average age was forty-eight. The first striking finding of this study was the very strong tendency of overweight children to be overweight adults. No less than 84 percent of markedly overweight children remained overweight as adults. In addition, 50 percent of the below average weight children were in either the adult average or overweight categories. Average weight children showed a similar tendency, with 40 percent moving into adult overweight categories and 60 percent of the moderately overweight children remaining overweight as adults. The second striking finding of this study was the relationship between changes in weight status and health. In this case the major health index to be measured was blood pressure. Three weight patterns are of particular interest:

1. Obese as children, obese as adults.

2. Obese as children, normal weight as adults.

3. Thin as children and obese as adults.

This latter pattern is the same as that of Stuchlíková's and Beauchene's healthy, long-lived rats and of Nolen's unhealthy, short-lived ones (Nolen, 1972; Stuchlíková et al., 1975; Beauchene, 1976).

Table IV shows the prevalence of hypertension by change in weight status from childhood to adulthood. It reveals that subjects whose weight status did not change during this interval showed a prevalence of hypertension of about 20 percent. It is noteworthy that obese children who remained obese as adults showed no greater prevalence of hypertension.

TABLE IV

Prevalence of Hypertension by Change in Weight Status From Childhood to Adulthood

	Weight		Percent	
	Childhood	Adulthood	Hypertensive	Number
Stable	Thin	Thin	21	112
	Normal	Normal	24	119
	Stout	Stout	23	52
	Obese	Obese	20	35
Decrease	Normal	Thin	16	94
	Stout & Obese	Normal	24	37
	Stout & Obese	Thin	0	12
Increase	Thin	Normal	31	64
	Thin	Stout	47	38
	Thin	Obese	75	8
	Normal	Stout	22	108
	Normal	Obese	36	36

(From Abraham *et al*., 1971.)

Those few children who had been either stout or obese and who had become thin adults showed a strikingly lower prevalence of hypertension than any of the other groups. Finally, the highest prevalence of hypertension was found among those persons who had increased their weight status as adults. In their greater incidence of disease, thus, these people are more like Nolen's than like Stuchlíková's and Beauchene's rats.

HUMAN STUDIES: RELATIONSHIP OF OBESITY TO CORONARY RISK FACTORS

The major age-associated affliction of humans is coronary heart disease, which was responsible for over half of all deaths in the United States during the past year. The relationship of nutrition and of obesity to coronary heart disease is still not fully understood. Indeed, there are those who assign relatively little importance to nutrition, and even less to obesity, as coronary risk factors (Mann, 1974). It must be acknowledged that the links between these factors are correlational and not causal. Nevertheless, these correlations are highly suggestive.

Studies of both populations and of individuals have established a very high correlation between the levels of serum cholesterol and coronary heart disease (Keys, 1970). Levels of serum cholesterol rise and fall in direct proportion to changes in body weight. Figure 8 shows the remarkably regular relationship between changes in weight and changes in serum cholesterol observed over a period of several years in a study population in Framingham, Massachusetts (Kagan et al., 1963). The Framingham study has shown, in addition, an accelerating increase in both heart disease and stroke with increasing degrees of overweight (Gordon and Kannel, 1973).

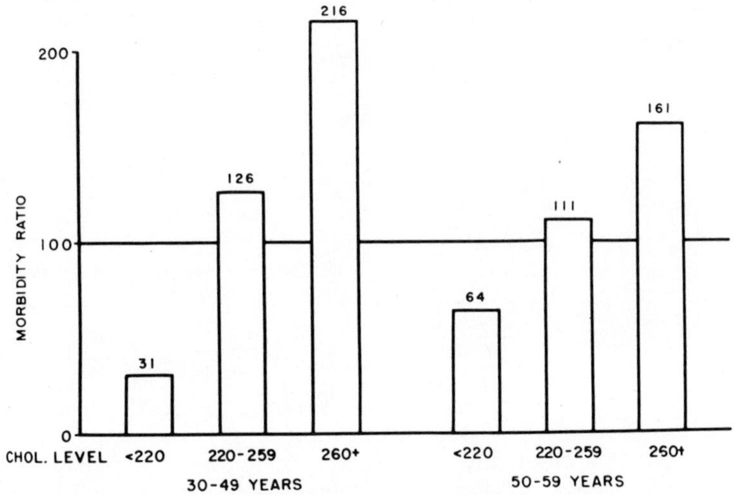

Pop. at Risk	720	534	281	262	195	135
Obs. Cases M.I.	4	13	12	10	13	13
Exp. Cases M.I.	13.0	10.3	5.6	15.7	11.7	8.1

Fig. 8 Risk of developing mild myocardial infarction in 8 years, according to initial serum cholesterol level. Data for men, aged 30 to 59 years, at entry into the Framingham study. (From Kagan et al., 1963.)

Figure 9 shows that an increase of no more than 50 percent over ideal weight increases the risk of these disorders among men by 100 percent and among women by an even greater percent. Two of the leading risk factors for coronary artery disease, hypertension and hypercholesterolemia, are similarly influenced by obesity. A recent review has described no less than 31 studies from all parts of the world which showed a positive correlation between overweight and hypertension and

19 that showed reduction in blood pressure consequent upon weight reduction (Chiang et al., 1969). Two excellent reports have similarly documented the relationship of obesity to diabetes with its attendant hypercholesterolemia (Bierman et al., 1968; Abrams et al., 1969).

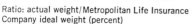

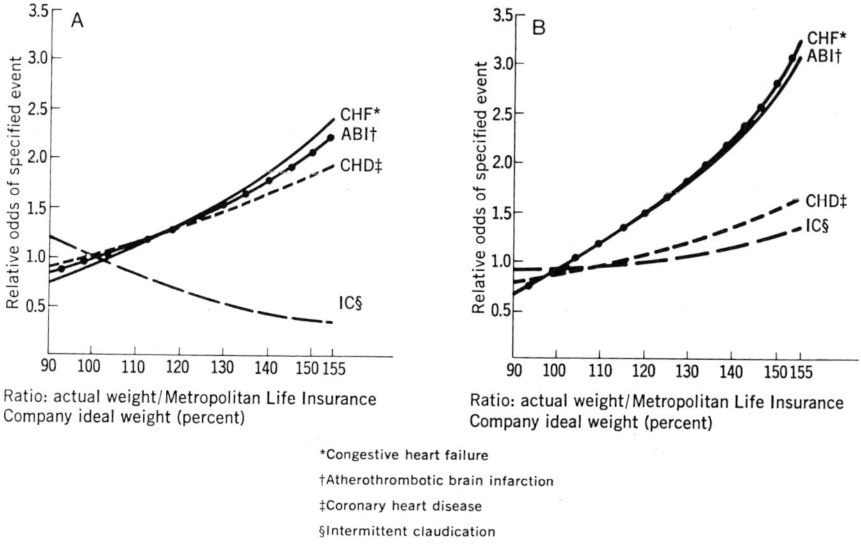

Fig. 9 Relationship of overweight to cardiovascular events. A. Odds according to relative weight: Men, Framingham study, 16 year follow-up. B. Odds according to relative weight: Women, Framingham study, 16 year follow-up. (From Gordon and Kannel, 1973.)

To these traditional evidences of the adverse consequences of obesity must be added a singularly persuasive study of the effects of weight reduction (Olefsky et al., 1974). This study is particularly credible, since its subjects showed only modest correlations between degree of obesity and metabolic indices. Its results thus do not depend upon any assumptions as to the effects of obesity upon these metabolic indices. It speaks to nothing more than the effects of weight reduction, pure and simple. The subjects were mildly overweight (21 percent) men and women, unselected except to exclude frank diabetics, who lose an average of 24 pounds, a figure comfortably within the range of the results of behavioral studies reviewed here. This modest weight loss had profound metabolic consequences. A well-established consequence is improvement in glucose tolerance. Figure 10 shows the effect of weight reduction on plasma glucose levels following a test dose of 40 gm/m^2 of body surface area. In this case, the improvement, a 12 percent decrease in the area under the curve, while statistically significant, is less than is usually found, and far less than would be the case had frank diabetics been included in the sample. Despite this small improvement in glucose tolerance, weight reduction produced a major decrease in insulin response to the glucose load. Figure 10 shows this striking 37 percent reduction in the area under the curve. Furthermore, the reduction in insulin response to a liquid meal, a closer approximation to real life than a glucose load, was a remarkable 48 percent!

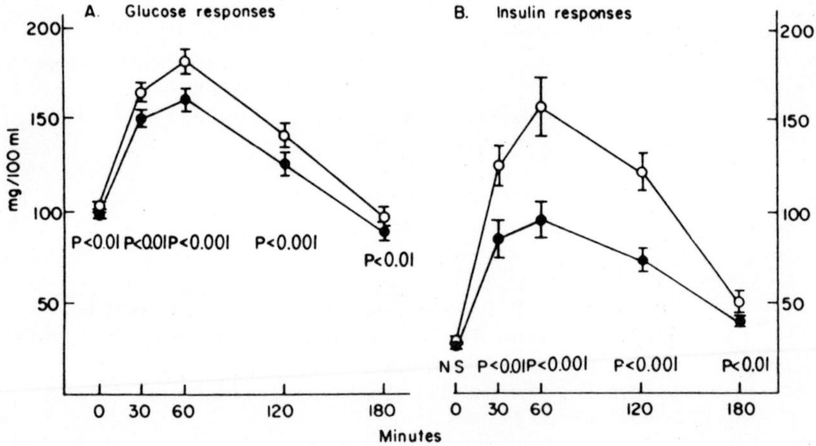

Fig. 10 Improved glucose tolerance and greatly improved insulin tolerance following weight loss of 24 pounds. (From Olefsky <u>et al</u>., 1974.)

Such hypersecretion of insulin, especially in response to carbohydrate ingestion, is believed to play a major role in the hyperlipemias associated with coronary artery disease. The effects of weight reduction upon the production of very low density lipoproteins was therefore assessed. Figure 11 shows the highly significant 40 percent decrease in the production of these lipoproteins, which are increasingly ascribed a critical role in coronary atherosclerosis.

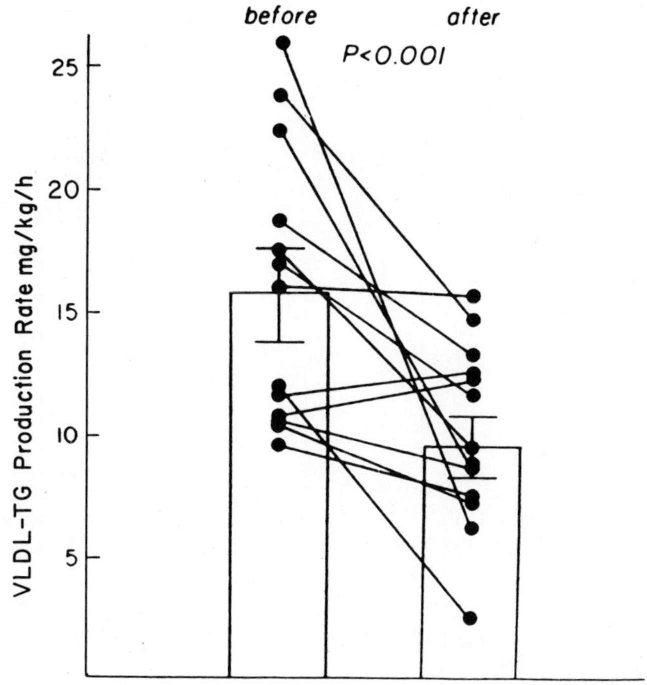

Fig. 11 Highly significant fall in very low density lipoproteins following a 24 pound weight loss. (From Olefsky et al., 1974.)

Finally, this modest weight reduction had a powerful impact upon plasma triglycerides and cholesterol. Figure 12 shows the fall in plasma triglyceride levels from 319 mg percent to 180 mg percent, a decrease of 44 percent. Plasma cholesterol levels fell from 282 mg percent to 223 mg percent, a decrease of 21 percent. Clearly, changes in nutrition and in body weight are closely linked to changes in coronary risk factors. The laborious task of proving that they also influence coronary heart disease has not yet been achieved. But this fact should not blind us to the very high probability that such a relationship exists. It seems desperately important that we be aware of these relationships, for they offer inviting prospects for therapeutic intervension by means of weight reduction. The question then arises, "What are the results of efforts at weight reduction?".

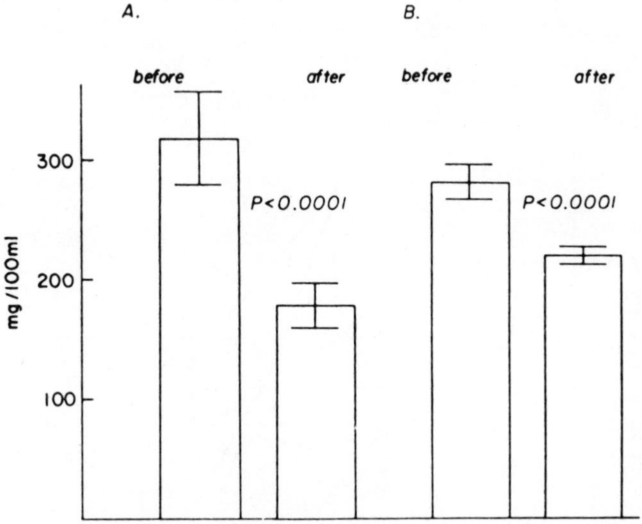

Fig. 12 Marked falls in serum triglyceride and cholesterol concentration following a 24 pound weight loss. (From Olefsky et al., 1974.)

HUMAN STUDIES: RESULTS OF EFFORTS AT WEIGHT REDUCTION

Only a little over fifteen years ago, the state of the art of weight reduction was summarized in the propositions that "most obese persons will not stay in treatment for obesity. Of those who stay in treatment, most will not lose weight, and of those who do lose weight, most will regain it" (Stunkard, 1958). During the past nine years new approaches to psychotherapy, which appear more effective than traditional ones in modifying several kinds of disturbed behavior, have been applied to the treatment of obesity. Obese patients have responded to behavior modification and experience has already been sufficient to permit the development and description of relatively specific behavioral programs for the control of obesity. These programs have been used to compare behavior modifications in a systematic manner with a variety of alternate treatment methods. Each of over twenty such studies has reported results favoring behavior modification, an unusual example of unaminity in this heterogeneous and complex disorder (Stunkard, 1975).

One of these controlled studies will be described briefly, for it is of interest on two counts (Penick et al., 1971).

First, it provides the first 5-year follow-up of treatment of obesity by behavior modification. Second, the therapeutic program used in this study has been applied in clinical practice to far larger numbers of patients, with equivalent losses of weight at the end of treatment and at six months follow-up (Westlake et al., 1974).

The treatment program consisted of elements which have become standard in the practice of behavior modification. They included a careful self-monitoring of food intake, far-reaching control of cues which stimulate eating, development of techniques to slow the speed of eating and prompt reinforcement of the foregoing behaviors. Control groups were treated by an internist with long experience in the treatment of obesity, who utilized all the traditional modalities of treatment.

The results of treatment are shown in Table V. In the behavior modification group half of the subjects lost more than twenty pounds and 13 percent lost more than forty pounds, results which are superior to those achieved by the control treatment and to those reported in the medical literature up to that time.

TABLE V

Results of Treatment
Percent of Groups Losing Specified Amounts of Weight

Weight Loss	After Treatment	1 Year	5 Years
	BEHAVIOR MODIFICATION		
More than 40 lb.	13	31	23
More than 20 lb.	53	61	31
n =	15	13	13
	TRADITIONAL THERAPY		
More than 40 lb.	0	12	14
More than 20 lb.	24	47	21
n =	17	15	14

Five-year follow-up of treatment for obesity by behavior modification and traditional therapy. Percent of groups losing specified amounts of weight are shown for three times: immediately after treatment, one year after treatment and five years after treatment.

Follow-up studies showed that 23 percent of subjects still alive at five years were more than forty pounds below their pre-treatment weight, although the difference in the results of behavioral and of traditional treatment became insignificant by the end of the first year.

These developments in the treatment of obesity give grounds for cautious optimism that such treatment can have a significant impact upon coronary risk factors and, perhaps, on the incidence of coronary artery disease itself. The weight reduction achieved in the foregoing study is sufficient to obtain the kinds of benefits in coronary risk reduction which were noted in the preceding section.

HUMAN STUDIES: EFFECTS OF DIETARY CHANGES UPON THE HEALTH OF PERSONS IN AN OLD AGE HOME

A comprehensive review of the English language literature has failed to reveal a controlled study of the effects of dietary intervention upon the health of adult humans. The discovery of such a study in the Spanish literature is, therefore, a happy event. It is made doubly so by the favorable consequences attributed to dietary restriction (Vallejo, 1957).

The study was carried out in an old age home in Madrid over a period of three years on a population of 120 men and women over the age of 65. Sixty control subjects received the standard institutional food with a daily intake of 2,300 calories, 50 grams of protein and 40 grams of fat. The experimental subjects received the same diet on even days of the month. On the odd days, their food was restricted to one liter of milk and 500 grams of fresh fruit. The nutritional value of this experimental diet appears to consist of 885 calories, 36 grams of protein and 40 grams of fat. During the three years of the study, subjects in the experimental group suffered six deaths and 123 days in the infirmary. The control group suffered thirteen deaths and 219 days in the infirmary. Table VI illustrates an attempt to estimate the statistical significance of the difference in days spent in the infirmary by the two groups. Well days were determined by subtracting from total days both sick days and days when subjects were not alive. The latter figure was determined by multiplying the number of deaths in each group by one half the number of days in the three years of the study. The difference between the experimental and control groups in days spent in the infirmary is statistically highly significant. The causes of death and the diagnoses of illness showed a preponderance of cardiovascular diseases in both the experimental and control groups.

TABLE VI

Effects of Dietary Restriction on Illness and Death in Older Persons

	Restricted	Control
Sick Days	123	219
Well Days	62,292	58,364
$X^2 = 33.1287$	$p < 0.001$	
Dead	6	13
Living	54	47
$X^2 = 2.3168$	$p < 0.2$	

(After Vallejo, 1957.)
Experimental (dietary-restricted) treatment is in the first column, control condition in the second. Number of sick days is shown in row one. Number of well days (estimated as described in text) is in the second row. The number of dead and living are shown in rows three and four.

Few details of the study are given and the opportunity for significant bias is great. For the author of the report apparently served both as medical consultant to the old age home and as director of the study. He would thus have been in a position to hospitalize members of the control group for less severe illnesses than persons in the experimental group. Despite this (and most likely other) flaws in this experiment, it still deserves careful attention, for it is the first controlled outcome study of the influence of a nutritional intervention upon health and survival of humans. It is perhaps a fitting study with which to end this review.

SUMMARY

This report began with a summary of the well known work of McCay and his collaborators which demonstrated that retardation of growth produced by restriction of food intake early in life leads to very pronounced increases in life span. It then reviewed the strong evidence, accumulated within the last five years, that the adoption of a regimen of dietary restriction after the attainment of maturity could also increase life span. However, such restriction in food intake produced far smaller increases in life span than restriction which had been begun earlier in life; moreover, it was far more often fraught with deleterious consequences. The influence of changes in dietary constituents was then examined, including, particularly, the well-established decrease in life span produced by high fat diets. A special aspect of the influence of nutrition upon life span is that of its influence upon tumors, overnutrition increasing tumor incidence to as high as 40 percent, and undernutrition restricting their development.

The review of animal experimentation closed with a consideration of the dramatic first results of the influence of dietary self-selection upon life span. Rats, permitted to choose freely among three different diets, selected precisely those combinations which maximized their incidence of degenerative disease and minimized their life span. Some even shifted dietary preferences during the course of life to select precisely those diets which were the most noxious at that particular time.

The second part of the review consisted of human investigation, beginning with an important and little known study which showed that obese adults who had been obese as children had a far lower prevalence of hypertension than did those who had been thin or normal weight as children. It then reviewed the converging evidence that obesity, acting primarily through its influence upon other coronary risk factors, markedly shortens life span. Weight reduction results in favorable reduction of these risk factors, and newer behavioral technologies give promise of wide applicability for this purpose. The review closes with the description of a Spanish study which strongly suggests that dietary restriction, even in old age, can reduce morbidity and probably mortality.

ACKNOWLEDGEMENT

I would like to thank Mrs. Marjorie Waxman and Dr. Morris Ross for their invaluable help in the preparation of this review.

REFERENCES

Abraham, S., Collins, G., and Nordsieck, M. (1971). HSMHA Health Rep. 86, 273.
Abrams, M.E., Jarrett, R.J., Keen, H., Boyns, D.R., and Crossley, J.N. (1969). Brit. Med. J. 1, 899.
Barelare, B., Jr., Holt, L.E., Jr., and Richter, C.P. (1938). Am. J. Physiol. 123, 7.
Barrows, C.H., Jr. (1972). Am. J. Clin. Nutr. 25, 829.
Barrows, C.H., Jr. (1976). Personal Communication.

Beauchene, R. (1976). Personal Communication.
Berg, B.N. and Simms, H.S. (1962). In "Biological Aspects of Aging" (N. Shock, ed.), pp. 35-37, Columbia University Press, New York.
Bierman, E.L., Bagdade, J.D., and Porte, D., Jr. (1968). Am. Med. J. Clin. Nutr. 20, 1431.
Cannon, W.B. (1939). "The Wisdom of the Body". W.W. Norton & Co., Inc., New York.
Chiang, B.N., Perlman, L.V., and Opstein, F.H. (1969). Circulation 39, 403.
French, C.R., Ingram, R.H., Uram, A.J., Barron, G.P., and Surf, R.W. (1953). J. Nutr. 51, 329.
Gordon, F. and Kannel, W. (1973). Geriatrics 28, 80.
Kagan, A., Kannel, W.B., Dowber, T.R., and Revotskie, N. (1963). Ann. N.Y. Acad. Sci. 97, 883.
Keys, A. (1970). Am. Health Assoc., Monograph #29.
Lane, P.W. and Dickie, M.M. (1958). J. Nutr. 64, 548.
Mann, G.V. (1974). N. Engl. J. Med. 291, 178.
Mayer, J., Dickie, M., Bates, M., and Vitale, J. (1951). Science 113, 745.
McCay, C.M. (1953). In "Cowdry's Problems of Ageing" (A. Lansing, ed.), pp. 139-203, Williams and Wilkins, Baltimore.
McCay, C.M., Dilley, W.E., and Crowell, T.F. (1929). J. Nutr. 1, 233.
McCay, C.M., Crowell, M.F., and Maynard, L.A. (1935). J. Nutr. 10, 63.
McCay, C.M., Sperling, G., and Barnes, L. (1939). J. Nutr. 18, 1.
McCay, C.M., Maynard, L.A., Sperling, G., and Osgood, H.S. (1941). J. Nutr. 21, 45.
Mickelsen, O., Takahashi, S., and Craig, C. (1955). J. Nutr. 57, 541.
Miller, D.S. and Payne, P. (1968). Exp. Gerontol. 3, 231.
Nolen, G. (1972). J. Nutr. 102, 1477.
Olefsky, J.M., Reaven, G.M., and Farquhar, J.W. (1974). J. Clin. Invest. 53, 64.
Penick, S.B., Filion, R.D.L., Fox, S., and Stunkard, A.J. (1971). Psychosom. Med. 33, 49.
Richter, C.P. (1936). Am. J. Physiol. 115, 155.
Richter, C.P. and Echert, J.F. (1937). Endocrinology 21, 50.
Richter, C.P., Holt, L.E., Jr., and Barelare, B., Jr. (1938). Am. J. Physiol. 122, 734.
Ross, M. (1961). Nutrition 75, 197.
Ross, M. (1969). J. Nutr. 97, 565.
Ross, M. (1972). Am. J. Clin. Nutr. 25, 834.
Ross, M. (1976). Personal Communication.

Ross, M. and Bras, G. (1965). Nutrition 87, 245.
Ross, M. and Bras, G. (1974). Nature 250, 263.
Ross, M. and Bras, G. (1975). Science 190, 165.
Schemmel, R., Mickelsen, O., and Tolgay, Z. (1969). Am. J. Physiol. 216, 373.
Silberberg, M. and Silberberg, R. (1954). Science 177, 23.
Stuchlíková, E., Juricava-Horakova, M., and Deyl, Z. (1975). Exp. Gerontol. 10, 141.
Stunkard, A.J. (1958). N.Y. J. Med. 58, 79.
Stunkard, A.J. (1975). Psychosom. Med. 37, 195.
Tannenbaum, A. (1942). Cancer Res. 2, 468.
Vallejo, E. (1957). Rev. Clin. Esp. 63, 25.
Westlake, R.J., Levitz, L.S., and Stunkard, A.J. (1974). Hosp. Community Psychiat. 25, 609.
White, F.R. (1961). Cancer Res. 21, 281.

A 6
B 7
C 8
D 9
E 0
F 1
G 2
H 3
I 4
J 5